T0263979

Comprehensive Management of Parotid Disorders

Editors

BABAK LARIAN
BABAK AZIZZADEH

OTOLARYNGOLOGIC CLINICS OF NORTH AMERICA

www.oto.theclinics.com

April 2016 • Volume 49 • Number 2

ELSEVIER

1600 John F. Kennedy Boulevard • Suite 1800 • Philadelphia, Pennsylvania, 19103-2899

http://www.oto.theclinics.com

OTOLARYNGOLOGIC CLINICS OF NORTH AMERICA Volume 49, Number 2
April 2016 ISSN 0030-6665, ISBN-13: 978-0-323-44756-0

Editor: Jessica McCool
Developmental Editor: Alison Swety

© **2016 Elsevier Inc. All rights reserved.**

This periodical and the individual contributions contained in it are protected under copyright by Elsevier, and the following terms and conditions apply to their use:

Photocopying
Single photocopies of single articles may be made for personal use as allowed by national copyright laws. Permission of the Publisher and payment of a fee is required for all other photocopying, including multiple or systematic copying, copying for advertising or promotional purposes, resale, and all forms of document delivery. Special rates are available for educational institutions that wish to make photocopies for non-profit educational classroom use. For information on how to seek permission visit www.elsevier.com/permissions or call: (+44) 1865 843830 (UK)/(+1) 215 239 3804 (USA).

Derivative Works
Subscribers may reproduce tables of contents or prepare lists of articles including abstracts for internal circulation within their institutions. Permission of the Publisher is required for resale or distribution outside the institution. Permission of the Publisher is required for all other derivative works, including compilations and translations (please consult www.elsevier.com/permissions).

Electronic Storage or Usage
Permission of the Publisher is required to store or use electronically any material contained in this periodical, including any article or part of an article (please consult www.elsevier.com/permissions). Except as outlined above, no part of this publication may be reproduced, stored in a retrieval system or transmitted in any form or by any means, electronic, mechanical, photocopying, recording or otherwise, without prior written permission of the Publisher.

Notice
No responsibility is assumed by the Publisher for any injury and/or damage to persons or property as a matter of products liability, negligence or otherwise, or from any use or operation of any methods, products, instructions or ideas contained in the material herein. Because of rapid advances in the medical sciences, in particular, independent verification of diagnoses and drug dosages should be made.

Although all advertising material is expected to conform to ethical (medical) standards, inclusion in this publication does not constitute a guarantee or endorsement of the quality or value of such product or of the claims made of it by its manufacturer.

Otolaryngologic Clinics of North America (ISSN 0030-6665) is published bimonthly by Elsevier, Inc., 360 Park Avenue South, New York, NY 10010-1710. Months of issue are February, April, June, August, October, and December. Business and Editorial Offices: 1600 John F. Kennedy Blvd., Suite 1800, Philadelphia, PA 19103-2899. Customer Service Office: 6277 Sea Harbor Drive, Orlando, FL 32887-4800. Periodicals postage paid at New York, NY and additional mailing offices. Subscription prices are $370.00 per year (US individuals), $765.00 per year (US institutions), $100.00 per year (US student/resident), $485.00 per year (Canadian individuals), $969.00 per year (Canadian institutions), $540.00 per year (international individuals), $969.00 per year (international institutions), $270.00 per year (international & Canadian student/resident). Foreign air speed delivery is included in all *Clinics'* subscription prices. All prices are subject to change without notice. **POSTMASTER:** Send address changes to *Otolaryngologic Clinics of North America*, Elsevier Health Sciences Division, Subscription Customer Service, 3251 Riverport Lane, Maryland Heights, MO 63043. **Telephone: 1-800-654-2452 (U.S. and Canada); 314-447-8871 (outside U.S. and Canada). Fax: 314-447-8029. E-mail: journalscustomerservice-usa@elsevier.com (for print support); journalsonlinesupport-usa@elsevier.com (for online support).**

Reprints. For copies of 100 or more of articles in this publication, please contact the Commercial Reprints Department, Elsevier Inc., 360 Park Avenue South, New York, NY 10010-1710. Tel.: 212-633-3874; Fax: 212-633-3820; E-mail: reprints@elsevier.com.

Otolaryngologic Clinics of North America is also published in Spanish by McGraw-Hill Interamericana Editores S.A., P.O. Box 5-237, 06500 Mexico D.F., Mexico.

Otolaryngologic Clinics of North America is covered in *MEDLINE/PubMed (Index Medicus), Current Contents/Clinical Medicine, Excerpta Medica, BIOSIS, Science Citation Index,* and *ISI/BIOMED.*

PROGRAM OBJECTIVE

The goal of the *Otolaryngologic Clinics of North America* is to provide information on the latest trends in patient management, the newest advances; and provide a sound basis for choosing treatment options in the field of otolaryngology.

LEARNING OBJECTIVES

Upon completion of this activity, participants will be able to:

1. Review the anatomy and common disorders of the parotid gland and facial nerve.
2. Discuss the diagnosis and management of malignant and benign parotid tumors.
3. Recognize and understand treatments for less common diseases and disorders of the parotid gland.

ACCREDITATION

The Elsevier Office of Continuing Medical Education (EOCME) is accredited by the Accreditation Council for Continuing Medical Education (ACCME) to provide continuing medical education for physicians.

The EOCME designates this enduring material for a maximum of 15 *AMA PRA Category 1 Credit*(s)™. Physicians should claim only the credit commensurate with the extent of their participation in the activity.

All other health care professionals requesting continuing education credit for this enduring material will be issued a certificate of participation.

DISCLOSURE OF CONFLICTS OF INTEREST

The EOCME assesses conflict of interest with its instructors, faculty, planners, and other individuals who are in a position to control the content of CME activities. All relevant conflicts of interest that are identified are thoroughly vetted by EOCME for fair balance, scientific objectivity, and patient care recommendations. EOCME is committed to providing its learners with CME activities that promote improvements or quality in healthcare and not a specific proprietary business or a commercial interest.

The planning committee, staff, authors and editors listed below have identified no financial relationships or relationships to products or devices they or their spouse/life partner have with commercial interest related to the content of this CME activity:

Babak Azizzadeh, MD, FACS; Carlos Busso, PhD; Adrianne Brigido; David M. Cognetti, MD, FACS; Jennifer R. Cracchiolo, MD; Terry A. Day, MD; Raymond S. Douglas, MD, PhD; Allen B. Flack, MD; Anjali Fortna; Michael A. Fritz, MD, FACS; Michele M. Gandolfi, MD; Stephen Hernandez, MD; Leslie E. Irvine, MD; Andrew W. Joseph, MD, MPH; Shannon S. Joseph, MD, MSc; Sobia F. Khaja, MD; Young J. Kim, MD; Amit Kochhar, MD; Edward C. Kuan, MD, MBA; Babak Larian, MD, FACS; Matthew K. Lee, MD; Aaron G. Lewis, MD; Ellie Maghami, MD; Jon Mallen-St. Clair, MD, PhD; Guy G. Massry, MD; Jessica McCool; Kevin M. Motz, MD; Premkumar Nandhakumar; Ravi S. Prasad, MD; Ali Razfar, MD; Bryan Nicholas Rolfes, MD; Akshay Sanan, MD; Ashok R. Shaha, MD; William Slattery III, MD; Maie A. St. John, MD, PhD; Megan Suermann; Tommy Tong, MD; Kevin Y. Zhan, MD.

The planning committee, staff, authors and editors listed below have identified financial relationships or relationships to products or devices they or their spouse/life partner have with commercial interest related to the content of this CME activity:

Rohan R. Walvekar, MD is a consultant/advisor for E. Benson Hood Laboratories, Inc., and Cook Medical, and receives royalties/patents from E. Benson Hood Laboratories, Inc.

UNAPPROVED/OFF-LABEL USE DISCLOSURE

The EOCME requires CME faculty to disclose to the participants:

1. When products or procedures being discussed are off-label, unlabelled, experimental, and/or investigational (not US Food and Drug Administration [FDA] approved); and
2. Any limitations on the information presented, such as data that are preliminary or that represent ongoing research, interim analyses, and/or unsupported opinions. Faculty may discuss information about pharmaceutical agents that is outside of FDA-approved labelling. This information is intended solely for CME and is not intended to promote off-label use of these medications. If you have any questions, contact the medical affairs department of the manufacturer for the most recent prescribing information.

TO ENROLL

To enroll in the *Otolaryngologic Clinics of North America* Continuing Medical Education program, call customer service at 1-800-654-2452 or sign up online at http://www.theclinics.com/home/cme. The CME program is available to subscribers for an additional annual fee of USD 260.

METHOD OF PARTICIPATION

In order to claim credit, participants must complete the following:

1. Complete enrolment as indicated above.
2. Read the activity.
3. Complete the CME Test and Evaluation. Participants must achieve a score of 70% on the test. All CME Tests and Evaluations must be completed online.

CME INQUIRIES/SPECIAL NEEDS

For all CME inquiries or special needs, please contact elsevierCME@elsevier.com.

Contributors

EDITORS

BABAK LARIAN, MD, FACS
Clinical Chief, Division of Otolaryngology, Head and Neck Surgery, Cedars-Sinai Medical Center; Department of Otolaryngology–Head and Neck Surgery, Assistant Clinical Professor of Surgery, David Geffen School of Medicine, University of California, Los Angeles, Los Angeles, California; Center for Advanced Parotid and Facial Nerve Surgery, Beverly Hills, California

BABAK AZIZZADEH, MD, FACS
Associate Clinical Professor, Department of Otolaryngology–Head and Neck Surgery, David Geffen School of Medicine, University of California, Los Angeles, Los Angeles, California; Center for Advanced Facial Plastic Surgery, Beverly Hills, California

AUTHORS

BABAK AZIZZADEH, MD, FACS
Associate Clinical Professor, Department of Otolaryngology–Head and Neck Surgery, David Geffen School of Medicine, University of California, Los Angeles, Los Angeles, California; Center for Advanced Facial Plastic Surgery, Beverly Hills, California

CARLOS BUSSO, PhD
Department of Otolaryngology–Head and Neck Surgery, Louisiana State University Health Sciences Center, New Orleans, Louisiana

DAVID M. COGNETTI, MD, FACS
Associate Professor, Department of Otolaryngology–Head and Neck Surgery, Thomas Jefferson University Hospital, Thomas Jefferson University, Philadelphia, Pennsylvania

JENNIFER R. CRACCHIOLO, MD
Head and Neck Service, Department of Surgery, Memorial Sloan Kettering Cancer Center, New York, New York

TERRY A. DAY, MD
Wendy and Keith Wellin Endowed Chair in Head and Neck Surgery, Professor and Director, Division of Head and Neck Oncologic Surgery, Vice Chair for Clinical Affairs, Department of Otolaryngology–Head and Neck Surgery, Medical University of South Carolina, Charleston, South Carolina

RAYMOND S. DOUGLAS, MD, PhD
Division of Oculoplastic Surgery, Department of Ophthalmology and Visual Sciences, University of Michigan Medical School, Ann Arbor, Michigan

ALLEN B. FLACK, MD
Department of Pathology, Medical University of South Carolina, Charleston, South Carolina

MICHAEL A. FRITZ, MD, FACS
Section Head of Facial Plastic and Reconstructive Surgery, Cleveland Clinic Head and Neck Institute, Cleveland, Ohio

MICHELE M. GANDOLFI, MD
House Clinic, Los Angeles, California

STEPHEN HERNANDEZ, MD
Department of Otolaryngology–Head and Neck Surgery, Louisiana State University Health Sciences Center, New Orleans, Louisiana

LESLIE E. IRVINE, MD
Caruso Department of Head and Neck Surgery, Keck School of Medicine, University of Southern California, Los Angeles, California

ANDREW W. JOSEPH, MD, MPH
Department of Otolaryngology–Head and Neck Surgery, Johns Hopkins University School of Medicine, Baltimore, Maryland

SHANNON S. JOSEPH, MD, MSc
Division of Oculoplastic Surgery, Department of Ophthalmology and Visual Sciences, University of Michigan Medical School, Ann Arbor, Michigan

SOBIA F. KHAJA, MD
Department of Otolaryngology–Head and Neck Surgery, Medical University of South Carolina, Charleston, South Carolina

YOUNG J. KIM, MD
Associate Professor, Otolaryngology–Head and Neck Surgery, Johns Hopkins Hospital, Baltimore, Maryland

AMIT KOCHHAR, MD
Department of Otolaryngology–Head and Neck Surgery, University of California, Los Angeles, Los Angeles, California

EDWARD C. KUAN, MD, MBA
Department of Head and Neck Surgery, University of California, Los Angeles (UCLA) Medical Center, Los Angeles, California

BABAK LARIAN, MD, FACS
Clinical Chief, Division of Otolaryngology, Head and Neck Surgery, Cedars-Sinai Medical Center; Department of Otolaryngology–Head and Neck Surgery, Assistant Clinical Professor of Surgery, David Geffen School of Medicine, University of California, Los Angeles, Los Angeles, California; Center for Advanced Parotid and Facial Nerve Surgery, Beverly Hills, California

MATTHEW K. LEE, MD
Division of Facial Plastic and Reconstructive Surgery, Stanford University School of Medicine, Palo Alto, California

AARON G. LEWIS, MD
Department of Surgery, City of Hope National Medical Center, Duarte, California

ELLIE MAGHAMI, MD
Associate Professor, Department of Surgery Chief, Division of Head and Neck Surgery, City of Hope National Medical Center, Duarte, California

JON MALLEN-ST. CLAIR, MD, PhD
Department of Head and Neck Surgery, University of California, Los Angeles (UCLA) Medical Center, Los Angeles, California

GUY G. MASSRY, MD
Ophthalmic Plastic and Reconstructive Surgery, Keck School of Medicine, University of Southern California, Beverly Hills, California

KEVIN M. MOTZ, MD
Otolaryngology–Head and Neck Surgery, Johns Hopkins Hospital, Baltimore, Maryland

RAVI S. PRASAD, MD
Department of Imaging, Cedars-Sinai Medical Center, Los Angeles, California

ALI RAZFAR, MD
Division of Facial Plastic and Reconstructive Surgery, University of Michigan School of Medicine, Ann Arbor, Michigan

BRYAN NICHOLAS ROLFES, MD
Department of Facial Plastic and Reconstructive Surgery, Boston Medical Center, Boston, Massachusetts

AKSHAY SANAN, MD
Resident Physician, Department of Otolaryngology–Head and Neck Surgery, Thomas Jefferson University Hospital, Thomas Jefferson University, Philadelphia, Pennsylvania

ASHOK R. SHAHA, MD
Head and Neck Service, Department of Surgery, Memorial Sloan Kettering Cancer Center, New York, New York

WILLIAM SLATTERY III, MD
House Clinic; Clinical Professor, University of Southern California; Clinical Professor, Department of Otolaryngology–Head and Neck Surgery, University of California, Los Angeles, California

MAIE A. ST. JOHN, MD, PhD
Department of Head and Neck Surgery; UCLA Head and Neck Cancer Program, Jonsson Comprehensive Cancer Center, University of California, Los Angeles (UCLA) Medical Center, Los Angeles, California

TOMMY TONG, MD
Department of Pathology, City of Hope National Medical Center, Duarte, California

ROHAN R. WALVEKAR, MD
Associate Professor and Director of Clinical Research, Department of Otolaryngology–Head and Neck Surgery, Louisiana State University Health Sciences Center, New Orleans, Louisiana

KEVIN Y. ZHAN, MD
Department of Otolaryngology–Head and Neck Surgery, Medical University of South Carolina, Charleston, South Carolina

Contents

This article provides an overview of important anatomic and functional anatomy associated with the parotid gland and facial nerve for the practicing otolaryngologist, head and neck surgeon, facial plastic surgeon, and plastic surgeon. The discussion includes the important anatomic relationships and physiology related to the parotid gland and salivary production. A comprehensive description of the path of facial nerve, its branches, and important anatomic landmarks also are provided.

In this article, various imaging modalities are discussed for evaluation of parotid disease, from congenital to inflammatory to neoplastic etiologies. Key imaging characteristics are outlined using case examples. Introduction to biological imaging is highlighted. Additionally, image-guided biopsy techniques are illustrated for sampling parotid and parapharyngeal space lesions in a minimally invasive manner.

The differential diagnosis of a parotid lesion is broad, and the otolaryngologist must consider inflammatory, neoplastic, autoimmune, traumatic, infectious, or congenital causes. A comprehensive history and physical examination, in conjunction with judicious use of radiographic imaging (MRI, computed tomography, ultrasonography, nuclear medicine studies), laboratory studies, and pathologic analysis (fine-needle aspiration, core biopsy, incisional biopsy), facilitates making an accurate diagnosis. This article reviews the key history and physical elements and adjunctive diagnostic tools available for working up parotid lesions.

This article reviews the epidemiology, embryology, risk factors, clinical presentation, diagnostic work-up, and basic management principles for the more common benign parotid neoplasms. The various histopathologies are also discussed and summarized.

> Malignant parotid tumors are heterogeneous and diverse. Accurate
> diagnosis requires a pathologist familiar with the various histologic sub-
> types, immunohistochemistry stains, and common translocations. Clinical
> course varies according to tumor subtype, ranging from indolent, slow-
> growing adenoid cystic carcinoma to rapidly progressive, often fatal,
> salivary ductal carcinoma. Histologic grade is important in prognosis
> and therapy. Surgery remains the mainstay of treatment when negative
> margins can be achieved. Radiation improves locoregional control of
> tumors with high-risk features. Chemotherapy for parotid tumors can
> be disappointing. Studies of new targeted therapies have not offered sig-
> nificant benefits.

 Video content accompanies this article at http://www.oto.theclinics.com

> Nonneoplastic disorders of the salivary glands involve inflammatory
> processes. These disorders have been managed conservatively with anti-
> biotics, warm compresses, massage, sialogogues, and adequate hydra-
> tion. Up to 40% of patients may have an inadequate response or
> persistent symptoms. When conservative techniques fail, the next step
> is operative intervention. Sialendoscopy offers a minimally invasive option
> for the diagnosis and management of chronic inflammatory disorders of
> the salivary glands and offers the option of gland and function preserva-
> tion. In this article, we review some of the more common nonneoplastic
> disorders of the parotid gland, indications for diagnostic and interventional
> sialendoscopy, and operative techniques.

> Parotidectomy for benign tumors is undergoing constant evolution. The
> potential for recurrence and malignant transformation of pleomorphic
> adenomas creates complexities that have forced head and neck surgeons
> to undertake more comprehensive parotid surgery with facial nerve
> dissection. This approach carries inherent morbidities, including facial
> nerve injury, Frey's syndrome, and facial asymmetry, that have to be
> addressed. Extracapsular dissection is compared with conventional
> superficial parotidectomy; surgical histologic findings are discussed as
> well as outcome data. More novel approaches are discussed as well.
> This article provides a systematic approach to benign parotid tumor
> surgery.

> Parotidectomy for parotid cancer includes management of primary sali-
> vary cancer, metastatic cancer to lymph nodes, and direct extension

from surrounding structures or cutaneous malignancies. Preoperative evaluation should provide surgeons with enough information to plan a sound operation and adequately counsel patients. Facial nerve sacrifice is sometimes required; but in preoperative functioning nerves, function should be preserved. Although nerve involvement predicts poor outcome, survival of around 50% has been reported for primary parotid malignancy. Metastatic cutaneous squamous cell carcinoma is a high-grade aggressive histology whereby local control for palliation with extended parotidectomy can be achieved; however, overall survival remains poor.

Various types of parotid gland tumors are discussed from nonneoplastic to both benign and malignant neoplasms. The anatomic relationship of the facial nerve is discussed as it exits the stylomastoid foramen and courses through the parotid gland. The effect of certain tumors on facial nerve function is also characterized. Details on which types of parotid tumors are more likely to affect facial nerve function and different prognostic predictors of return to function are evaluated. In addition, the prognostic value of tumor size and histologic type of parotid tumor is included.

Parotidectomy for benign and malignant tumors often results in conspicuous contour abnormalities and soft tissue defects. Immediate reconstruction leads to improved patient satisfaction and local or regional flaps can be used for reconstruction in most cases. This article provides a systematic approach to parotid reconstruction.

Parotidectomy is a commonly performed procedure for both benign and malignant lesions. When a significant portion of the gland is resected and the lost tissue volume is not replaced, a disfiguring contour defect can result. This defect can be disfiguring and have a profound impact on quality of life. Large defects are best replaced with vascularized tissue to provide stable volume.

Facial nerve paralysis is a devastating condition arising from several causes with severe functional and psychological consequences. Given the complexity of the disease process, management involves a multi-specialty, team-oriented approach. This article provides a systematic approach in addressing each specific sequela of this complex problem.

OTOLARYNGOLOGIC CLINICS
OF NORTH AMERICA

THE CLINICS ARE AVAILABLE ONLINE!
Access your subscription at:
www.theclinics.com

Preface

Comprehensive Management of Parotid Disorders

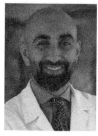 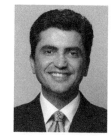

Babak Larian, MD, FACS   Babak Azizzadeh, MD, FACS
Editors

Many texts have been written about salivary disease as a collective, but the parotid gland deserves special distinction. The parotid gland is anatomically unique in its intimate relationship with the facial nerve. It is subject to a wide range of diseases from neoplastic to obstructive, infectious, and inflammatory. It develops more neoplasms than all remaining salivary glands combined. There has also been advancement in treatment of both neoplastic diseases of the parotid gland and sialolithiasis.

Historically, aggressive treatment of parotid gland disease was thought to be the most appropriate choice; yet, as in other fields, our understanding of the disease process is improving and our interventions are becoming less radical. In the case of salivary stone, sialoendoscopy has revolutionized treatment. It has also allowed us to offer treatments for processes that were previously untreatable, such as radioactive iodine–induced parotitis. In terms of benign salivary neoplasms, the approach to surgery has become more catered to benign disease and distinguished from surgical treatment of malignant diseases. What was once an acceptable morbidity of superficial parotidectomy is now addressed and prevented. Collaboration of head and neck surgeons, otologists, and reconstructive surgeons has allowed for a more comprehensive approach and improved outcomes. The contributing authors of this text are world-class experts in the field. They have put forth great effort in preparing exceptional articles with cutting-edge treatments. We hope you enjoy this issue of *Otolaryngologic Clinics of North America* and find it useful.

Our deepest gratitude to our parents for a lifetime of support, enthusiasm, and encouragement; our wives, Maryam and Jessica, for being loving and invaluable partners in our lives; and our beloved children, Kylie, Logan, Ava, and Daara. We would like

Otolaryngol Clin N Am 49 (2016) xv–xvi
http://dx.doi.org/10.1016/j.otc.2016.01.001
0030-6665/16/$ – see front matter © 2016 Published by Elsevier Inc.

oto.theclinics.com

to thank the exceptional editorial team at Elsevier. Jessica McCool, Alison Swety, and Santha Priya were instrumental in making this issue of *Otolaryngologic Clinics of North America* come to fruition.

Babak Larian, MD, FACS
Division of Otolaryngology, Head and Neck Surgery
Cedars-Sinai Medical Center
David Geffen School of Medicine
University of California, Los Angeles
9401 Wilshire Boulevard, Suite 650
Beverly Hills, CA 90212, USA

Babak Azizzadeh, MD, FACS
Center for Advanced Facial Plastic Surgery
9401 Wilshire Boulevard, Suite 650
Beverly Hills, CA 90212, USA

E-mail addresses:
dr@larianmd.com (B. Larian)
MD@FacialPlastics.info (B. Azizzadeh)

Facial Nerve and Parotid Gland Anatomy

 CrossMark

Amit Kochhar, MD[a], Babak Larian, MD[a,b], Babak Azizzadeh, MD[a,b,*]

KEYWORDS

- Parotid gland • Facial nerve • Salivary gland anatomy and physiology
- Parotidectomy • Facial paralysis

KEY POINTS

- This article provides an overview of important anatomic and functional anatomy associated with the parotid gland and facial nerve for the practicing otolaryngologist–head and neck surgeon, facial plastic surgeon and plastic surgeon.
- The discussion includes the important anatomic relationships and physiology related to the parotid gland and salivary production.
- A comprehensive description of the path of the facial nerve, its branches, and important anatomic landmarks also are provided.

INTRODUCTION

The parotid gland and facial nerve have a unique anatomic and functional relationship. The parotid gland is the largest of 3 paired major salivary glands in the head and neck. The major function of the parotid and other salivary glands is to secrete saliva, which plays a significant role in lubrication, digestion, immunity, and the overall maintenance of homeostasis within the human body. The facial nerve (CN VII) originates in the brainstem and travels through the temporal bone before exiting the stylomastoid foramen. The extratemporal branches of the facial nerve are located within the body of the parotid gland and divide it into superficial and deep lobes before innervating the muscles of facial expression (**Fig. 1**). A thorough understanding of the anatomy of the parotid gland and facial nerve is essential for safe management of related pathology.

Disclosures: The authors have no disclosures.
Conflict of interest: The authors have no conflicts of interest.
[a] Department of Otolaryngology–Head and Neck Surgery, University of California, Los Angeles, 200 UCLA Medical Plaza #550, Los Angeles, CA 90095, USA; [b] Center for Advanced Facial Plastic Surgery, 9401 Wilshire Boulevard, Suite 650, Beverly Hills, CA 90212, USA
* Corresponding author. Center for Advanced Facial Plastic Surgery, 9401 Wilshire Boulevard, Suite 650, Beverly Hills, CA 90212.
E-mail address: drazizzadeh@gmail.com

Otolaryngol Clin N Am 49 (2016) 273–284
http://dx.doi.org/10.1016/j.otc.2015.10.002
0030-6665/16/$ – see front matter © 2016 Elsevier Inc. All rights reserved.

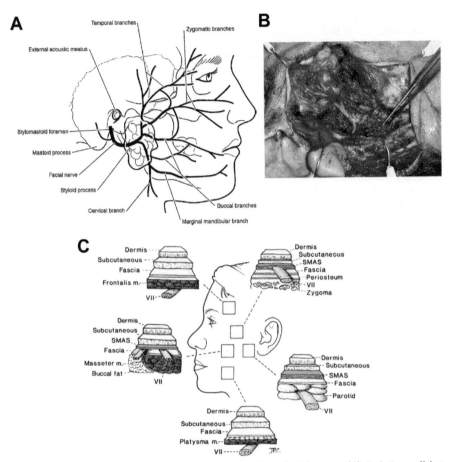

Fig. 1. Parotid gland and extratemporal branches of the facial nerve. (*A*) Artist's rendition. (*B*) Surgical image of facial nerve dissection. (*C*) Cross-sectional relationships of the facial nerve to various layers of the face in each repair. (*From* [*A*] Holsinger FC. Anatomy, function, and evaluation of the salivary glands. Springer; 2007, with permission; and [*C*] May M, Sobol SM, Mester SJ. Managing segmental facial nerve injuries by surgical repair. Laryngoscope 1990;100:1062–7, with permission.)

THE PAROTID GLAND
Anatomy

The paired parotid glands are the largest of the major salivary glands. They are each located in the preauricular region and span from the masseter to the posterior surface of the mandible. The gland is divided into superficial and deep lobes by the facial nerve. The superficial lobe is defined as the part of the gland lateral to the nerve and overlies the lateral surface of the masseter muscle. The deep lobe is located medial to the facial nerve and lies between the mastoid process of the temporal bone and the mandibular ramus with deep margins resting in the prestyloid compartment of the parapharyngeal space (PPS).

Most benign neoplasms are found within the superficial lobe and can be removed with a superficial parotidectomy. A tumor of the deep lobe may go unnoticed, as it does not displace the overlying superficial lobe until it extends laterally and causes displacement of the overlying superficial lobe. These deep lobe tumors lie within the PPS and typically grow into a dumbbell shape, because their growth is directed through the stylomandibular tunnel.[1]

The superior boundary of the parotid gland is the zygomatic arch. Inferiorly, the tail of the parotid gland extends down to the sternocleidomastoid muscle (SCM). The tail of the parotid gland extends posteriorly over the superior border of the SCM toward the mastoid tip and the deep lobe lies within the PPS.[2]

Accessory parotid tissue is present in approximately 20% of the population. It is generally found approximately 6 mm anterior to the main parotid gland and is usually adjacent to the parotid duct (Stensen duct) as it passes over the masseter. Multiple accessory glands may be present. Accessory glandular tissue is histologically distinct from parotid tissue in that it may contain mucinous acinar cells in addition to the serous acinar cells generally found in the parotid gland.[3,4]

The parotid fascia, or parotidomasseteric fascia, forms a dense inelastic capsule over the parotid gland and deeply covers the masseter muscle. This facia should not be confused with the superficial musculoaponeurotic system (SMAS), which is continuous with the platysma inferiorly, and the superficial temporal fascia superiorly. Rather, the parotid fascia is a continuation of the deep cervical fascia as it travels superiorly. Once it reaches the parotid gland, this fascia splits into superficial and deep layers to encase the parotid gland. The superficial fascia is thicker and extends superiorly from the masseter and SCM to the zygomatic arch, where it attaches to the root of the zygoma. The thinner, deep layer extends to the stylomandibular ligament, which is an important surgical landmark when considering the resection of deep lobe tumors.[5,6]

Within close proximity to the parotid gland are 2 nerves that deserve mentioning. The great auricular nerve, a branch of the cervical plexus, runs parallel to the external jugular vein along the lateral surface of the SCM toward the tail of the parotid gland. It then divides into an anterior and posterior branch to provide sensation to posterior portion of the pinna and the lobule. If injured during parotidectomy, it can result in long-term sensory loss. It may also serve as a suitable nerve graft and can be easily harvested for facial nerve grafting when needed for reanimation purposes. The auriculotemporal nerve is a branch of the mandibular nerve, the third inferior subdivision of the trigeminal nerve (V3). After exiting the foramen ovale, the nerve travels superiorly to innervate the skin and scalp immediately anterior to the ear. It runs parallel to the superficial temporal vessels and anterior to the external auditory canal.[6]

Ductal Organization

Ductal organization of the parotid gland can be divided into 2 parts: proximal and distal. Proximally, when traveling from the Stensen duct toward the terminal acini, a treelike branching pattern develops and the ducts become progressively smaller, with more numerous branches. Distally, the Stensen duct exits the anterior border of the parotid gland and travels 1 cm inferior and parallel to the zygoma in an anterior direction across the masseter muscle. It then turns and pierces the buccinator muscle to enter the oral cavity opposite the second upper molar.

The main excretory ducts of the parotid gland lead into the striated ducts, the intercalated ducts, and the terminal acini (**Fig. 2**).[7,8] There is rich adipose tissue present in the parotid parenchyma, with a ratio of adipose-to-glandular tissue of 1:1.[6] Sebaceous elements are uncommon, but may be found in the parotid gland and are believed to explain the sebaceous differentiation that may be seen in some salivary tumors.

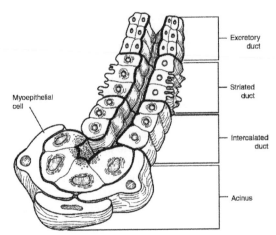

Excretory duct

Striated duct

Myoepithelial cell

Intercalated duct

Acinus

Fig. 2. Schematic representation of a normal secretary unit. (*From* Holsinger FC. Anatomy, function, and evaluation of the salivary glands. Springer; 2007; with permission.)

Vascular Supply and Lymphatic Drainage

The external carotid artery (ECA) provides arterial blood supply to the parotid gland. From the carotid bifurcation, the ECA travels superiorly and parallel to the mandible before going medial to the posterior belly of the digastric muscle. Once the artery is medial to the parotid gland it divides into its 2 terminal branches, the superficial temporal (STA) and maxillary arteries (MA). The STA runs superiorly from the superior portion of the parotid gland to the scalp within the pretragal region. The MA exits the medial portion of the parotid to supply the infratemporal fossa and the pterygopalatine fossa. Controlling the MA is required when performing a radical parotidectomy, especially when marginal or segmental mandibulectomy is also performed. The transverse facial artery is a branch off the STA and runs anteriorly between the zygoma and parotid duct to supply the parotid gland, parotid duct, and the masseter muscle.[2]

Venous outflow occurs through the retromandibular vein, which is formed by the maxillary and superficial temporal veins. The retromandibular vein travels through the parotid gland just deep to the facial nerve to join the external jugular vein and may have extremely variable anatomy. For instance, it may bifurcate into an anterior and posterior branch. The anterior branch can join the posterior facial vein to form the common facial vein. The posterior facial vein lies immediately deep to the marginal mandibular branch of the facial nerve and is therefore often used as a landmark for identification of the nerve branch. The posterior branch of the retromandibular vein may also combine with the postauricular vein above the SCM and then drain into the external jugular vein.[6,9]

There is a high density of lymph nodes within and around the parotid gland. The parotid is the only salivary gland with 2 nodal layers, both of which drain into the superficial and deep cervical lymph systems.[6] Approximately 90% of the nodes are located in the superficial layer between the glandular tissue and its capsule. The parotid gland, external auditory canal, pinna, scalp, eyelids, and lacrimal glands are all drained by these superficial nodes. The deep layer of nodes drains the gland, external auditory canal, middle ear, nasopharynx, and soft palate.[10]

Autonomic Innervation

The glossopharyngeal nerve (CN IX) provides innervation required for secretion of saliva to the parotid gland. CN IX carries preganglionic parasympathetic fibers from the medulla (inferior salivatory nucleus) through the jugular foramen (**Fig. 3**). Distal to the inferior ganglion, a small branch of CN IX, the Jacobsen nerve, reenters the skull through the inferior tympanic canaliculus to form the tympanic plexus within the middle ear. The preganglionic fibers then become the lesser petrosal nerve and travel into the middle cranial fossa. After exiting from the foramen ovale, they synapse in the otic ganglion with postganglionic parasympathetic fibers. These fibers then exit the otic ganglion beneath the mandibular nerve and join the auriculotemporal nerve in the infratemporal fossa. These fibers will innervate the parotid gland for the secretion of saliva.[6]

Within the gland, the neurotransmitter acetylcholine (ACh) binds muscarinic receptors to stimulate both acinar activity and ductal transport. This leads to vasodilation of the glands and contraction of the myoepithelial cells. Production of inositol trisphosphate leads to increased calcium concentrations within the cell, which significantly increase salivary volume secretion by second messenger activity.[6,11] Acetylcholinesterases, which inhibit the breakdown of ACh, may be released and allow for continued

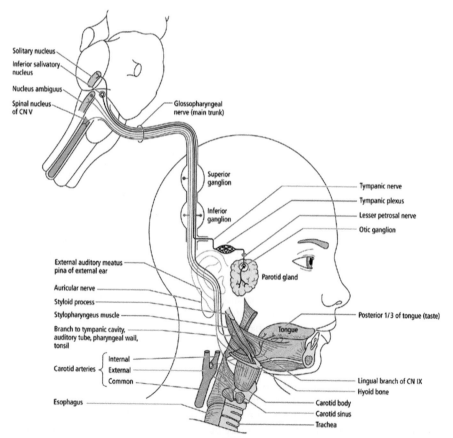

Fig. 3. Parasympathetic innervation of the salivary glands. (*From* Patestas MA, Gartner LP. A textbook of neuroanatomy. Blackwell Publishing; 2006; with permission.)

secretion of saliva. Atropine, the muscarinic antagonist, decreases salivation by competing with ACh for the salivary receptor site.[6]

The neurotransmitter norepinephrine, mediates the effects of the sympathetic nervous system via postganglionic sympathetic fibers that innervate salivary glands, sweat glands, and cutaneous blood vessels. These fibers travel through the external carotid plexus from the superior cervical ganglion via the thoracic spinal nerves. Binding of norepinephrine to beta-adrenergic receptors results in activation of the adenylate cyclase second messenger system, which then results in formation of 3′,5′-cyclic adenosine monophosphate (cAMP). cAMP leads to phosphorylation of various proteins and activation of different enzymes.[6,11]

Interestingly, ACh can serve as a neurotransmitter for both postganglionic sympathetic and parasympathetic fibers.[2] This is believed to contribute to "gustatory sweating" (Frey syndrome) in some patients following parotidectomy.[12,13] Regeneration of parasympathetic fibers to the sweat glands leads to aberrant autonomic reinnervation and patients can then develop sweating and flushing of the skin overlying the parotid region during eating.

Functional Anatomy and Physiology

The purpose of the parotid and other salivary glands is to produce saliva. Saliva has several very important functions related to digestion, immunity, and homeostasis. It is involved in the digestion of carbohydrates and fats, and protects mucosa from the deleterious effects of microbial toxins, noxious stimuli, and minor trauma. The salivary mucins (glycoproteins) also act as lubricants for mastication, swallowing, speech, and taste.[8,14] Secretory immunoglobulin A, enzymes (lysozyme, peroxidase, alpha-amylase, and lactoferrin), and ions, such as thiocyanate and hydrogen, are found within saliva and also contribute to its antibacterial activity.

Saliva is 99.5% water with the remainder is composed of proteins and electrolytes. Its specific gravity is 1.002 to 1.012. Salivary pH ranges from 5.6 to 7.0 (average 6.7) and varies directly with the blood pH.[8,14,15] One to 1.5 L of saliva are produced daily from all salivary glands and the parotid glands contribute approximately 45% (450–675 mL) of the total secretions.[14] During the resting state, one-fourth of saliva is produced by the parotid gland and most (two-thirds) is from the submandibular gland. However, during stimulation (presence of food in the mouth, mastication, and nausea), the relative amounts are reversed and two-thirds of secretion comes from the parotid gland.

The basic secretory unit of the parotid gland consists of an acinus, a secretory duct, and a collecting duct (see **Fig. 2**). Acinar cells are extremely polarized and are bounded by a plasma membrane with 2 distinct domains, a basolateral domain and an apical domain, that are separated by tight junctions that link adjacent cells. The parotid gland consists of serous acini that contain pyramidal-shaped cells with round basal nuclei surrounding the lumen and secretory granules at the apex. Each acinus is surrounded by a layer of myoepithelial cells, which in turn is bordered by a distinct basement membrane layer. Myoepithelial cells are elongated or star-shaped nonsecreting cells with long-branching processes that surround the acinus and proximal ducts. They have been found to possess adenosine triphosphate (ATP) activity, have intercellular gap junctions, and contain myofilaments. These properties are believed to provide myoepithelial cells with contractile function that assists in expelling secretions.[16–18]

The intercalated ducts lie next to the acinus. They are hollow structures lined by a single layer of small cuboidal cells. The intercalated ducts continue as intralobular striated ducts and together form the secretory duct. Striated ducts are lined by columnar cells with a brush border composed of microvilli on their luminal surface. Striated ductal cells are rich in mitochondria. They are thought to be involved with the transport of ions and water. Excretory ducts extend from the striated ducts and are lined by 2 layers of epithelium, a layer of flat cells surrounding the ductal lumen, and an outer layer of columnar cells.[19,20]

Throughout the secretory unit, active transport processes occur that alter the composition of saliva into a complex mixture of electrolytes and macromolecules (**Table 1**). All fluid is produced in the acinus and most protein secretion also occurs here.[20] The fluid is derived from the highly permeable local vascular bed in the form of an isotonic solution and is secreted into the acinar lumen before traveling through the ductal system before emptying into the mouth. Unlike the water-permeable cells of the acinus, ductal cells are impermeable to water. Most of the sodium and chloride in the primary secretion is reabsorbed in the duct, and a small amount of potassium and bicarbonate is secreted. In addition, some proteins are added to the salivary fluid as it traverses the secretory duct. By the time the saliva enters the mouth, it has generally been rendered hypotonic. The electrolyte composition of saliva, however, can be influenced by salivary flow rates. The reabsorption of salivary sodium and chloride is directly related to these rates, with decreased reabsorption and increased salivary concentrations of electrolytes with increasing salivary flow rates but potassium reabsorption is independent of flow rates.[21,22]

THE FACIAL NERVE
Intratemporal Anatomy

The facial nerve is composed of approximately 10,000 fibers. These fibers are predominantly myelinated and innervate the muscles of facial expression (**Fig. 4**) as

Table 1 Flow rates of saliva within the parotid gland in healthy adults	
Stimulated flow rate, mL/min/gland	0.7
Inorganic constituents, mEq/L	
K^+	20
Na^+	23
Cl^-	23
HCO_3	20
Ca^{++}	2
Mg^{++}	0.2
HPO_4^{-2}	6
Organic constituents, mg/dL	
Urea	15
Ammonia	0.3
Uric acid	3
Glucose	<1
Cholesterol	<1
Fatty acids	1
Total lipids	2–6
Amino acids	1.5
Protein	250

Adapted from Mandel ID. Sialochemistry in diseases and clinical situations affecting salivary glands. Crit Rev Clin Lab Sci 1980;12:321; with permission.

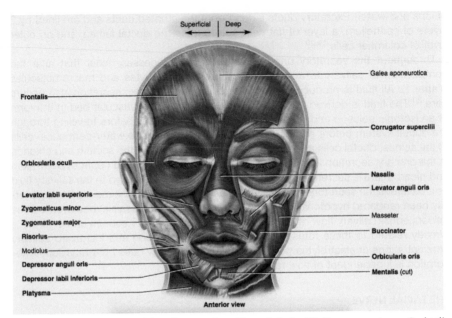

Fig. 4. The paired muscles of facial expression. (*From* Saladin KS. Human anatomy. 2nd edition. McGraw Hill; 2008; with permission.)

well as the posterior belly of the digastric, stylohyoid, and stapedius muscles.[23] The remaining fibers contribute to taste sensation, through neuronal projections from the nervus intermedius, (via afferent fibers from the anterior two-thirds of the tongue), cutaneous sensation to the external ear, lacrimation, and salivation via secretory fibers. **Table 2** outlines the subdivisions and functions of the facial nerve.

The primary somatomotor cortex of the facial nerve is located in the precentral gyrus of the frontal lobe. Corticobulbar fibers project from the precentral gyrus to the facial nucleus with most crossing over to contribute to the contralateral side. As a result, crossed and uncrossed fibers are found in each nucleus and the facial nucleus can

Table 2
Subdivisions and functions of the facial nerve

Subdivision	Function
Branchial (special visceral efferent)	Motor innervation of muscles of facial expression, stylohyoid, stapedius, posterior belly of digastric
Visceral motor (general visceral efferent)	Preganglionic parasympathetic innervation of sublingual/submandibular gland, lacrimal gland, nasal mucosa/mucous membrane
Special sensory (special afferent)	Provides taste from the anterior two-thirds of the tongue via the chorda tympani nerve
General sensory (general somatic afferent)	Provides sensory input from the auricular concha, portions of external auditory canal, and tympanic membrane

Adapted from Chu EA, Byrne PJ. Treatment considerations in facial paralysis. Facial Plast Surg 2008;24:164–9; with permission.

be divided into 2 parts: (1) the upper part, which receives corticobulbar projections bilaterally and later courses to the upper parts of the face, including the forehead, and (2) the lower part, with principally crossed projections that supply innervation to lower facial muscles. Efferent fibers from the facial nucleus run from its origin at the ventral aspect of the pontomedullary junction of the brainstem to the porus acusticus of the internal auditory meatus. Sensory and parasympathetic fibers of the facial nerve originate in the nervus intermedius and exit the brainstem adjacent to the motor branch of the facial nerve. As the facial nerve approaches the internal auditory meatus, it is joined by these additional sensory fibers.

The facial nerve courses through the temporal bone (**Fig. 5**) and may be further subdivided into 4 segments: the meatal, the labyrinthine, the tympanic, and the mastoid segments. The meatal foramen, the narrowest portion of the fallopian canal, measures on average 0.68 mm. It has been implicated in the etiology of Bell palsy, as the narrow diameter and bony confines leave little room for expansion due to edema or inflammation.[24,25] The labyrinthine segment measures approximately 4 mm and extends perpendicular to the temporal bone axis. The tympanic segment of the fallopian canal extends approximately 1 cm and runs in a horizontal manner. Dehiscence of the

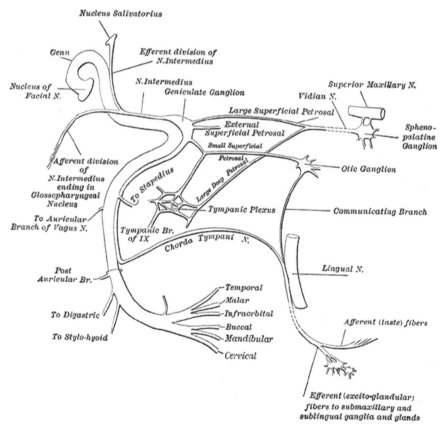

Fig. 5. The intratemporal and extratemporal course of the facial nerve. (*From* Gray H. Gray's anatomy: anatomy of the human body. 20th edition, thoroughly rev. and reedited by Warren H. Lewis.)

Table 3
Anatomic landmarks for identification of distal facial nerve branches

Branch	Location
Frontal	Follows a line from 0.5 cm below the tragus to 1.5 cm above the lateral brow,[27,28] multiple rami present crossing central zygomatic arch.[29,30]
Zygomatic/ buccal	Identified at the midway point on a line drawn from the root of the helix and the lateral commissure of the mouth.[31]
Marginal mandibular	Closely associated with the inferior border of the mandible where it crosses the facial vessels.[32]

Data from Refs.[27–32]

tympanic segment may occur in up to 30% of normal facial nerves and may be at increased risk during middle ear surgery or in severe otologic infection.[26] The mastoid, or vertical, segment extends approximately 1.5 cm and the nerve exits the fallopian canal through the stylomastoid foramen.

Extratemporal Anatomy

The course and branching pattern of the extratemporal facial nerve has significant variability. Several anatomic landmarks are noted in **Table 3**. Commonly, the main trunk of the facial nerve, the pes anserinus, will divide into 2 trunks: (1) an upper trunk that gives rise to the frontal, zygomatic, and buccal branches, and (2) a lower trunk that terminates in the marginal mandibular and cervical branches. The frontal branch parallels the superficial temporal vessels and runs across the central portion of the zygoma to supply the frontal belly of the occipitofrontalis muscle, the orbicularis oculi, the corrugator supercilii, and the anterior and superior auricular muscles.[27–30] The zygomatic branch travels directly over the periosteum of the zygomatic arch to innervate the zygomatic, orbital, and infraorbital muscles. The buccal branch travels with the Stensen duct anteriorly over the masseter muscle to supply the buccinator, upper lip, and nostril muscles.[31] The marginal mandibular branch runs along the inferior border of the parotid gland to innervate the lower lip and chin muscles. It lies in close proximity to the inferior border of the mandible and superficial to the posterior facial vein and retromandibular veins in the plane of the deep cervical fascia directly beneath the platysma muscle. The cervical branch innervates the platysma muscle and, like the marginal mandibular nerve, is located within the plane of the deep cervical fascia directly underneath the platysma. All muscles of facial expression are innervated on their deep surface except for the mentalis, levator anguli oris, and buccinator muscles.[32] Interconnections exist between the branches with the highest frequency of collateral branches between the zygomatic and buccal branches. This may explain why there is a higher rate of recovery of function in distal injuries in this region, as well as the high rate of synkinesis that accompanies recovery of a proximal injury.[26]

SUMMARY

The parotid gland and facial nerve anatomy compose a critically important aspect of head and neck anatomy. Understanding the anatomic and functional relationships between the 2 systems is very important for the practicing otolaryngologist–head and neck surgeon to diagnose and treat underlying pathology.

REFERENCES

1. Davis RA, Anson BJ, Budinger JM, et al. Surgical anatomy of the facial nerve and parotid gland based upon a study of 350 cervicofacial halves. Surg Gynecol Obstet 1956;102(4):385–412.
2. Grant J. An atlas of anatomy. 6th edition. Baltimore (MD): Williams & Wilkins; 1972.
3. Frommer J. The human accessory parotid gland: its incidence, nature, and significance. Oral Surg Oral Med Oral Pathol 1977;43(5):671–6.
4. Gray H. Anatomy of the human body. In: Goss C, editor. Philadelphia.
5. Orabi AA, Riad MA, O'Regan MB. Stylomandibular tenotomy in the transcervical removal of large benign parapharyngeal tumours. Br J Oral Maxillofac Surg 2002; 40(4):313–6.
6. Holsinger FC, Bui DT. Anatomy, function, and evaluation of the salivary glands. In: Myers EN, Ferris RL, editors. Salivary gland disorders. Springer; 2007. p. 1–16.
7. Batsakis J. Tumor of the head and neck: clinical and pathological considerations. 2nd edition. Baltimore (MD): Williams & Wilkins; 1979.
8. Mason D, Chisholm D. Salivary glands in health and disease. London: WB Saunders; 1975.
9. Bhattacharyya N, Varvares MA. Anomalous relationship of the facial nerve and the retromandibular vein: a case report. J Oral Maxillofac Surg 1999;57(1):75–6.
10. Garatea-Crelgo J, Gay-Escoda C, Bermejo B, et al. Morphological study of the parotid lymph nodes. J Craniomaxillofac Surg 1993;21(5):207–9.
11. Elluru R. Physiology of the salivary glands. In: Flint P, Haughey B, Quatela V, et al, editors. Cummings otolaryngology. 6th edition. Philadelphia: Saunders; 2015. p. 1202–12.
12. Myers EN, Conley J. Gustatory sweating after radical neck dissection. Arch Otolaryngol 1970;91(6):534–42.
13. Roark DT, Sessions RB, Alford BR. Frey's syndrome—a technical remedy. Ann Otol Rhinol Laryngol 1975;84(6):734–9.
14. Wotson S, Mandel I. The salivary secretions in health and disease. In: Rankow R, Polayes I, editors. Diseases of the salivary glands. Philadelphia: WB Saunders; 1976. p. 32–53.
15. Taybi H, Lachman R. Radiology of syndromes, metabolic disorders, and skeletal dysplasias. St Louis (MO): CV Mosby; 1996.
16. Nagato T, Tandler B. Gap junctions in rat sublingual gland. Anat Rec 1986;214(1): 71–5.
17. Palmer RM. The identification of myoepithelial cells in human salivary glands. A review and comparison of light microscopical methods. J Oral Pathol 1986; 15(4):221–9.
18. Shear M. The structure and function of myoepithelial cells in salivary glands. Arch Oral Biol 1966;11(8):769–80.
19. Nachlas N, Johns M. Physiology of the salivary glands. In: Otolaryngology: basic science and related principles. 3rd edition. Philadelphia: WB Saunders; 1991.
20. Baum BJ. Principles of saliva secretion. Ann N Y Acad Sci 1993;694:17–23.
21. Polak JM, Bloom SR. Neuropeptides in salivary glands. J Histochem Cytochem 1980;28(8):871–3.
22. Turner RJ. Mechanisms of fluid secretion by salivary glands. Ann N Y Acad Sci 1993;694:24–35.
23. Limb C, Niparko J. The acute facial palsies. In: Jackler R, Brackmann D, editors. Neurotology. Philadelphia: The Curtis Center; 2005. p. 1230–57.

24. Schwaber MK, Larson TC 3rd, Zealear DL, et al. Gadolinium-enhanced magnetic resonance imaging in Bell's palsy. Laryngoscope 1990;100(12):1264–9.

25. Wilson DF, Talbot JM, Hodgson RS. Magnetic resonance imaging-enhancing lesions of the labyrinth and facial nerve. Clinical correlation. Arch Otolaryngol Head Neck Surg 1994;120(5):560–4.

26. Moore GF. Facial nerve paralysis. Prim Care 1990;17(2):437–60.

27. Furnas DW. Landmarks for the trunk and the temporofacial division of the facial nerve. Br J Surg 1965;52:694–6.

28. Pitanguy I, Ramos AS. The frontal branch of the facial nerve: the importance of its variations in face lifting. Plast Reconstr Surg 1966;38(4):352–6.

29. Zani R, Fadul RJ, Da Rocha MA, et al. Facial nerve in rhytidoplasty: anatomic study of its trajectory in the overlying skin and the most common sites of injury. Ann Plast Surg 2003;51(3):236–42.

30. Gosain AK. Surgical anatomy of the facial nerve. Clin Plast Surg 1995;22(2):241–51.

31. Dorafshar AH, Borsuk DE, Bojovic B, et al. Surface anatomy of the middle division of the facial nerve: Zuker's point. Plast Reconstr Surg 2013;131(2):253–7.

32. Dingman RO, Grabb WC. Surgical anatomy of the mandibular ramus of the facial nerve based on the dissection of 100 facial halves. Plast Reconstr Surg Transplant Bull 1962;29:266–72.

Parotid Gland Imaging

Ravi S. Prasad, MD

KEYWORDS

- Parotid imaging • Pleomorphic adenoma • Biologic imaging • Image-guided biopsy
- Parapharyngeal space

KEY POINTS

- Ultrasound is a readily available initial imaging modality for the workup of parotid space tumors in the pediatric population.
- Computed tomography and MRI are essential for characterization of parotid space lesions and certain features may provide clues to the underlying histology.
- Biologic imaging is a new frontier that can offer insight into the behavioral characteristics of tumors.
- Image-guided biopsies offer a minimally invasive approach for histologic diagnosis.

INTRODUCTION

Given the location and anatomy of the parotid gland, lesions in the parotid gland can often remain indolent. This is true of lesions in the deep portion of the parotid gland or exophytic lesions extending into the paraphayrngeal space. As a result, many parotid lesions are incidental findings on imaging for other causes (neck trauma, headaches). The workup of incidental parotid lesions and patients presenting with specific symptoms related to their parotid gland, that is, facial pain or cheek mass, are some of the reasons for dedicated parotid gland imaging.

IMAGING MODALITIES
Conventional Radiographs

The use of plain radiographs and sialography are nearly obsolete in the current era of modern imaging. Only 60% of parotid calculi are seen on radiographs and determining whether they are parenchymal versus ductal is very limited.[1] Computed tomography (CT) had a nearly 10-fold increased sensitivity to sialolith detection over conventional radiographs.[2]

Sialography

Before cross-sectional imaging, siolograms were important for identifying lesions based on displacement of the ductal system and for assessing processes resulting

---

Disclosure: The author has nothing to disclose.
Department of Imaging, Cedars Sinai Medical Center, 8700 Beverly Boulevard, Suite M–335, Los Angeles, CA 90048, USA
E-mail address: Ravi.Prasad@cshs.org

Otolaryngol Clin N Am 49 (2016) 285–312
http://dx.doi.org/10.1016/j.otc.2015.10.003
0030-6665/16/$ – see front matter © 2016 Elsevier Inc. All rights reserved.

oto.theclinics.com

```
Abbreviations
ADC   Apparent Diffusion Coefficient
BV    Blood Volume
CP    Capillary Permeability
CT    Computed Tomography
CTP   Computed Tomography Perfusion
FNA   Fine-Needle Aspiration
PPS   Parapharyngeal Space
US    Ultrasonography
```

in ductal obstruction. After the advent of CT, sialograms played a role in differentiating subacute and chronic sialdenitis and autoimmune causes such as Sjögren syndrome.[3] Serology has superseded the diagnostic accuracy of conventional sialography.[2]

MR Sialography

MR sialography is a useful alternative to sialograms. It is performed with a heavily T2-weighted high-resolution fast spin echo sequence (TR 3600/TE 800) with fat suppression with a 4- to 6-cm slab thickness and a surface coil or multichannel head coil.[4] This technique offers a noninvasive means of assessing the ductal anatomy with comparable sensitivity to conventional sialography for large stone detection. Small stones, those approximately 3 mm, are more difficult to identify on MRI. MRI is also limited by the time required for the single sequence acquisition and the susceptibility to motion degradation for this sequence. For select cases, MR sialography can be added to the MRI parotid study.

Ultrasound

Another noninvasive tool for examining the parotid gland is high-resolution ultrasonography (US). In the United States, US is underused,[5] whereas in Europe and Asia it is often the first diagnostic test for parotid pathology workup.[6,7] Given that the bulk of the parotid gland is superficial, US serves as a readily available screening test for parotid pathology. Because most clinicians are familiar with cross-sectional anatomy, a sound understanding of the ultrasonographic appearance of the parotid space and spatial relationships is necessary for successful imaging of the parotid gland. For pediatric patients, it is the preferred diagnostic test given the concerns for radiation exposure and the low incidence of primary tumors in this population.[2,8]

Wide-band linear transducers of 5 to 12 MHz are used for examination.[9] Most superficial lesions are best evaluated with frequency probes greater than 7.5 MHz with evaluation of the deeper portions of the gland best evaluated with lower linear frequency probes (5-7 MHz) given the need for deeper penetration. This also forms a significant limitation for parotid US because lesions in the deep portion of the parotid gland, at the stylomandibular notch, or parapharyngeal space are obscured by the mandible. For these lesions, cross-sectional imaging is recommended[10,11] (**Fig. 1**).

Conventional Angiography

Catheter-based angiography has limited role in workup of parotid region tumors. Aside from the rare instances of a large arteriovenous malformation or hemangiomas that may require preoperative embolization, most parotid space tumors are not excessively hypervascular. With the advent of high resolution multislice CT scans, preoperative planning can be performed adequately with cross-sectional imaging. Even for the aforementioned hypervascular lesions, a CT angiography is adequate for preoperative

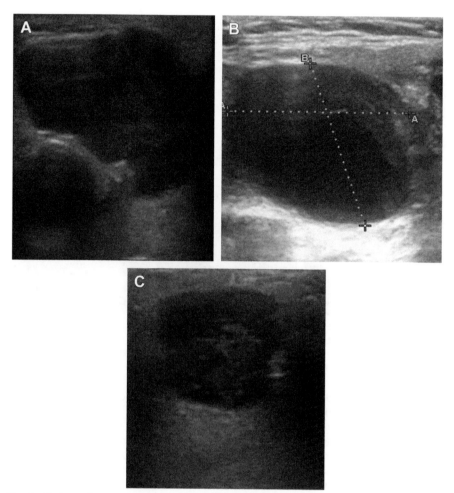

Fig. 1. High-resolution ultrasound of typical parotid masses. (*A*) Pleomorphic adenoma. Typically-well circumscribed hypoechoic lesion with slight lobulations. (*B*) Branchial cleft cyst. Hypoechoic–anechoic well circumscribed mass with some internal echoes representing debris and posterior acoustic enhancement. (*C*) Warthin's tumor. Hypoechoic and sharply defined mass.

planning and adds the benefit of providing better spatial resolution than conventional angiography.[12]

Computed Tomographic Imaging of the Parotid Gland

In the normal adult parotid gland, the gland is fatty with Hounsfield units of 15 to 25.[13] On CT imaging, this translates into attenuation that is slightly darker than muscle but brighter than subcutaneous fat (**Fig. 2**). In the pediatric population, the fat content is smaller and hence the gland is often brighter. A denser gland can mask small intra-glandular lesions. For inflammatory disease or sialadenitis, CT is the preferred imaging modality given its spatial resolution and sensitivity to calcification.[2] Limitations of CT include extensive dental artifacts that cannot be avoided with angled axial imaging, contrast contraindications in densely glandular tissue where an intraglandular

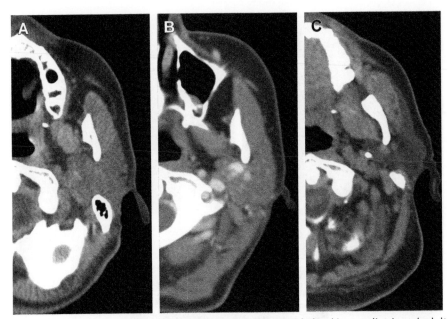

Fig. 2. Normal computed tomography (CT) scan of the parotid gland in a pediatric and adult patient. (*A*) Noncontrast CT. (*B*) Contrast-enhanced CT. Notice the enhancement of the gland, which can mask small tumors. (*C*) Noncontrast CT in a 65-year-old male. Notice the increased fat content of the gland.

neoplasm is suspected, assessment of perineural spread of disease, and radiation concerns in the pediatric population.

With the advent of multidetector CT scans, most parotid space imaging would include thin section acquisition (≤2.5 mm) from the inferior orbits through the mandible. If the entire neck is scanned (for workup of malignant lymphadenopathy), scanning through the aortic arch should be included. Nonionic iodinated contrast is helpful for evaluation for lesion conspicuity, assessment of lymph nodes, evaluation of the extent of inflammation in infectious etiology, and for understanding the vascularity of the lesions. Care should be made to avoid the orbits if possible and to use iterative reconstructive dose reduction techniques to minimize radiation exposure, especially in the pediatric population.[14] Rarely should a noncontrast and contrast CT be performed.

A clear advantage of CT scan is exact localization of the facial nerve in the mastoid bone and position of the stylomastoid foramen. This information is useful in cases of tumors invading the mastoid, and tumors that abut the skull base adjacent to the stylomastoid foramen in assessing their relationship to the facial nerve.

MRI of the Parotid Gland

The normal adult parotid gland has a high T1-weighted signal and low to intermediate T2-weighted signal on conventional MRI. As in CT, the fat content of the parotid gland makes it ideal for MRI. Aside from lipomas, most lesions within the parotid gland stand out on precontrast T1-weighted imaging. Additionally, the ability to follow abnormal enhancement along the nerves and assessment of the regional vasculature makes parotid space imaging ideal with MRI[5] (**Fig. 3**). Contrast can be helpful in lesions that are inconspicuous on T1-weighted imaging or for characterization of nodal spread.[15]

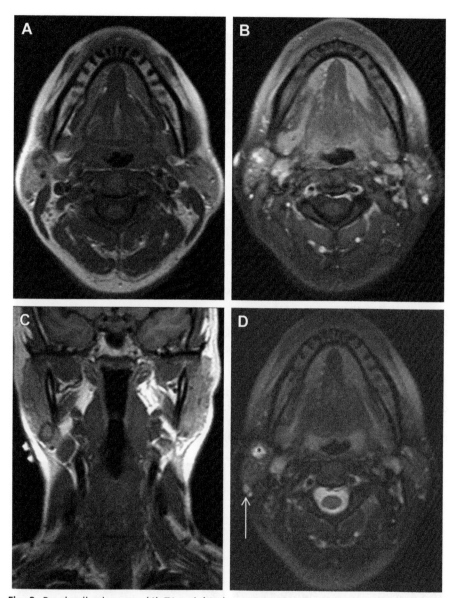

Fig. 3. Basal cell adenoma. (*A*) T1-weighted precontrast image. (*B*) T1-weighted fat-suppressed post contrast image. (*C*) Coronal T1-weighted precontrast image. (*D*) T2-weighted fat-suppressed image. The lesion (denoted by the *asterisk*) is more conspicuous on the precontrast T1 owing to inherent macroscopic fat within the gland. The lesion is well seen on the T2 images. Incidental note of an intraparotid lymph node (*arrow*).

Although imaging protocols vary from center to center, most protocols will include T1-weighted imaging in 3 planes, T2-wegithed imaging with fat suppression to highlight nodal disease and lesion conspicuity, and fat-suppressed postcontrast T1-weighted imaging. The area of coverage should include the base of the mastoid through the mandible for adequate inclusion of parotid glands of varying size. High field strength MRI such as 3T MRI, when available, offers greater signal to noise ratio with a shorter acquisition time.[16] In the pediatric population and the claustrophobic population, this can often shorten the duration of sedation.

BIOLOGIC IMAGING OF PAROTID SPACE TUMORS
Radionuclide Imaging

Radionuclide salivary studies are also available as a mode of evaluating both the parenchymal and excretory functions of the gland.[17] The parotid glands normally concentrate ^{99m}Tc-pertechnetate, so most lesions within the parotid gland are difficult to identify with scintigraphic studies compared with cross-sectional studies. Single photon emission CT–CT is more promising for its spatial resolution.[2] Radioactive tracers are hypersecreted in cases of acute sialadenitis, lymphoma, and sialosis in addition to tumors such as Warthin's tumors and oncocytomas.[18] Diminished radionuclide excretory activity is commonly seen in Sjögren syndrome or chronic parotitis.[19,20] One study comparing ^{99m}Tc and ^{201}Tl single photon emission CT with CT/MRI imaging demonstrated the ability to differentiate Warthin's tumors from other major salivary gland tumors with greater sensitivity than conventional CT/MRI imaging.[21] Nonetheless, aside from nonoperative patients, surgical excision is still recommended for these tumors, regardless of histology. The subsequent treatment options and outcomes are only then affected by the histology.[21]

PET Imaging

PET imaging has had little role in initial workup of parotid tumors. The cost of the test, the time involved, and its low specificity preclude routine use of this test.[22] Furthermore, normal activity in the parotid gland may mask an underlying lesion.[23] Both malignant and benign parotid space tumors have increased glucose metabolism and even some inflammatory processes can demonstrate increased uptake. Specificity can be increased by using multiple tracers however these are tracers that are not routinely readily available.[24] There is a role for PET surveillance for recurrent disease or for assessing distant metastases (**Fig. 4**).

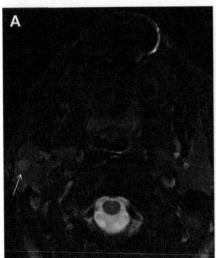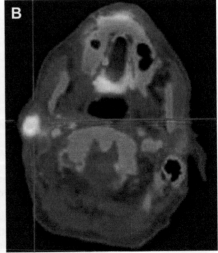

Fig. 4. Pleomorphic adenoma. (*A*) Axial T2 fat-suppressed image. (*B*) Axial fused 18-FDG PET-computed tomography scan. Well-circumscribed superficial parotid lobe lesion (*arrow*) demonstrates increased metabolic activity on subsequent PET study.

Proton MR Spectroscopy

MR spectroscopy has a unique ability to examine a tumor at the metabolic level. Its limitations relate to the minimum voxel size necessary for spectral analysis in tumors that are often small and irregular and the low signal-to-noise ratios obtained from head and neck imaging.[25] Despite these restrictions, by assessing ratios of metabolites, a predictor of malignancy and cellular turnover can be made. In a study by King and colleagues,[26] the choline to creatine ratio was examined between benign and malignant tumors and between Warthin's tumor and pleomorphic adenoma. Ratios of greater than 2.4 were predictive of a benign tumor and those greater than 4.5 had a 71% positive predictive value of being a Warthin's tumor. Spectral analysis, however, has yet to be proven effective in predicting outcome or evaluating treatment efficacy. King and colleagues[27] showed that the choline values on the pretreatment scans and posttreatment studies are not predictive of treatment response.

Computed Tomography Perfusion

CT perfusion (CTP) is a reproducible examination that examines the microvascularity of tumors. With dynamic acquisitions over the tumor region, certain characteristics such as blood volume (BV), blood flow, capillary permeability (CP), and mean transit time can be calculated mathematically. Malignant tumors demonstrate increased BV, blood flow, and CP with a diminished mean transit time.[28,29] For treatment response and outcomes prediction, studies have shown a role for CTP. Most tumors with early therapeutic response exhibit diminished BV and CP on posttherapy studies and nonresponders showed increased BV and CP. Additionally, marked elevated BV on baseline studies were more predictive of short-term response.[30,31]

Perfusion-Weighted MRI

Like CTP, perfusion-weighted MRI examines the vascular infrastructure of tumors. Unlike CTP, there are variations in how the images are acquired as well as dependent on which vascular model is applied for determination of BV and permeability. Additionally, perfusion MR acquisitions require more time for scanning. These have generally limited its use to a few centers. Recent studies have looked at permeability on the pretreatment studies. As in CTP, an increased permeability in the treatment responders was higher than in nonresponders on the baseline study.[32]

Diffusion-Weighted MRI

Diffusion-weighted imaging looks at water molecule motion through the cell membranes of the tissues in the scan field. When the NA–K pumps fail or when the extracellular space is minute, there is increased in diffusion restriction of the water molecules (shown as increased DW signal and low apparent diffusion coefficient [ADC] values). Diffusion-weighted imaging has been introduced into many head and neck MRIs owing to its short acquisition time and its reproducibility. In parotid imaging, restricted diffusion with low ADC values are predictive of tumor malignancy.[33,34] Most studies have shown ADC values below 0.9 to 1.3×10^{-3} mm^2/s are typical for malignant tumors or metastatic lymph nodes. Values greater than 1.8×10^{-3} mm^2/s have a high positive predictive value for pleomorphic adenomas.[35–37] Diffusion-weighted imaging is another biological imaging tool to predict tumor behavior (**Fig. 5**).

A combination of dynamic contrast-enhanced MR and ADC is another preoperative tool to assess benignity of parotid tumors. Yabuuchi and colleagues[38] classified parotid tumors based on their time–intensity curves. Tumors with flat contrast enhancement and gradual contrast enhancement were highly predictive of benign tumors.

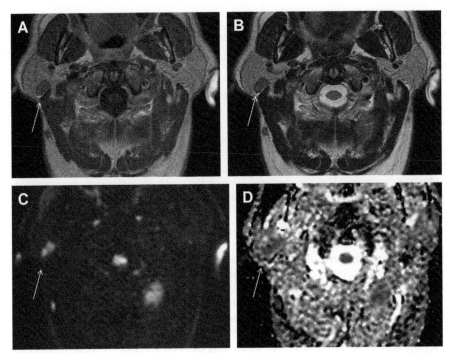

Fig. 5. Warthin's tumor. (*A*) Axial T1-weighted image. (*B*) Axial T2-weighted image. (*C*) Axial diffusion-weighted imaging. (*D*) Axial apparent diffusion coefficient (ADC) image. Well-circumscribed lesion (*white arrow*) in the superficial parotid gland with increased diffusion signal and diminished ADC signal.

Those tumors with rapid peak enhancement but gradual washout were suggestive of malignancy and those tumors with rapid peak enhancement but steep washout were more suggestive of benign histology. These last 2 categories often had overlap. Adding the cutoff ADC values of 1.4×10^{-3} mm²/s between pleomorphic adenomas and malignant tumors and 1.0×10^{-3} mm²/s between Warthin's and malignant tumors further helped to accurately identify tumors preoperatively (accuracy 82% vs 94%; positive predictive value 67% vs 92%).[39]

Furthermore, functionality of the gland can be assessed by looking at the ADC values. In normal parotid tissue, during the early gustatory stimulation, there are low ADC values that steadily increase over time. In a gland previously treated with radiotherapy, this gradual increase to greater than the baseline value is not seen; the ADC values remain increased at baseline and after stimulation.[40]

PICTORIAL ESSAY OF PAROTID SPACE LESIONS
Lipoma

Lipoma of the parotid space accounts for 10% of all parotid lesions. Clinically, lipomas are found either incidentally or from painless swelling. There is no predilection for malignant transformation and surgical excision is reserved for cosmetic purposes. On US, lipomas are compressible, echogenic lesions without posterior acoustic shadowing. On CT, they have Hounsfield units of -20 to -100 with possible thin rim of enhancement. No nodularity is noted. They are T1 and T2 hyperintense on MRI, similar to subcutaneous fat with complete fat suppression. CT/MRI is helpful to examine the extent of lipomatous infiltration and to assess for any nodularity suggestive of sarcomatous degeneration[41] (**Fig. 6**).

Intraparotid Lymph Nodes

Intraparotid lymph nodes are normally seen within the parotid glands. Approximately 20 lymph nodes reside within the parotid space owing to late embryologic encapsulation.[2] Intraglandular lymph nodes are not seen in the other salivary glands. They serve as the primary lymphatic drainage of the external auditory canal, pinna, and regional scalp (see **Fig. 3**A, D).

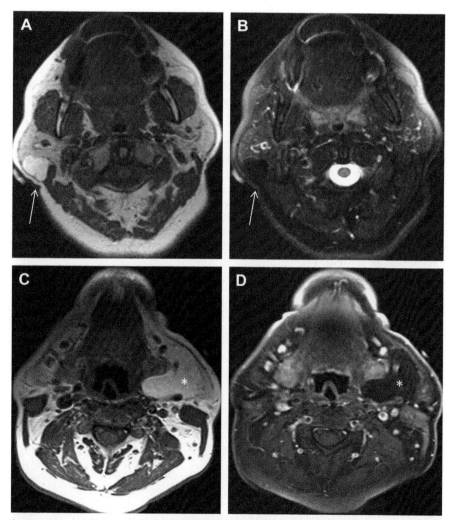

Fig. 6. Lipoma. (*A*) Axial T1-weighted image. (*B*) Axial T2 fat-suppressed image. (*C*) Axial T1-weighted image. (*D*) Axial T1 fat-suppressed post contrast image. In (*A, B, white arrow*), lesion in the posterior right parotid gland is seen, which suppresses with fat suppression. In (*C, D, asterisk*), the large lesion infiltrates through the inferior parotid gland. No nodular enhancement is seen on postcontrast imaging.

Branchial Cleft Cyst (Types I and II)

First branchial cleft cysts are usually periaricular or periparotid/intraparotid. These latter cysts/sinus tracts are classified as type II and are the most common 1st branchial cleft cyst.[42] On US, they are usually solitary anechoic masses with posterior acoustic shadowing. On CT, they are well-circumscribed, rim-enhancing lesions within the substance of the parotid, periparotid space or parapharyngeal space. They are hyperintense on T2-weighted imaging and hypointense on T1-weighted imaging. A thickened rim is suggestive of acute/chronic infection.[43] (**Fig. 7**) In contrast, a second branchial cleft cyst is often seen deep to platysma, anterior to the sternocleidomastoid muscle, posterior to the submandibular gland, and lateral to the carotid sheath.[44] It often lies inferior to the parotid gland (**Fig. 8**).

Parotitis

Parotitis is often a clinical diagnosis; the majority of these cases have a viral etiology. They tend to be bilateral with glandular enlargement, whereas bacterial parotitis is uninlateral with associated cellulitis with or without abscess. Autoimmune parotitis is often difficult to distinguish from viral parotitis because it is often bilateral. Periglandular inflammation is less common. Serology is often required for diagnosis[45] (**Fig. 9**).

Sarcoidosis

Parotid sarcoidosis is rare to only manifest in the parotid space. Additional salivary glands or systemic symptoms are presenting symptoms[46] (**Fig. 10**).

Sialadenitis

Sialolithiasis is most common in the submandibular gland with approximately 10% to 20% occurring in the parotid gland with 32% being multiple. Of parotid stones, 60% are radiopaque.[47,48] CT is the preferred imaging modality for evaluation of sialoliths. Imaging is helpful for assessing calculus size, abscess formation, and changes of chronic sialadenitis (**Fig. 11**).

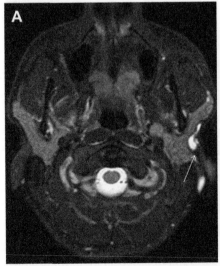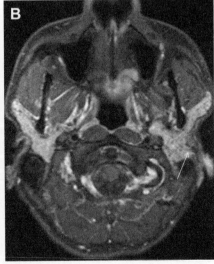

Fig. 7. First Branchial cleft cyst (*white arrow*). (*A*) T2-weighted, fat-suppressed image. (*B*) T1-weighted fat-suppressed post contrast image. T2-weighted image of a bright cystic lesion in the left periparotid space without enhancement or fat suppression.

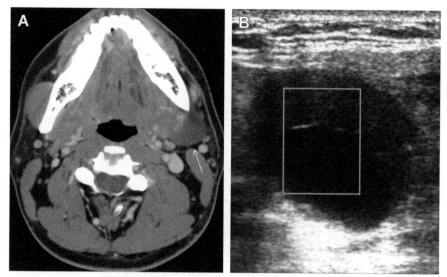

Fig. 8. Second branchial cleft cyst (*white arrow*). (*A*) Contrast-enhanced computed tomography (CT) scan. (*B*) Ultrasound (US) image of a cystic lesion medial to the parotid tail. US-guided fine-needle aspiration biopsy was performed owing to solid component on CT scan (not shown). Cyst contents demonstrated blood products and no nodular components were seen.

Lymphoepithelial Cysts

Lymphoepithelial lesions are typically found in immunocompromised patients and those with human immunodeficiency virus infection. They present with painless bilateral parotid swelling and can often regress with antiretroviral therapy. There is a very small risk of transformation to B-cell lymphoma.[49] On imaging, there are multiple cystic and solid masses within the parotid gland. Imaging from the base of skull to the thoracic inlet also shows constellation of lymphoid hyperplasia and cervical lymphadenopathy. Some variants have multiple solid masses that can mimic intraparotid

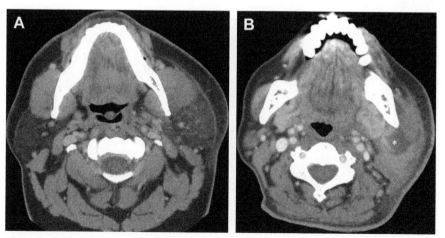

Fig. 9. Parotitis. (*A*) Contrast-enhanced computed tomography (CT) scan with enlarged left parotid gland and periglandular inflammatory changes. (*B*) Contrast-enhanced CT with left parotitis and intraparotid abscess (*asterisk*).

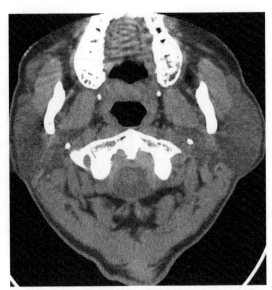

Fig. 10. Sarcoidosis. Noncontrast computed tomography scan showing subtle bilateral enlargement of bilateral parotid glands in a patient with known sarcoidosis.

neoplasia. In contrast, cysts associated with Sjögren syndrome are usually smaller and uniform in size. The parotid glands progress from normal, to enlarged, to atrophy with disease progression[2] (**Fig. 12**).

Congenital Capillary Hemangiomas

Hemangiomas in the pediatric group are most typically of a capillary subtype. These mesenchymal tumors are lobular and demonstrate enhancement on CT. On MRI, they can have heterogenous signal on T1 precontrast owing to prior hemorrhage, fluid–fluid levels, and are bright on T2-weighted imaging with variable enhancement[50] (**Fig. 13**).

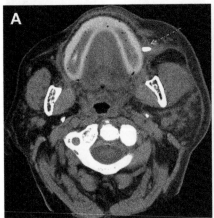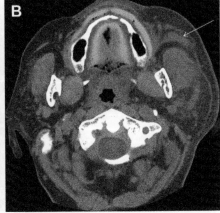

Fig. 11. Sialolith with sialadenitis. (*A*) Noncontrast computed tomography scan demonstrating sialolith (*dashed arrow*) in the distal left Stentson's duct. (*B*) Notice periglandular stranding, enlargement, and ipsilateral Stenson's duct enlargement (*arrow*).

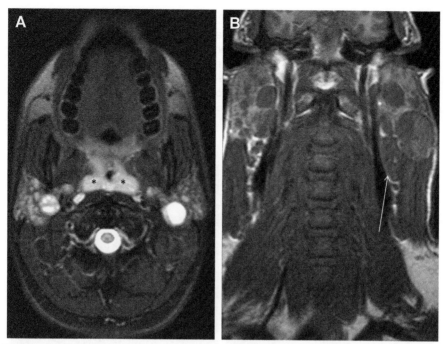

Fig. 12. Lymphoepithelial cysts. (*A*) Axial T2-wegithed fat-suppressed image. (*B*) Coronal T1-weighted image. Notice the bilateral cystic lesions of mixed signal intensity and size. The (*asterisks*) represent lymphoid hyperplasia and the (*arrow*) denotes enlarged cervical lymph nodes in this patient with human immunodeficiency virus infection.

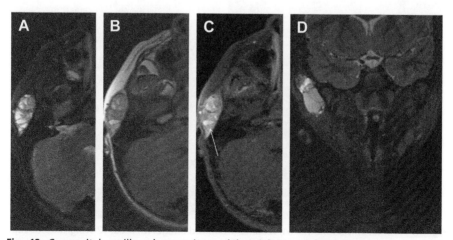

Fig. 13. Congenital capillary hemangioma. (*A*) Axial T1-weighted image. (*B*) Axial T1-weighted fat-suppressed postcontrast image. (*C*) Axial T2-weighted fat-suppressed image. Notice the blood–fluid level (*arrow*). (*D*) Coronal T2-weighted fat-suppressed image. Multilobulated T2-weighted bright and precontrast T1-weighted image of a heterogenous lesion with some enhancement.

Pleomorphic Adenoma

Benign mixed tumors of the parotid gland account for 80% of the salivary gland tumors. Ninety percent occur lateral to the plane of the facial nerve.[51] They demonstrate slow growth and have a 2% to 5% risk of malignant degeneration. Unlike Warthin's tumors, 0.5% are multicentric.[52] When these tumors undergo malignant transformation, they often present with rapid growth, pain, and facial nerve paralysis. On imaging, benign mixed tumors are hypoechoic on US and hypovascular on angiography.

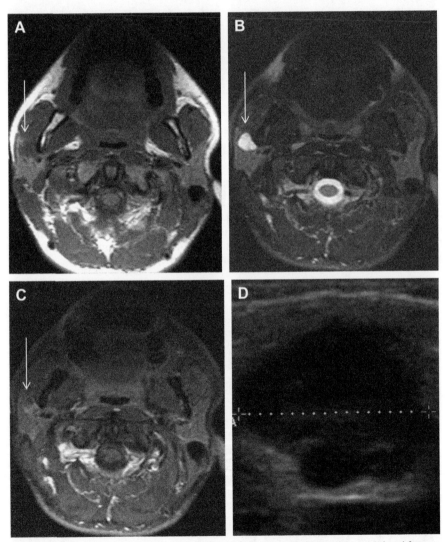

Fig. 14. Pleomorphic adenoma. (*A*) Axial T2-weighted image. (*B*) Axial T2-weighted fat-suppressed image. (*C*) Axial T1-weighted fat-suppressed postcontrast image. (*D*) Ultrasound image. There is a well-circumscribed T1-weighted hypointense, T2-weighted hyperintense lesion in the anterior superficial aspect of the right parotid gland (*arrow*). The lesion demonstrates heterogeneous enhancement. On ultrasonography, the lesion is a lobulated hypoechoic solid mass.

They are cold on Tc^{99m}-pertechnetate scans. They are well-demarcated on CT/MRI with variable enhancement, depending on underlying necrosis. They may rarely contain calcifications. Smaller lesions are more likely to be homogenously enhancing. On MRI, they are well-demarcated on T2 imaging with intermediate to high signal internally with typically hypointense peripheral rim. They demonstrate higher ADC values than other parotid tumors. Generally, pleomorphic adenomas have shown quick contrast uptake with a gradual plateau representing contrast retention[39] (**Fig. 14**).

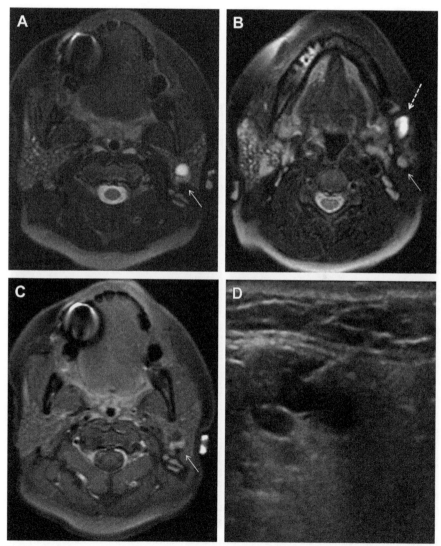

Fig. 15. Warthin's tumor. (*A*) Axial T2-weighted fat-suppressed image. (*B*) Axial T2-weighted fat-suppressed image. (*C*) Axial T1-weighted fat-suppressed postcontrast image. (*D*) Ultrasound (US). There is a mixed cystic and solid lesion seen in the posterior left parotid gland (*arrow*) with a second cystic lesion seen in the anterior aspect of the gland (*dashed arrow*). On US before fine-needle aspiration, the lesion is partially cystic with a solid component.

Warthin's Tumor

Warthin's tumors are the second most common tumor of the parotid gland (4%–10%) with lesions more commonly seen in the parotid tail. Ninety percent are found in smokers, 20% are bilateral, and 30% are cystic; 2.7% to 12% may arise in extraparotid tissue such as periparotid lymph nodes. These, like pleomorphic adenomas, are slow growing with 1% risk of malignant degeneration into either carcinoma or lymphoma.[2] Unlike benign mixed tumors, Warthin's tumors demonstrate increased uptake on Tc99m-pertechnetate scans and PET scan. On CT/MR, they are well-defined lesions, with variable enhancement (**Fig. 15**). They demonstrate intermediate to high T2 signal and have lower ADC values as compared with pleomorphic adenoma. Additionally, on perfusion imaging, there is rapid contrast uptake with rapid contrast washout.[39]

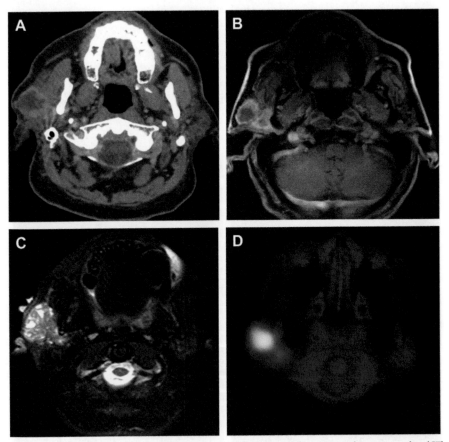

Fig. 16. Mucoepidermoid carcinoma. (*A*) Contrast-enhanced computed tomography (CT) scan. (*B*) Postcontrast T1-weighted fat-suppressed image. (*C*) T1-weighted fat-suppressed image. (*D*) PET-CT scan. *A, B,* A heterogeneously enhancing, partially cystic, multilobulated tumor in the superficial right parotid gland. *C,* Classic heterogenous appearance with low T2 signal compared with typical pleomorphic adenomas. This lesion demonstrated increased metabolic activity on the PET study (*D*).

Mucoepidermoid Tumor

Mucoepidermoid carcinoma (MEC) is the most common primary parotid malignancy. They present as a firm mass with facial pain/otalgia, and possible cranial neuropathies. Recurrence rate depends on histologic grade. Assessment of the facial nerve and mandibular division of the trigeminal nerve (commonly for lesions in the deep portion of the parotid gland) are necessary. MEC can invade into the mandible and deep facial spaces and metastasize to regional lymph nodes (level IIA nodes most common). Low-grade MECs are well-circumscribed with variable enhancement if cystic components are present (**Fig. 16**). They are usually lower in T2 signal than pleomorphic adenomas and demonstrate lower ADC values (similar to Warthin's tumors). Higher grade MECs have associated lymphadenopathy.[53]

Adenoid Cystic Carcinoma

Adenoid cystic carcinoma is the second most common parotid malignancy with the greatest propensity for perineural spread. Thirty-three percent of these lesions present with facial nerve paralysis with painful hard mass. They have poor prognosis for late recurrence and commonly metastasizes to the lungs and bone preferably over first-order lymph nodes. These tumors, unlike MECs, are homogenously enhancing. High-grade adenoid cystic carcinoma have infiltrative margins, lower ADC values than pleomorphic adenomas, and perineural spread of cranial nerve VII. They tend to be intermediate signal on T2-weighted imaging, higher than MEC. Imaging of the facial nerve is crucial to assess perineural disease[54] (**Fig. 17**).

Lymphoma

Primary parotid lymphoma accounts for 2% to 5% of all parotid tumors. Systemic non-Hodgkin lymphoma involves the parotid in 1% to 8% of cases. On US, multiple

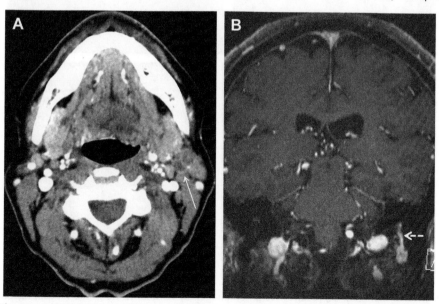

Fig. 17. Adenoid cystic carcinoma. (*A*) Contrast-enhanced computed tomography scan. (*B*) Coronal fat-suppressed T1 postcontrast image. Notice the heterogenous lesion in the left parotid gland (*arrow*). Perineural spread of tumor along the descending segment of the left facial nerve is seen (*dashed arrow*).

hypoechoic masses with internal increased vascularity are noted. On CT/MRI, multiple homogenously enhancing masses are seen with additional lymph nodes seen in the cervical neck.[55] Primary parenchymal lymphoma, on the other hand, presents as an infiltrative mass of the parotid gland with both solid/cystic components. Additionally, primary lymphoma of the parotid is best appreciated on T2-weighted fat-suppressed images or T1-weighted precontrast images (**Fig. 18**).

Metastatic Disease

Metastatic disease to the parotid gland accounts for 4% of all parotid tumors. The breast and lung are most common systemic malignancies.[56] MRI is helpful to assess for perineural spread if there is extracapsular tumor in the parotid gland. PET scan is the imaging modality of choice for tumor burden assessment. Metastatic disease from skin cancers can spread to the parotid owing to intrinsic parotid nodes and

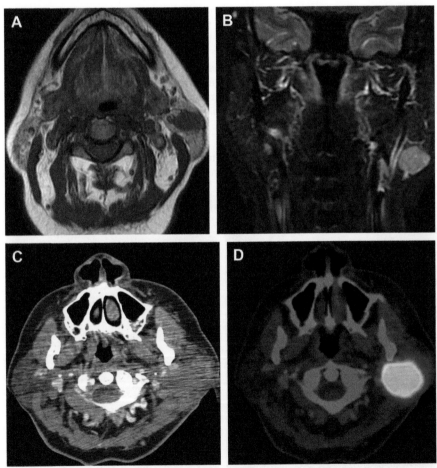

Fig. 18. Lymphoma. (*A*) Axial T1-weighted image. (*B*) Coronal T2-weighted fat-suppressed image. (*C*) Contrast-enhanced computed tomography (CT) scan. (*D*) PET-CT. Notice how the tumor is readily distinguishable in (*A*) and (*B*); (*C*) and (*D*) are images 1 month later demonstrating interval growth of tumor. The lesion is more infiltrative and less discernible on CT than on MRI.

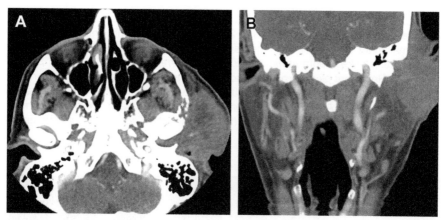

Fig. 19. Metastatic squamous cell cancer to the parotid. (*A*) Contrast-enhanced computed tomography (CT) scan. (*B*) Coronal contrast-enhanced CT scan. Notice the erosion of the zygomatic arch (*asterisk*). The lesion is infiltrative into the superficial and deep portions of the gland as well as the temporalis muscles.

regional spread. Sixty percent represent squamous cell cancer of the scalp or ear with 15% representing melanoma.[57] CT and MRI including the ear and extending through the external auditory canal and temporal scalp is helpful for identifying the original site and extent of the disease (**Fig. 19**). Imaging is also helpful to determine if there is skull base involvement and facial nerve involvement, which can change surgical options for the patient.

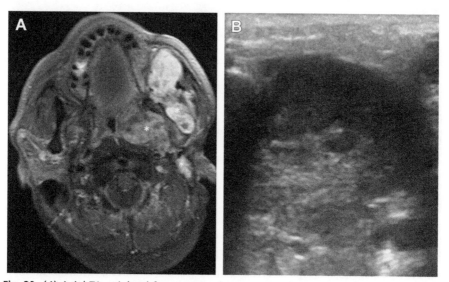

Fig. 20. (*A*) Axial T1-weighted fat-suppressed postcontrast image demonstrating recurrent pleomorphic adenomas. There are 3 distinct areas of recurrence (denoted by *asterisk*) in a patient with multiple previous parotid surgeries for tumor removal. (*B*) Ultrasound image of an acinic cell carcinoma.

Miscellaneous Disease

Basal cell adenoma accounts for 1% to 2% of all parotid tumors and has a very low risk of malignant transformation. They are usually less than 3 cm and have a slow growth rate. Unlike pleomorphic adenomas, recurrence rates are up to 25%.[58] (see **Fig. 3**) Recurrent pleomorphic adenomas are rare with rates of 1% to 4% in current literature with recent smaller studies showing minimal to no recurrence rates[59,60] (**Fig. 20**A). Acinic cell carcinoma of the parotid gland are the third most common primary parotid malignancy (5%–17%), often considered a low grade

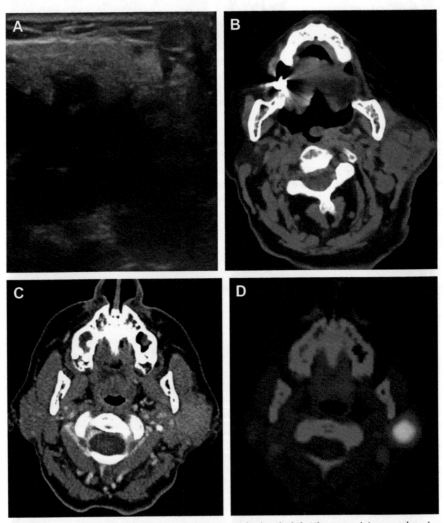

Fig. 21. Squamous cell carcinoma of the parotid gland. (*A*) Ultrasound image showing heterogenous mixed echogenic mass with infiltrative border. (*B*) Noncontrast computed tomography (CT) scan showing multiple masses with some ill-defined borders. Undifferentiated carcinoma of the parotid gland. (*C*) Contrast-enhanced CT scan. (*D*) PET scan showing avid uptake within the lesion.

tumor. Lesions are usually homogenous in enhancement but can be partially cystic[61] (see **Fig. 20**B).

Squamous cell carcinoma of the parotid gland are rare malignancies. On imaging, they are often infiltrative and may contain necrotic areas (**Fig. 21**A, B). **Fig. 21**C, D demonstrates an example of undifferentiated carcinoma of the parotid gland, which is FDG avid on PET imaging.

Facial nerve schwannomas are often homogenously enhancing and well-circumscribed (**Fig. 22**A). If they occur proximally, they can enlarge the stylomastoid foramen. Patients often present with slow growing cheek mass without facial nerve palsy. Lesions larger than 2 cm may contain intratumoral cysts.[62] Plexiforma neurofibromas are typically seen in the setting of neurofibromatosis type I. They can lobular or infiltrative and can be multiple. They will often have avid yet variable enhancement and are often bright on T2-weighted imaging (see **Fig. 22**B). Epithelioma–myoepithelial carcinoma is a rare parotid tumor with high rate of recurrence (60%) even years after resection. On imaging, they are nonspecific in appearance but are usually well-circumscribed with cystic changes. Given its appearance, they are difficult to distinguish from a Warthin's tumor[63] (see **Fig. 22**C).

Parapharyngeal Space Lesions

Parapharygeal lesions can vary from benign etiologies, such as asymmetric pterygoid venous plexus to carcinomatous lesions. Lesions within the parapharyngeal space are often extension from the surrounding structures however distinct lesions such as lymphatic malformations, minor salivary gland tumors, or lipomas can occur here.[2,64] **Fig. 23** illustrates a variety of lesions that occur in the parapharyngeal space.

IMAGE-GUIDED INTERVENTION

Once a parotid gland lesion is identified, tissue diagnosis can be obtained percutaneously through fine-needle aspiration or through core biopsies. Tissue sampling may be obtained by palpation, US guidance, or CT guidance.[65,66] MR guidance, given the acquisition time and equipment limitations, are not a preferred choice for tissue biopsy.[67]

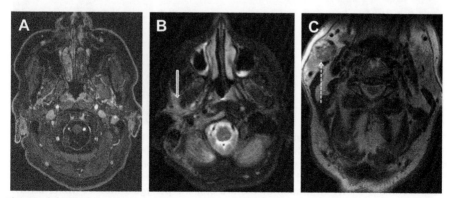

Fig. 22. (*A*) Facial nerve schwannoma. Axial T1-weighted fat-suppressed postcontrast image demonstrates enlargement of the left facial nerve at the stylomastoid foramen (*asterisk*). (*B*) Axial T2-weighted fat-suppressed image demonstrating a plexiform neurofibroma infiltrating through the right parotid gland (*white arrow*). (*C*) Axial T2-weighted image demonstrating a heterogenous lesion in the anterior superficial right parotid gland with some small internal cystic components (*dotted white line*). The lesion is well-circumscribed and multilobulated, typical of this lesion.

Percutaneous Ultrasound Interventions

For image-guided interventions, US is the most common modality used. Fine-needle aspiration is a well-accepted method with an average specificity for detecting malignant parotid tumors of 96%. Sensitivity does vary depending on the study with an average 79%.[68,69] Operator experience, presence of a cytopathologist, tumor composition, and location within the parotid gland are all factors affecting the sensitivity.[70] Most FNA are performed with 22-G needles with suction applied to each passes; 1 to 5 passes are usually attempted[2] (**Fig. 24**). Recent studies have shown an increase in sensitivity with the addition of core biopsies. This technique provides larger tissue sample with preserved architecture for further immunochemical staining, increasing

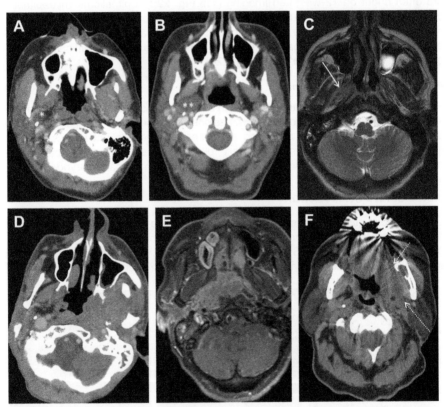

Fig. 23. (*A*). Schwannoma. Axial contrast-enhanced computed tomography (CT) scan shows nonenhancing cystic lesion in the right parapharyngeal space (PPS; *single asterisk*). (*B*) Pleomorphic adenoma. Axial contrast-enhanced CT scan shows nonenhancing lesion exophytic from the right deep space of the parotid gland (*double asterisk*). (*C*) Lymphoma. Axial T2-weighted image shows infiltration of the PPS and the pterygoid muscles (*white arrow*). (*D*) Metastatic squamous cell carcinoma. Axial contrast-enhanced CT scan shows infiltrative mass in the left PPS with involvement of the pterygoid muscles and the pharyngeal mucosal space. The patient had a history of recurrent squamous cell cancer of the tongue. (*E*) Nasopharyngeal cancer. Axial T1-weighted fat-suppressed postcontrast image demonstrates heterogeneous enlarged enhancing mass of the nasopharynx with right lateral extension into the PPS. (*F*) Adenoid cystic carcinoma. Axial noncontrast CT scan shows infiltrative mass in the left PPS and pterygoid muscles.

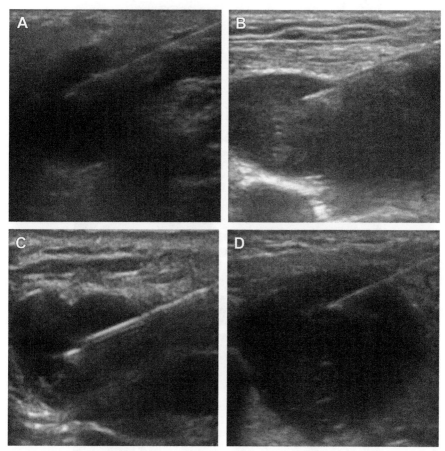

Fig. 24. Ultrasound-guided biopsies. (*A*) Fine-needle aspiration (FNA) of Warthin's tumor. (*B*) FNA of infected branchial cleft cyst. (*C*) Core biopsy of intraparotid lymphoma. (*D*) FNA of squamous cell cancer of the parotid.

the sensitivity to 96% and specificity to 100%.[71] The risks of facial nerve injury, especially for deep parotid space lesions and patient discomfort, need to be weighed when determining biopsy techniques. In a recent study, Eoma and colleagues[72] described the efficacy of core needle biopsies in 282 patients with no complications of facial nerve injury or hematoma. Patient selection and proper technique are key for successful core biopsies. The authors even showed that core biopsies are often less susceptible to operator experience given the larger tissue sample. Seeding of the biopsy tract, unfortunately, has not been evaluated in a large population study.

Percutaneous Computed Tomography-Guided Interventions

A CT-guided intervention is the preferred modality for percutaneous biopsies of deep parotid space masses and parapharyngeal space masses.[73] There are multiple approaches that can be used for access depending on lesion location. Biopsies are performed using a coaxial technique with the outer 18- to 19-G guide needle placed at the lesion periphery (**Fig. 25**). Either FNA or core biopsies are then performed with a 20- to 22-G needle into the lesion. This technique avoids unnecessarily passing through

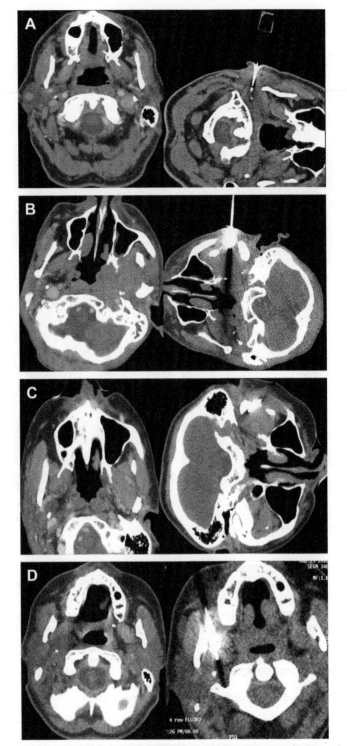

Fig. 25. Computed tomography (CT)-guided biopsies. (*A*) Transparotid approach to a pleomorphic adenoma. (*B*) Transmastoid approach to metastatic squamous cell carcinoma of the tongue to the parapharyngeal space (PPS). (*C*) Transzygomatic approach to a right PPS schwannoma. (*D*) Transbuccal approach to a right PPS pleomorphic adenoma.

normal overlying tissues, decreases scan time and radiation exposure, and decreases patient discomfort.[74] The most common approaches for parotid space and parapharyngeal space access include the subzygomatic,[75] retromandibular,[76] and transbuccal[77] approaches with the trajectory depending on the location of the lesions, patient cooperation level, and regional neurovascular structures.

SUMMARY

There are many tools available for parotid space imaging. Cross-sectional studies including CT and MRI are the workhorses for most tumor characterization with US being used as a first line tool especially in the pediatric population and acutely symptomatic patients (abscesses, cysts). Although in its infancy, biological imaging can hint at the underlying histology of parotid space tumors and can offer insight into tumor behavior and treatment efficacy. Finally, minimally invasive options are available for accessing parotid tumors to provide additional information before definitive surgical excision.

REFERENCES

1. Kraaij S, Karagozoglu KH, Forouzanfar T, et al. Salivary stones: symptoms, aetiology, biochemical composition and treatment. Br Dent J 2014;217(11):E23.
2. Som PM, Brandwein MS. Salivary glands: anatomy and pathology. In: Som PM, Curtin HD, editors. Head and neck imaging. 4th edition. St Louis (MO): Mosby; 2003. p. 2005–134.
3. Som P, Shugar J, Train J, et al. Manifestations of parotid gland enlargement: radiologic, pathologic and clinical correlations, part I: the autoimmune pseudosialectasias. Radiology 1981;141:415–9.
4. Jungehulsing M, Fischback R, Schroder U, et al. Magnetic resonance sialography. Otolaryngol Head Neck Surg 1999;121(4):488–94.
5. Yousem DM, Kraut MA, Chalian AA. Major salivary gland imaging. Radiology 2000;216:19–29.
6. Alyas F, Lewis K, Williams M, et al. Diseases of the submandibular gland as demonstrated using high resolution ultrasound. Br J Radiol 2005;78:362–9.
7. Howlett DC, Kesse KW, Hughes DV, et al. The role of imaging in the evaluation of parotid disease. Clin Radiol 2002;57:692–701.
8. Gritzmann N, Rettenbacher T, Hollerweger A, et al. Sonography of the salivary glands. Eur Radiol 2003;13:964–75.
9. Bialek EJ, Jakubowski W, Zajkowski P, et al. US of the major salivary glands: anatomy and spatial relationships, pathologic conditions, and pitfalls. Radiographics 2006;26(3):745–63.
10. Koischwitz D, Gritzmann N. Ultrasound of the neck. Radiol Clin North Am 2000; 38:1029–45.
11. Candiani F, Martinoli C. Salivary glands. In: Solbiati L, Rizzatto G, editors. Ultrasound of superficial structures. Edinburgh (United Kingdom): Churchill Livingstone; 1995. p. 125–39.
12. Achache M, Fakhry N, Varoquaux A, et al. Prise en charge des malformations vasculaires de la region parotidienne. Annales françaises d'oto-rhino-laryngologie et de pathologie cervico-faciale 2013;130(2):60–5.
13. Bryan R, Miller R, Ferreyro R, et al. Computed tomography of the major salivary glands. AJR Am J Roentgenol 1982;139:547–54.
14. Vachha B, Brodoefel H, Wilcox C, et al. Radiation dose reduction is soft tissue neck CT using adaptive statistical iterative reconstruction (ASIR). Eur J Radiol 2013;82(12):2222–6.

15. Chaudhuri R, Gleeson M, Graves P, et al. MR evaluation of the parotid gland using STIR and gadolinium-enhanced imaging. Eur Radiol 1992;2:357–64.
16. Stern JS, Ginat DT, Nicholas JL, et al. Imaging of pediatric head and neck masses. Otolaryngol Clin North Am 2015;48(1):225–46.
17. Klutmann S, Bohuslavizki KH, Kroger S, et al. Quantitative salivary gland scintigraphy. J Nucl Med Technol 1999;27:20–6.
18. Brandwein M, Huvos A. Oncocytic tumors of major salivary glands. A study of 68 cases with follow-up of 44 patients. Am J Surg Pathol 1991;15:514–28.
19. Pretorius D, Taylor A. The role of nuclear scanning in head and neck surgery. Head Neck Surg 1982;4:427–32.
20. Schall G. The role of radionuclide scanning in the evaluation of neoplasms in the salivary glands: a review. J Surg Oncol 1971;3:699–714.
21. Arbab AS, Koizumi K, Toyama K, et al. Various imaging modalities for the detection of salivary gland lesions: the advantages of 201Tl SPECT. Nucl Med Commun 2000;21:277–84.
22. Strauss LG. Fluorine-18 deoxyglucose and false-positive results: a major problem in the diagnostics of oncological patients. Eur J Nucl Med 1996;23:1409–15.
23. Roh JL, Ryu CH, Choi SH, et al. Clinical utility of 18F-FDG PET for patients with salivary gland malignancies. J Nucl Med 2007;48(2):240–6.
24. Okamura T, Kawabe J, Koyama K, et al. Fluorine-18 fluorodeoxyglucose positron emission tomography imaging of parotid mass lesions. Acta Otolaryngol Suppl 1998;538:209–13.
25. Shah GV, Gandhi D, Mukherji SK. Magnetic resonance spectroscopy of head and neck neoplasms. Top Magn Reson Imaging 2004;15:87–94.
26. King AD, Yeung DK, Ahuja AT, et al. Salivary gland tumors at in vivo proton MR spectroscopy. Radiology 2005;237(2):563–9.
27. King AD, Yeung DK, Yu KH, et al. Pretreatment and early intratreatment prediction of clinicopathologic response of head and neck cancer to chemoradiotherapy using 1H-MRS. J Magn Reson Imaging 2010;32:199–203.
28. Gandhi D, Hoeffner EG, Carlos RC, et al. Computed tomography perfusion of squamous cell carcinoma of the upper aerodigestive tract: initial results. J Comput Assist Tomogr 2003;27:687–93.
29. Rumboldt Z, Al-Okaili R, Deveikis JP. Perfusion CT for head and neck tumors: pilot study. AJNR Am J Neuroradiol 2005;26:1178–85.
30. Bisdas S, Rumboldt Z, Surlan-Popovic K, et al. Perfusion CT in squamous cell carcinoma of the upper aerodigestive tract: long-term predictive value of baseline perfusion CT measurements. AJNR Am J Neuroradiol 2010;31:576–81.
31. Surlan-Popovic K, Bisdas S, Rumboldt Z, et al. Changes in perfusion CT of advanced squamous cell carcinoma of the head and neck treated during the course of concomitant chemoradiotherapy. AJNR Am J Neuroradiol 2010;31:570–5.
32. Srinivasana A, Mohana S, Mukherji SK. Biologic imaging of head and neck cancer: the present and the future. AJNR Am J Neuroradiol 2012;33:586–94.
33. Eida S, Sumi M, Sakihama N, et al. Apparent diffusion coefficient mapping of salivary gland tumors: prediction of the benignancy and malignancy. AJNR Am J Neuroradiol 2007;28:116–21.
34. Srinivasan A, Dvorak R, Perni K, et al. Differentiation of benign and malignant pathology in the head and neck using 3T apparent diffusion coefficient values: early experience. AJNR Am J Neuroradiol 2008;29:40–4.
35. Wang J, Takashima S, Takayama F, et al. Head and neck lesions: characterization with diffusion-weighted echo-planar MR imaging. Radiology 2001;220:621–30.

36. Motoori K, Iida Y, Nagai Y, et al. MR imaging of salivary duct carcinoma. AJNR Am J Neuroradiol 2005;26:1201–6.
37. Ikeda M, Motoori K, Hanazawa T, et al. Warthin tumor of the parotid gland: diagnostic value of MR imaging with histopathologic correlation. AJNR Am J Neuroradiol 2004;25:1256–62.
38. Yabuuchi H, Fukuya T, Tajima T, et al. Salivary gland tumors: diagnostic value of gadolinium-enhanced dynamic MR imaging with histopathologic correlation. Radiology 2003;226(2):345–54.
39. Yabuuchi H, Matsuo Y, Kamitani T, et al. Parotid gland tumors: can addition of diffusion-weighted MR imaging to dynamic contrast-enhanced MR imaging improve diagnostic accuracy in characterization? Radiology 2008;249(3):909–16.
40. Dirix P, De Keyzer F, Vandecaveye V, et al. Diffusion-weighted magnetic resonance imaging to evaluate major salivary gland function before and after radiotherapy. Int J Radiat Oncol Biol Phys 2008;71:1365–71.
41. Holweg-Majert B, Metzger MC, Dueker J, et al. Salivary gland lipomas: ultrasonographic and magnetic resonance imaging. J Craniofac Surg 2007;18(6):1464–6.
42. Ankur G, Bhalla AS, Sharma R. First branchial cleft cyst (type II). Ear Nose Throat J 2009;88(11):1194–5.
43. Mukherji SK, Tart RP, Slattery WH, et al. Evaluation of first branchial cleft anomalies by CT and MR. J Comput Assist Tomogr 1993;17(4):576–81.
44. Benson MT, Dalen K, Mancuso AA, et al. Congenital anomalies of the branchial apparatus: embryology and pathologic anatomy. Radiographics 1992;12(5):943–60.
45. McQuone SJ. Acute viral and bacterial infections of the salivary glands. Otolaryngol Clin North Am 1999;32(5):793–811.
46. Mandel L, Surattanont F. Bilateral parotid swelling: a review. Oral Surg Oral Med Oral Pathol Oral Radiol Endod 2002;93(3):221–37.
47. Moss-Salentijn L, Moss M. Development and functional anatomy. In: Rankow R, Polayes I, editors. Diseases of the salivary glands. Philadelphia: WB Saunders; 1976. p. 17–31.
48. Rabinov K, Weber A. Radiology of the salivary glands. Boston: G Hall; 1985. p. 1–221.
49. Craven DE, Duncan RA, Stram JR, et al. Response of lymphoepithelial parotid cysts to antiretroviral treatments in HIV-infected adults. Ann Intern Med 1998;128(6):455–9.
50. Touloukian R. Salivary gland diseases in infancy and childhood. In: Rankow R, Polayes I, editors. Diseases of the salivary glands. Philadelphia: WB Saunders; 1976. p. 284–303.
51. Peel R, Gnepp D. Diseases of the salivary glands. In: Leon Barnes, editor. Surgical pathology of the head and neck. New York: Marcel Dekker; 1985. p. 533–645.
52. Som P, Shugar J, Sacher M, et al. Benign and malignant parotid pleomorphic adenomas: CT and MR studies. J Comput Assist Tomogr 1988;12:65–9.
53. Freling NJ, Molenaar WM, Vermey A, et al. Malignant parotid tumors: clinical use of MR imaging and histologic correlation. Radiology 1992;185(3):691–6.
54. Bradley PJ. Adenoid cystic carcinoma of the head and neck: a review. Curr Opin Otolaryngol Head Neck Surg 2004;12(2):127–32.
55. Aiken AH, Glastonbury C. Imaging Hodgkin and non-Hodgkin lymphoma in the head and neck. Radiol Clin North Am 2008;46(2):363–78.
56. Hisa Y, Tatemoto K. Bilateral parotid gland metastases as the initial manifestation of a small cell carcinoma of the lung. Am J Otolaryngol 1998;19:140–3.

57. del Charco J, Mendenhall W, Parsons J. Carcinoma of the skin metastatic to the parotid area lymph nodes. Head Neck 1998;20:369–73.
58. Nagao K, Matsuzaki O, Saiga H. Histopathologic studies of basal cell adenoma of the parotid gland. Cancer 1982;50:736–45.
59. Leverstein H, van der Wal JE, Tiwari RM, et al. Surgical management of 246 previously untreated pleomorphic adenomas of the parotid gland. Br J Surg 1997;84: 399–403.
60. Zernial O, Springer IN, Warnke P, et al. Long-term recurrence rate of pleomorphic adenoma and postoperative facial nerve paresis (in parotid surgery). J Craniomaxillofac Surg 2007;35(3):189–92.
61. Al-Zaher N, Obeid A, Al-Salam S, et al. Acinic cell carcinoma of the salivary glands: a literature review. Hematol Oncol Stem Cell Ther 2009;2(1):259–64.
62. Ma Q, Song H, Zhang P, et al. Diagnosis and management of intraparotid facial nerve schwannoma. J Craniomaxillofac Surg 2010;38(4):271–3.
63. Savera A, Sloman A, Huvos A, et al. Myoepithelial carcinoma of the salivary glands: a clinicopathologic study of 25 patients. Am J Surg Pathol 2000;24: 761–74.
64. Zhi K, Ren W, Zhou H, et al. Management of parapharyngeal-space tumors. J Oral Maxillofac Surg 2009;67(6):1239–44.
65. Mann W, Wachter W. Ultrasonic diagnosis of the salivary glands. Laryngol Rhinol Otol (Stuttg) 1988;67:197–201 [in German].
66. Abemayor E, Ljung B, Ward P, et al. CT-directed aspiration biopsies of masses in the head and neck. Laryngoscope 1985;95:1382–6.
67. Lufkin R, Teresi L, Hanafee W. New needle for MR-guided aspiration cytology of the head and neck. AJR Am J Roentgenol 1987;149:380–2.
68. Schmidt RL, Hall BJ, Wilson AR, et al. A systematic review and meta-analysis of the diagnostic accuracy of fine-needle aspiration cytology for parotid gland lesions. Am J Clin Pathol 2011;136:45–59.
69. Aversa S, Ondolo C, Bollito E, et al. Preoperative cytology in the management of parotid neoplasms. Am J Otolaryngol 2006;27:96–100.
70. Izquierdo R, Arekat MR, Knudson PE, et al. Comparison of palpation-guided versus ultrasound-guided fine-needle aspiration biopsies of thyroid nodules in an outpatient endocrinology practice. Endocr Pract 2006;12:609–14.
71. Taki S, Yamamoto T, Kawai A, et al. Sonographically guided core biopsy of the salivary gland masses: safety and efficacy. Clin Imaging 2005;29:189–94.
72. Eoma HJ, Leea JH, Kob MS, et al. Comparison of fine-needle aspiration and core needle biopsy under ultrasonographic guidance for detecting malignancy and for the tissue-specific diagnosis of salivary gland tumors. AJNR Am J Neuroradiol 2015;36:1188–93.
73. Gupta S, Henningsen JA, Wallace MJ, et al. Percutaneous biopsy of head and neck lesions with CT guidance: various approaches and relevant anatomic and technical considerations. Radiographics 2007;27(2):371–90.
74. Mukherji SK, Turetsky D, Tart RP, et al. A technique for core biopsies of head and neck masses. AJNR Am J Neuroradiol 1994;15:518–20.
75. Abrahams JJ. Mandibular sigmoid notch: a window for CT-guided biopsies of lesions in the peripharyngeal and skull base regions. Radiology 1998;208:695–9.
76. Yousem DM, Sack MJ, Scanlan KA. Biopsy of parapharyngeal space lesions. Radiology 1994;193:619–22.
77. Tu AS, Geyer CA, Mancall AC, et al. The buccal space: a doorway for percutaneous CT-guided biopsy of the parapharyngeal region. AJNR Am J Neuroradiol 1998;19:728–31.

Evaluation of Parotid Lesions

Edward C. Kuan, MD, MBA[a], Jon Mallen-St. Clair, MD, PhD[a],
Maie A. St. John, MD, PhD[a,b],*

KEYWORDS

- Parotid • Mass • Malignancy • Radiology • Biopsy

KEY POINTS

- When working up a parotid lesion, the otolaryngologist must consider inflammatory, neoplastic, autoimmune, traumatic, infectious, or congenital etiologies.
- A complete history should be elicited, including onset, laterality, changes, and associated symptoms (pain, facial weakness, drainage).
- A thorough physical examination is critical, and should include examination of bilateral parotid regions, oral cavity and oropharynx, facial nerve function, and neck.
- Laboratory studies are helpful in the work-up of nonneoplastic, noninfectious parotid lesions, whereas imaging, particularly MRI, remains the gold standard for evaluating neoplastic lesions.
- FNA biopsy, core biopsy, and intraoperative frozen analysis are all acceptable methods of obtaining an accurate tissue diagnosis. Image guidance may enhance biopsy accuracy.

INTRODUCTION

The parotid gland is the largest major salivary gland and is anatomically located anterior to the external auditory canal, overlying the level of the zygoma superiorly, and the ramus of the mandible laterally. Anteriorly, it extends over the masseter muscle, and overlies the sternocleidomastoid muscle posteriorly. A small area of extension posterior to the angle of the mandible is conventionally dubbed the tail of the parotid. The extratemporal facial nerve (ie, distal to the stylomastoid foramen) and its branches divide the parotid gland into its superficial and deep lobes. The differential diagnosis

Conflicts of Interest: None.
Financial Disclosures: None.
[a] Department of Head and Neck Surgery, University of California, Los Angeles (UCLA) Medical Center, Los Angeles, CA, USA; [b] UCLA Head and Neck Cancer Program, Jonsson Comprehensive Cancer Center, University of California, Los Angeles (UCLA) Medical Center, Los Angeles, CA, USA
* Corresponding author. UCLA Department of Head and Neck Surgery, 10833 Le Conte Avenue, 62-132 CHS, Los Angeles, CA 90095.
E-mail address: MstJohn@mednet.ucla.edu

for a parotid mass is extensive, and includes inflammatory, neoplastic, autoimmune, traumatic, infectious, or congenital lesions. Because of its unique location in the head and neck, it is critical for the clinician to properly diagnose a parotid mass as actually within the parenchyma of the gland (as opposed to a nearby facial or neck mass).

The parotid gland is comprised of multiple tissue morphologies, including secretory units (acinar cells, intercalated ducts, striated ducts, and excretory ducts), intraparenchymal lymphoid tissue, and myoepithelial cells. Dysfunction of any of these components may manifest clinically as a parotid mass. Accordingly, parotid masses from disparate histologic origins are managed differently. Several large series have demonstrated that roughly 70% of parotid masses are neoplastic,[1,2] 75% to 80% of these parotid tumors are benign, and it is thus important to exclude nonneoplastic conditions to avoid unnecessary operations. Specifically, it is important to exclude congenital, granulomatous, and inflammatory etiologies of parotid enlargement, which may be amenable to primary medical therapy.

A systematic approach to the diagnosis of a parotid mass is of utmost importance, because the differential diagnosis is broad (**Table 1**). The process begins with a complete history and physical examination. Imaging studies, laboratory tests, and pathologic analyses (ie, biopsies) play complementary roles in determining the nature of a parotid mass, and all factors taken together are essential for guiding management.

HISTORY

Any patient presenting with a parotid mass should undergo a comprehensive history and physical examination. It is crucial to delineate how long the mass has been present, and whether its onset was acute or gradual. It is also important to ascertain changes in size over time, and laterality of the lesion (unilateral or bilateral). Associated symptoms including pain, facial weakness, overlying skin changes (eg, erythema, edema, drainage), xerostomia, dry eyes, purulent or thick drainage from within the mouth, or fevers and chills should also be elucidated. If there is facial nerve weakness, it is important to understand the time course of the paresis, because malignancy must be considered high on the differential for patients with gradually deteriorating facial nerve function. In contrast, acute onset facial palsy is more suggestive of a nonneoplastic cause, such as Bell palsy. Exacerbating and alleviating factors for each associated symptom should be elicited. A recent history of trauma, when applicable, is important to note.

The history should also include a list of the patient's medical problems, past surgeries (especially of the face, neck, and ears), current medications (eg, anticholinergics), immunizations (ie, patients with suspected mumps), history of head and neck radiation therapy (ie, radioactive iodine), and social history (including sexual history and a history of eating disorders, such as bulimia nervosa). In patients presenting with suspected parotitis, the clinician should focus on the patient's nutritional status, fluid intake, and hydration habits. A thorough review of systems should be performed. Many parotid lesions are actually otolaryngologic manifestations of systemic diseases, where the first clinical presentation may be as a parotid mass (discussed later).

PHYSICAL EXAMINATION

In a large proportion of cases, a complete physical examination of the parotid mass, in conjunction with a solid history, is sufficient to make a diagnosis.[3] Examination of the mass involves delineating its physical characteristics and anatomic relationships. Is the lesion a discrete mass or diffuse swelling? Is the mass soft and compressible, or firm? Is the mass tender with manipulation and/or associated with overlying skin

Table 1
Differential diagnosis of parotid lesion

Diagnosis	Laterality	Pain	Pearls
Atypical mycobacterial infection	Bilateral	Possible	May only be diagnosed through acid-fast bacilli culture (negative skin test and gamma-interferon test) Cervical lymphadenopathy, possible draining fistula
Benign neoplasm	Unilateral	No (unless advanced)	FNA to establish diagnosis, ± imaging Warthin tumor may be multifocal and bilateral
Bulimia nervosa	Bilateral	Possible	Eating disorder Check serum electrolytes
Hematoma	Unilateral	Yes	History of trauma or recent parotid surgery, coagulopathy, antiplatelet therapy
HIV	Bilateral	Possible	ELISA (screening), Western blot (confirmation), HIV viral load (progression), CD4 count Lymphoepithelial cysts
IgG4-related disease	Bilateral	Possible	Elevated serum IgG4 and IgG4/IgG ratio >40% Chronic sclerosing sialadenitis of submandibular gland, cholangitis, autoimmune pancreatitis
Lymphoma	Unilateral	No	Core biopsy sufficient for diagnosis Parotidectomy not indicated
Metastatic lymphadenopathy	Unilateral	No	May have concurrent cervical lymphadenopathy May have known diagnosis of head and neck cancer
Mumps	Bilateral	Yes	Immunization status Antimumps IgM may establish diagnosis in acute infection Pancreatitis, orchitis/oophoritis
Primary parotid malignancy	Unilateral	Possible	FNA to establish diagnosis Imaging usually required for staging and determining resectability Special attention to facial nerve function Consider intraoperative frozen sections
Reactive lymphadenopathy	Bilateral	Yes	Recent history of respiratory illness
Sarcoidosis	Bilateral	Possible	Elevated ACE and calcium levels (serum and urine), chest radiography Noncaseating granulomas on biopsy Bilateral hilar adenopathy, uveitis, peripheral skin lesions (erythema nodosum, arthritis, tenosynovitis), facial weakness (Heerfordt syndrome)
Sialoadenitis	Unilateral	Yes	Dehydration, malnutrition, poor oral hygiene, history of external-beam radiation or radioactive iodine If suppurative, may express purulent discharge from Stensen duct
Sialolithiasis	Unilateral	Yes	Dehydration, malnutrition, poor oral hygiene May be visualized on CT scan

(continued on next page)

Table 1
(continued)

Diagnosis	Laterality	Pain	Pearls
Sjögren syndrome	Bilateral	Possible	Anti-Ro/SSA and anti-La/SSB antibiotics helpful but nondiagnostic Minor salivary gland biopsy for diagnosis Possible overlap with other autoimmune conditions (secondary Sjögren syndrome) Keratoconjunctivitis sicca, xerostomia, lymphoepithelial cysts
Tuberculosis	Bilateral	Possible	Tuberculin test, indirect antigen challenge/gamma-interferon test, respiratory culture Pulmonary involvement most likely site

Abbreviations: ACE, angiotensin-converting enzyme; CT, computed tomography; ELISA, enzyme-linked immunosorbent assay; FNA, fine-needle aspiration; HIV, human immunodeficiency virus.

changes? Is the mass mobile or fixed? In patients with a unilateral parotid lesion, the clinician should palpate the side with the lesion and compare it with the uninvolved side.

Next, the clinician should examine the oral cavity and oropharynx. The finding of trismus in the setting of a parotid mass is suggestive of malignancy, indicating possible pterygoid musculature invasion. Stensen duct drains into the buccal mucosa opposite to the second maxillary molar, and the duct orifice should be examined while the ipsilateral parotid gland is being massaged or bimanually palpated (**Fig. 1**). Saliva or even small stones may be expressed. In many cases of parotitis, this maneuver may actually be therapeutic as thick and purulent discharge is evacuated. Deep parotid lobe or parapharyngeal tumors may cause bulging of the ipsilateral tonsillar fossa, so asymmetries of the oropharynx should be noted.

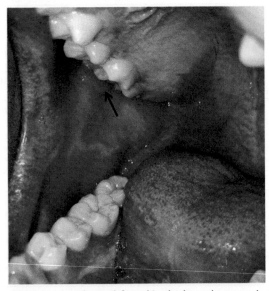

Fig. 1. The orifice of Stensen duct (*arrow*) found in the buccal mucosa just opposite the second maxillary molar.

Facial nerve function should be assessed. Progressive unilateral facial weakness in the setting of a parotid mass is suggestive of malignancy, and baseline facial nerve function should be documented before any intervention.

Finally, palpation of the cervical lymph nodes for lymphadenopathy may provide additional diagnostic information. For instance, tender lymphadenopathy may suggest an infectious or inflammatory, whereas nontender or fixed lymph nodes may indicate metastatic disease.

IMAGING STUDIES

Given the anatomic complexity of the parotid gland and its relationship to the facial nerve, imaging plays a helpful role in the work-up of a parotid mass, although it may be unnecessary in many cases.[3] Imaging is particularly important when malignancy is suspected, or in cases of suspected or confirmed recurrent disease after surgical treatment of a previous neoplasm. Additionally, imaging studies are required to determine involvement of the parapharyngeal space, or to determine if a mass is resectable (ie, significant carotid encasement, skull base invasion).

Although of historical importance, conventional sialography is rarely performed today for the evaluation of parotid lesions, because cross-sectional imaging and sialoendoscopy have replaced its role in evaluation of the intraglandular ductal system.[4] More recently, magnetic resonance sialography has emerged as a potentially useful tool for the evaluation of the intraglandular ductal system, although its utility in the evaluation of parotid parenchymal lesions has not been explored.[5,6]

MRI

MRI is generally considered to be the imaging modality of choice for parotid masses.[7] MRI provides superior soft tissue definition, allows for the identification of deep lobe tumors that otherwise may not be fully delineated on examination, and enables determination of perineural and marrow invasion.[8]

There are several distinguishing features of benign parotid neoplasms on MRI. Pleomorphic adenomas tend to be well-circumscribed, homogenous (unless large), intermediate or hypointense on T1, hyperintense on T2, and enhance with gadolinium (**Figs. 2** and **3**).[9] Warthin tumors may be cystic, multiple and bilateral, intermediate intensity on T1, hyperintense on T2 centrally, and do not enhance with contrast.[9] There is no characteristic appearance of malignant lesions, but infiltrative, poorly defined borders and perineural invasion may suggest this diagnosis.[9,10]

The retromandibular vein, or posterior facial vein, normally passes through the parotid gland and divides the parotid into the superficial and deep lobes radiographically. The retromandibular vein has been traditionally thought of as being anatomically related to the facial nerve; however, a recent anatomic study found that the facial nerve was just lateral to the vein in 65% of cases,[11] lower than previously accepted.[12] Other work, such as the study by Imaizumi and colleagues,[13] has demonstrated that the retromandibular vein correctly predicted the location of the parotid mass within the corresponding lobe (as confirmed intraoperatively) in 81% of cases. As such, the retromandibular vein is not a perfect anatomic landmark for facial nerve location, but may be helpful in preoperative planning.

Computed Tomography

Computed tomography (CT) scans also provide valuable information, and are especially useful in identifying bony erosion or invasion (**Fig. 4**). CT is also excellent for visualization of sialoliths. Other indications for obtaining a CT scan in these patients

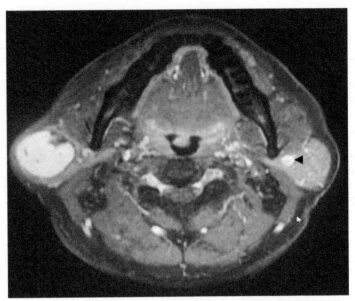

Fig. 2. Axial view of gadolinium-enhanced MRI of the face demonstrates a hyperintense, well-circumscribed, mostly homogenous mass of the right superficial parotid. Pathologic analysis was consistent with pleomorphic adenoma. The arrowhead in the left parotid gland points to the retromandibular vein, which serves as the division between the superficial and deep lobes.

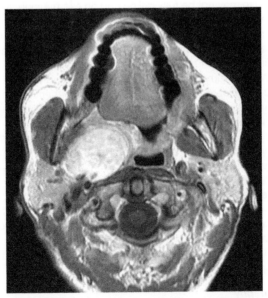

Fig. 3. MRI of the face demonstrating a right parapharyngeal mass in patient who presented with painless, gradually increasing parotid and neck fullness. Pathologic analysis was consistent with pleomorphic adenoma. Complete surgical resection was achieved via a transcervical approach.

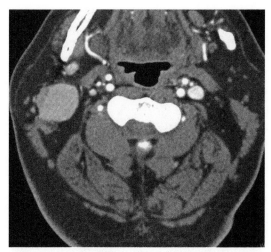

Fig. 4. Axial view of contrast-enhanced CT of the face demonstrating a right deep lobe of parotid mass. A parotidectomy was performed, with pathology consistent with oncocytoma.

include diffuse enlargement of the parotid gland, deep extension of tumors, facial nerve weakness, trismus, fixation to adjacent structures, and when MRI cannot be performed (eg, patients with certain metallic implants and pacemakers).[14] Despite the time and cost-effectiveness of CT scan compared with MRI, MRI ultimately provides superior visualization of the parotid region and is not associated with radiation exposure.

Ultrasonography

Ultrasound provides limited assessment of the deep lobe of the parotid and parapharyngeal space, but provides a low-cost alternative for lateral lobe lesions and can improve the accuracy of biopsies (discussed later).[15,16] There is currently some interest in using ultrasound in the diagnosis of Sjögren syndrome, although the results are still being validated at this time.[17-19]

PET

PET scans are rarely used for the initial assessment of parotid lesions given the lack of sensitivity and specificity, because inflammatory and infectious processes and benign and malignant neoplasms may all demonstrate fluorodeoxyglucose (FDG) uptake.[20] However, there is use in obtaining PET scans in the setting of known malignancies with possible metastases. The resolution is improved when a CT scan is performed concurrently, because areas of FDG uptake may be radiographically matched to an overlapping anatomic area.

In performing whole-body PET/CT scans (ie, for cancer staging), there is the rare (2.1% in a recent study) possibility of uncovering an incidental parotid lesion with increased FDG uptake (**Fig. 5**).[21] The bilateral parotid glands, at baseline, demonstrate symmetric, physiologic FDG uptake.[22] As such, unilateral avid FDG uptake especially corresponding to a mass lesion should be worked up with further imaging studies. In a study by Seo and colleagues[21] examining 1342 patients with known head and neck malignancies undergoing PET/CT for staging, one-third of incidental parotid masses found on PET/CT represented metastatic disease to the parotid, whereas another

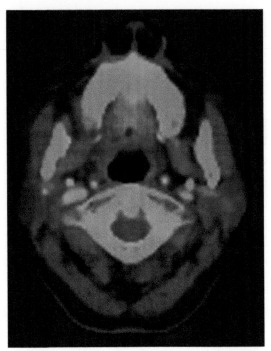

Fig. 5. Axial view of whole-body PET/CT scan at the level of the bilateral parotids. The patient originally had the scan performed for a mandibular neoplasm, but an incidental left parotid mass with mildly increased FDG uptake was noted. A parotidectomy was performed at the time of his mandibular surgery, which was consistent with pleomorphic adenoma.

one-third of masses were histologically confirmed to be benign primary parotid neoplasms.

LABORATORY STUDIES

Generally, laboratory testing is not required for the diagnosis of neoplastic disease. Serum electrolytes, particularly renal function tests, may be useful in cases of parotitis secondary to dehydration. If a patient presents with purulent discharge at Stensen duct, a culture of the discharge may be taken and sent for microbial analysis, which may guide targeted antibiotic therapy. Patients in whom viral parotitis, or mumps, is suspected should undergo serologic testing against paromyxovirus. Patients with clinical features of mumps who test positive for serum antimumps IgM antibodies, or who have a four-fold increase in serum antimumps IgG antibodies, are considered to have a positive diagnostic test.[23]

Laboratory investigations should be performed to exclude nonneoplastic, noninfectious causes of parotid swelling. In general, nonneoplastic, noninfectious causes of parotid enlargement are often bilateral in nature, and tend to be associated with pain on presentation. These include granulomatous diseases, such as sarcoidosis and tuberculosis; autoimmune diseases, such as Sjögren syndrome and IgG4-related disease; or infectious causes, such as bacterial parotitis or human immunodeficiency virus (HIV) infection.

Sarcoidosis is associated with elevated levels of angiotensin-converting enzyme, hypercalcemia (10%), and hypercalciuria (30%), because the characteristic noncaseating granulomas secrete 1,25-dihydroxyvitamin D.[24] Tuberculosis may be diagnosed through tuberculin skin testing, indirect testing for gamma-interferon release to *Mycobacterium tuberculosis* challenge, or acid-fast bacilli respiratory culture; atypical mycobacterial infections can only be diagnosed through culture.

Laboratory tests can also be useful in distinguishing between different causes of parotid enlargement that present similarly clinically. In particular, Sjögren syndrome and HIV are associated with the formation of lymphoepithelial cysts, which typically present with bilateral nodular parotid involvement. The work-up in this case is to determine the HIV status to initiate proper referral and/or timely antiretroviral therapy, if indicated.

When autoimmune causes of parotid enlargement are suspected, it is important to determine the presence of markers of autoimmune disease, including rheumatoid factor, antinuclear antibodies, sedimentation rate, and complete blood count. Anti-Ro/SSA and anti-La/SSB antibodies are present in 60% to 80% of cases of Sjögren syndrome, although serum positivity is not diagnostic, because these antibodies may be present in other autoimmune conditions.[25] IgG4-related diseases of the head and neck may be diagnosed through elevated serum levels of IgG4-positive plasma cells and an IgG4/total IgG ratio of greater than 40%.[26]

Patients who have parotid swelling caused by repeated episodes of emesis, as in the case of bulimia nervosa, should have serum electrolytes checked, with special attention to the presence of hypokalemia.[27]

PATHOLOGY
Fine-Needle Aspiration Biopsy

Fine needle aspiration (FNA) biopsy plays an important role in the work-up of parotid masses, especially when a neoplastic process is suspected. FNA may be used to distinguish between neoplastic and nonneoplastic processes.[28] Before any surgical planning, a FNA biopsy is instrumental in obtaining a tissue diagnosis. Part of the challenge of obtaining an accurate diagnosis is that a parotid mass is heterogeneous in content, and that tumor may not always be sampled within a given pass of the needle. Ultrasound-guided biopsies can improve the likelihood of an accurate biopsy, and may be useful for deeper tumors.[9,29] A systematic review and meta-analysis on the diagnostic accuracy of FNA for benign parotid neoplasms reported high sensitivity (96%) and specificity (98%), and high positive (100%) and negative (81%) predictive value.[30] For malignancies, the sensitivity and specificity were lower, at 79% and 96%, respectively.[30] For tissue diagnosis for treatment planning, we recommend starting with FNA for all superficial, readily palpable lesions, and reserving ultrasound-guided FNA for deeper lesions revealed on imaging.

Core Needle Biopsy

Another technique for obtaining a tissue diagnosis for parotid lesions is through a core biopsy. Core biopsies have the advantage of obtaining a larger sample of tissue with preserved architecture, although at the risk of transecting a larger area of normal tissue given the increased needle size. Despite being performed with a larger needle, the rate of complications, namely hematoma, remains acceptably low (1.4% in one study).[31] When performed under ultrasonic guidance, core biopsies have been shown in meta-analyses to have high sensitivity and specificity (92%–96% and 96%–100%, respectively) in the work-up of malignancies.[31–33] However, because FNA has been shown to have comparable diagnostic accuracy, we recommend reserving core biopsies for masses that are nondiagnostic on FNA, and when there is a clinical suspicion of a hematologic malignancy requiring fresh tissue analysis (ie, lymphoma).

Tumor Seeding?

With any form of needle biopsy of a neoplastic mass, there is the theoretic concern of tumor seeding. Several large-scale studies have examined this possibility, but overall the rate of tumor seeding has been nonexistent to extremely low, especially with the specific needle sizes used for each technique (18-gauge for core, 21-gauge for FNA).[31,32] The only reports within the literature that demonstrate tumor seeding include one case of parotid carcinoma sampling using a 14- to 16-gauge needle[34] and two cases of seeding after FNA.[35,36]

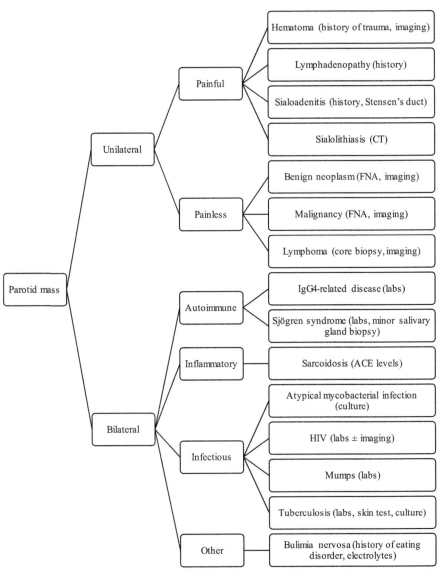

Fig. 6. Suggested approach to the parotid mass, including differential diagnosis and work-up strategies.

Incisional Biopsy and Frozen Section Analysis

More invasive, open biopsies are generally contraindicated given the potential morbidity of the procedure (ie, risk to facial nerve) and increased theoretic risk of tumor seeding,[9] although it has been reported as a means of providing a definitive diagnosis in the rare cases when FNA and core biopsies are nondiagnostic.[37] The exception is intraoperative frozen section analysis. A meta-analysis by Schmidt and colleagues[38] demonstrated that frozen section analysis had a sensitivity of 90% and a specificity of 99%. The choice of performing frozen section analysis with or without a preoperative tissue diagnosis is based on surgeon preference.[39–41] The main advantage of this technique is the ability to perform all necessary procedures under one surgical encounter (eg, deep lobe dissection, neck dissection, facial nerve sacrifice and reanimation). In a series of 1339 patients who underwent parotidectomy for a known parotid mass, Olsen and colleagues[42] found only one case of overtreatment and three cases of undertreatment based on discrepancies between frozen sections and permanent analysis, with overall sensitivity and specificity for diagnosing malignancy at 98.5% and 99%, respectively.

SUMMARY

The differential diagnosis of the parotid mass is broad, but a systematic, thoughtful approach to ordering imaging, laboratory studies, and pathologic analysis coupled to a comprehensive history and physical, allows the otolaryngologist to ascertain the proper diagnosis (**Fig. 6**).

REFERENCES

1. Eveson JW, Cawson RA. Salivary gland tumours. A review of 2410 cases with particular reference to histological types, site, age and sex distribution. J Pathol 1985;146(1):51–8.
2. Spiro RH. Salivary neoplasms: overview of a 35-year experience with 2,807 patients. Head Neck Surg 1986;8(3):177–84.
3. Carlson ER, Webb DE. The diagnosis and management of parotid disease. Oral Maxillofac Surg Clin North Am 2013;25(1):31–48, v.
4. Som PM, Curtin HD. Head and neck imaging. 5th edition. St Louis (MO): Mosby; 2010.
5. Ohbayashi N, Yamada I, Yoshino N, et al. Sjogren syndrome: comparison of assessments with MR sialography and conventional sialography. Radiology 1998; 209(3):683–8.
6. Wada A, Uchida N, Yokokawa M, et al. Radiation-induced xerostomia: objective evaluation of salivary gland injury using MR sialography. AJNR Am J Neuroradiol 2009;30(1):53–8.
7. Adelstein DJ, Rodriguez CP. What is new in the management of salivary gland cancers? Curr Opin Oncol 2011;23(3):249–53.
8. Lee YY, Wong KT, King AD, et al. Imaging of salivary gland tumours. Eur J Radiol 2008;66(3):419–36.
9. Howlett DC, Kesse KW, Hughes DV, et al. The role of imaging in the evaluation of parotid disease. Clin Radiol 2002;57(8):692–701.
10. Vogl TJ, Dresel SH, Spath M, et al. Parotid gland: plain and gadolinium-enhanced MR imaging. Radiology 1990;177(3):667–74.
11. Toure G, Vacher C. Relations of the facial nerve with the retromandibular vein: anatomic study of 132 parotid glands. Surg Radiol Anat 2010;32(10):957–61.

12. Laing MR, McKerrow WS. Intraparotid anatomy of the facial nerve and retromandibular vein. Br J Surg 1988;75(4):310–2.
13. Imaizumi A, Kuribayashi A, Okochi K, et al. Differentiation between superficial and deep lobe parotid tumors by magnetic resonance imaging: usefulness of the parotid duct criterion. Acta Radiol 2009;50(7):806–11.
14. Bussu F, Parrilla C, Rizzo D, et al. Clinical approach and treatment of benign and malignant parotid masses, personal experience. Acta Otorhinolaryngol Ital 2011; 31(3):135–43.
15. Brennan PA, Herd MK, Howlett DC, et al. Is ultrasound alone sufficient for imaging superficial lobe benign parotid tumours before surgery? Br J Oral Maxillofac Surg 2012;50(4):333–7.
16. Mann W, Wachter W. Ultrasonic diagnosis of the salivary glands. Laryngol Rhinol Otol (Stuttg) 1988;67(5):197–201 [in German].
17. Hammenfors DS, Brun JG, Jonsson R, et al. Diagnostic utility of major salivary gland ultrasonography in primary Sjogren's syndrome. Clin Exp Rheumatol 2015;33(1):56–62.
18. Das S, Huynh D, Yang H, et al. Salivary gland ultrasonography as a diagnostic tool for secondary Sjogren syndrome in rheumatoid arthritis. J Rheumatol 2015; 42(7):1119–22.
19. Delli K, Dijkstra PU, Stel AJ, et al. Diagnostic properties of ultrasound of major salivary glands in Sjogren's syndrome: a meta-analysis. Oral Dis 2015;21(6): 792–800.
20. Lee SK, Rho BH, Won KS. Parotid incidentaloma identified by combined 18F-fluorodeoxyglucose whole-body positron emission tomography and computed tomography: findings at grayscale and power Doppler ultrasonography and ultrasound-guided fine-needle aspiration biopsy or core-needle biopsy. Eur Radiol 2009;19(9):2268–74.
21. Seo YL, Yoon DY, Baek S, et al. Incidental focal FDG uptake in the parotid glands on PET/CT in patients with head and neck malignancy. Eur Radiol 2015;25(1): 171–7.
22. Basu S, Houseni M, Alavi A. Significance of incidental fluorodeoxyglucose uptake in the parotid glands and its impact on patient management. Nucl Med Commun 2008;29(4):367–73.
23. Fiebelkorn AP, Barskey A, Hickman C, et al. Mumps (October 2012). Chapter 9. In: Roush SW, Baldy LM, editors. Manual for the surveillance of vaccine-preventable diseases. Atlanta (GA): Centers for Disease Control and Prevention; 2012. p. 1–18.
24. Sharma OP. Vitamin D, calcium, and sarcoidosis. Chest 1996;109(2):535–9.
25. Harley JB, Sestak AL, Willis LG, et al. A model for disease heterogeneity in systemic lupus erythematosus. Relationships between histocompatibility antigens, autoantibodies, and lymphopenia or renal disease. Arthritis Rheum 1989;32(7): 826–36.
26. Deshpande V. IgG4 related disease of the head and neck. Head Neck Pathol 2015;9(1):24–31.
27. Mehler PS. Clinical practice. Bulimia nervosa. N Engl J Med 2003;349(9):875–81.
28. Sharma G, Jung AS, Maceri DR, et al. US-guided fine-needle aspiration of major salivary gland masses and adjacent lymph nodes: accuracy and impact on clinical decision making. Radiology 2011;259(2):471–8.
29. Bajaj Y, Singh S, Cozens N, et al. Critical clinical appraisal of the role of ultrasound guided fine needle aspiration cytology in the management of parotid tumours. J Laryngol Otol 2005;119(4):289–92.

30. Schmidt RL, Hall BJ, Wilson AR, et al. A systematic review and meta-analysis of the diagnostic accuracy of fine-needle aspiration cytology for parotid gland lesions. Am J Clin Pathol 2011;136(1):45–59.
31. Witt BL, Schmidt RL. Ultrasound-guided core needle biopsy of salivary gland lesions: a systematic review and meta-analysis. Laryngoscope 2014;124(3): 695–700.
32. Novoa E, Gurtler N, Arnoux A, et al. Role of ultrasound-guided core-needle biopsy in the assessment of head and neck lesions: a meta-analysis and systematic review of the literature. Head Neck 2012;34(10):1497–503.
33. Schmidt RL, Hall BJ, Layfield LJ. A systematic review and meta-analysis of the diagnostic accuracy of ultrasound-guided core needle biopsy for salivary gland lesions. Am J Clin Pathol 2011;136(4):516–26.
34. Yamaguchi KT, Strong MS, Shapshay SM, et al. Seeding of parotid carcinoma along Vim-Silverman needle tract. J Otolaryngol 1979;8(1):49–52.
35. Shinohara S, Yamamoto E, Tanabe M, et al. Implantation metastasis of head and neck cancer after fine needle aspiration biopsy. Auris Nasus Larynx 2001;28(4): 377–80.
36. Supriya M, Denholm S, Palmer T. Seeding of tumor cells after fine needle aspiration cytology in benign parotid tumor: a case report and literature review. Laryngoscope 2008;118(2):263–5.
37. Gross M, Ben-Yaacov A, Rund D, et al. Role of open incisional biopsy in parotid tumors. Acta Otolaryngol 2004;124(6):758–60.
38. Schmidt RL, Hunt JP, Hall BJ, et al. A systematic review and meta-analysis of the diagnostic accuracy of frozen section for parotid gland lesions. Am J Clin Pathol 2011;136(5):729–38.
39. Zbaren P, Nuyens M, Loosli H, et al. Diagnostic accuracy of fine-needle aspiration cytology and frozen section in primary parotid carcinoma. Cancer 2004;100(9): 1876–83.
40. Fakhry N, Santini L, Lagier A, et al. Fine needle aspiration cytology and frozen section in the diagnosis of malignant parotid tumours. Int J Oral Maxillofac Surg 2014;43(7):802–5.
41. Zbaren P, Guelat D, Loosli H, et al. Parotid tumors: fine-needle aspiration and/or frozen section. Otolaryngol Head Neck Surg 2008;139(6):811–5.
42. Olsen KD, Moore EJ, Lewis JE. Frozen section pathology for decision making in parotid surgery. JAMA Otolaryngol Head Neck Surg 2013;139(12):1275–8.

Benign Parotid Tumors

Kevin Y. Zhan, MD[a], Sobia F. Khaja, MD[a], Allen B. Flack, MD[b],
Terry A. Day, MD[c],*

KEYWORDS

- Benign parotid tumors • Parotid neoplasms • Pleomorphic adenoma
- Parotidectomy • Warthin tumor

KEY POINTS

- Most parotid tumors are benign, with pleomorphic adenoma and Warthin tumors accounting for up to 94% of all tumors.
- Evaluation of a parotid mass should be done to rule out malignancy and should include a fine-needle aspiration biopsy and imaging studies as indicated.
- Accurate preoperative diagnosis is critical for surgical planning and appropriate management in adequate tumor removal and preventing complications.
- Despite the myriad of histologies, surgical excision via parotidectomy is the most common treatment.
- Local recurrences are often related to subtotal tumor excision.

EPIDEMIOLOGY

Primary parotid tumors are rare and account for approximately 1% to 3% of all head and neck tumors.[1] Fortunately, most (75%–85%) are benign.[1–3] The annual age-adjusted incidence of benign parotid tumors in the United States is approximately 3.8 per 100,000 per year,[2] with roughly 1300 to 1600 diagnosed cases each year.[4] Worldwide, incidence varies by geography, with reports of 5.3 to 6.2 per 100,000 in the United Kingdom[2] and 1.35 per 100,000 in Poland. Japan and Malay report an incidence of 1.3 and 1.1 for all benign salivary neoplasms.[5] Unlike their malignant counterparts, no national registries exist for benign diseases, making true incidence difficult to ascertain.

No disclosures.
[a] Department of Otolaryngology – Head and Neck Surgery, Medical University of South Carolina, 135 Rutledge Avenue, MSC 550, Charleston, SC 29425, USA; [b] Department of Pathology, Medical University of South Carolina, 171 Ashley Avenue, MSC 908, Charleston, SC 29425, USA; [c] Division of Head & Neck Oncologic Surgery, Department of Otolaryngology – Head and Neck Surgery, Medical University of South Carolina, 135 Rutledge Avenue, MSC 550, Charleston, SC 29425, USA
* Corresponding author.
E-mail address: headneck@musc.edu

Otolaryngol Clin N Am 49 (2016) 327–342
http://dx.doi.org/10.1016/j.otc.2015.10.005
0030-6665/16/$ – see front matter © 2016 Elsevier Inc. All rights reserved.

oto.theclinics.com

Salivary tumor classification schemes include benign versus malignant, major (parotid, submandibular, sublingual) and minor salivary glands, and by individual histopathology.[4] The 2005 World Health Organization's classification contains 24 malignant salivary histopathologies and 11 benign, excluding hematolymphoid and secondary tumors.[4] Of parotid tumors, the most common benign and malignant tumors are pleomorphic adenoma (PA) and mucoepidermoid carcinoma, respectively.[1] This article is limited to benign parotid neoplasms and does not address malignancies or tumors that primarily occur in the submandibular, sublingual, or minor salivary glands. Many clinicians use the 80/20 rule for salivary gland neoplasms: 80% benign, 80% occur in the parotid, and 80% are PA. However, variations in certain proportions and relative incidences exist. A Ugandan study reported only 29% of benign tumors occur in the parotid gland, with 53.8% of parotid tumors being malignant. Zero cases of Warthin tumors (WTs) were found, a paucity also described in other African studies. Underreporting may be an issue in resource-poor areas, as adequate therapy may not be sought for non–life-threatening diseases.[6] These issues highlight the variations in incidence reporting for benign parotid tumors.

By age, incidence of benign parotid tumors steadily increases starting at 15 to 25 years of age, with a peak in 65 to 74 years of age.[7] There is a female sex preference overall (1.46:1.0) for benign parotid tumors and a racial difference favoring Caucasian patients over African American.[2,7] Males (ratio 2.31:1) are more affected in WTs (presumably because of historically higher rates of smoking) and parotid malignancies (ratio 3.47:1) overall. PA and WTs combine to make up 83% to 93% of benign parotid tumors.[2] More detailed epidemiologic variables will be forthcoming for individual histopathologies (**Table 1**).

EMBRYOLOGY AND HISTOGENESIS

Understanding parotid embryology is important as several theories propose an etiopathogenesis based on salivary cell types and tumor cell origin. All salivary glands derive from ingrowths of oral epithelium, with parotid anlage starting to appear at 4 to 6 weeks of development.[8] Lymphoid tissue develops before the encapsulation of the parotid

Table 1 Benign salivary tumors and masses	
Epithelial Tumors	**Soft Tissue Masses**
PA	Hemangioma
Myoepithelioma	Vascular malformations
Basal cell adenoma	Benign lymphoepithelial cysts
WT	Lipoma
Oncocytoma	Lymph node
Canalicular adenoma	Cystic hygroma
Sebaceous adenoma/lymphadenoma	Congenital anomalies
Inverted ductal papilloma	—
Intraductal papilloma	—
Sialadenoma papilliferum	—
Cystadenoma	—

Data from Thompson L. World Health Organization classification of tumours: pathology and genetics of head and neck tumours. Ear Nose Throat J 2006;85(2):74.

gland begins but after the encapsulation of both submandibular and sublingual glands, thus explaining the lack of lymphoid tissue in the latter. Because of concomitant parotid encapsulation and lymphatic development, salivary cells sometimes appear within the intraparotid and periparotid lymph nodes.[9]

The most basic secretory unit, the acinus, is formed from acinar cells and is surrounded by contractile myoepithelial cells. Acini drain into intercalated ducts, followed by striated intralobular ducts, and finally intralobular and main excretory ducts (**Figs. 1–3**). Acinar cells are exclusively of the serous type in the parotid gland. Noncontractile basal cells line the most distant ducts. Intraparotid and periparotid lymph nodes that may give rise to lymphoma are a part of the lymphatic drainage pathway of cancers from the scalp and face or other distant sites.

Controversies exist regarding salivary gland histogenesis. For decades, a bicellular theory of histogenesis was dominant, suggesting that the varied salivary cell types were products of differentiation from 2 stem cell progenitors: excretory duct reserve cells and intercalated reserve cells.[10] Therefore, mucoepidermoid, ductal, and adenocarcinomas arose from proximal excretory cells, whereas the remainder arose from more terminal, intercalated cells. However, animal and human models have demonstrated that even differentiated cells, such as acinar cells, can cycle between one another and any cell could be a potential target of neoplastic processes.[11]

The multicellular theory of histogenesis assumes numerous cell types can contribute to tumorigenesis, even highly differentiated acinar cells. Such a varied input of histogenesis may account for the wide spectrum of pathologies that exist. More recent work has been in classification of tumors by morphologic features regardless of cell origins: tumor organization, types of cell differentiation, materials produced by tumor cells, and so forth.[12] All of these issues place credence to the complex and relatively unknown pathogenesis of parotid tumors.

CAUSE AND RISK FACTORS

Despite the poorly understood histogenesis of parotid tumors, several environmental variables have been associated with parotid gland tumors. However, conclusive evidence demonstrating causal relationships is lacking.[13] A Japanese study of atomic bomb survivors found a 3.5% and 11.0% relative risk increase for radiation and

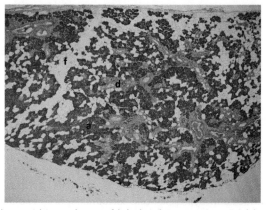

Fig. 1. The normal parotid is made up of lobules that contain acini (a), ducts (d), and adipose tissue (f) (hematoxylin-eosin, original magnification ×20).

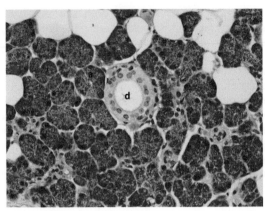

Fig. 2. Serous-type acinar cells (a) and ducts (d) make up the functional unit of the parotid (hematoxylin-eosin, original magnification ×200).

salivary gland tumors, with WT being most associated with radiation risk.[14] Another study found a 2.6-fold increased incidence of parotid tumors with head and neck scalp irradiation after a 2-decade latency period.[15] Studies looking at cell phone radiation and tumor risk have found mixed results, though a 2008 Israeli study found a 1.58 increased odds ratio for tumors only in a specific subgroup of the very highest cell phone users.[16]

Cigarette smoking is strongly associated with WTs[17]; certain occupational exposures, such as heavy metals,[18] and hormonal factors[19] (eg, early menarche) have also been associated with an increased risk of salivary tumors.

Advancements in genetic sequencing technologies have allowed for easier identification and discovery of distinct genetic translocations, of which we now know of 6. These translocations include PLAG1 and HMGA2 rearrangements in PA, CRCT1-MAML2 found in mucoepidermoid carcinoma and WT, and 4 others. Some may serve as prognostic markers, but more investigation is needed.[20] Recent work on single nucleotide polymorphism analysis on a genome-wide level shows promise in finding new genetic markers.[13] However, the genetic basis to parotid tumorigenesis is still largely unknown.

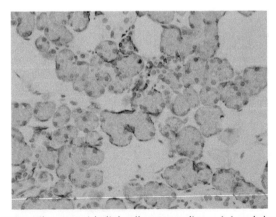

Fig. 3. The flat, contractile myoepithelial cells surrounding acini and ducts are difficult to appreciate with standard hematoxylin and eosin stains, better appreciated with calponin staining (*brown*) (calponin, original magnification ×200).

CLINICAL ANATOMY FOR BENIGN NEOPLASMS

For more detailed discussion of parotid gland and facial nerve anatomy, see Chapter 1 of this text.

The paired parotid glands are the largest salivary glands and weigh, on average, 15 to 30 g. The parotid gland is bounded superiorly by the zygomatic arch and inferiorly by the anteromedial margin of the sternocleidomastoid muscle. The posterior extent can reach the external auditory meatus and mastoid tip. The superficial portion may cover a small portion of the masseter muscle anteriorly. The deep portion of the gland wraps around the mandibular ramus and rests on the surface of the posterior digastric muscle, styloid process, and stylohyoid muscle.[8] Any mass in these areas should be considered neoplastic until proven otherwise.

The facial nerve divides the parotid gland into 2 lobes, superficial (lateral) and deep (medial).[21] This distinction is critical for surgical planning as PAs represent most deep lobe and parapharyngeal space tumors. Surgery of deep lobe tumors has a markedly increased rate of facial nerve injury and operative time.[22] This increased rate is due to the frequent need to expose, mobilize, and retract the facial nerve in order to access these tumors.

Ichihara and colleagues[21] recently reviewed 425 cases of benign parotid tumors and proposed instead a 3-category clinical classification scheme: superficial tumors, deep tumors, and lower pole tumors, defined as the region inferior to marginal mandibular nerve. They found distinct characteristics for lower pole tumors. Compared with superficial tumors, lower pole tumors had older patients on average (57.4 vs 52.2 years), more males (ratio 1.6:1), and more WT compared with PA (ratio 2.5:1). More importantly, the investigators concluded that nerve dissection for deep, lower pole tumors could safely be limited to the marginal mandibular nerve in place of a true deep dissection, highlighting the importance of preoperative localization. This method allowed for a faster, safer, and easier dissection relative to a regular deep parotid dissection.

The accessory parotid gland is a tiny 0.5- to 1.0-cm gland found in 21% to 56% of people based on cadaveric studies. It is usually located 6 mm anterior to the main gland, adjacent to Stenson's duct as it passes over the masseter muscle. Accessory gland lesions make up 1% to 8% of parotid lesions and up to half are malignant.[23] With accessory gland tumors, patients may present with a midcheek mass.

CLINICAL PRESENTATION

Benign parotid tumors classically present with a painless, slow-growing, preauricular or upper-neck swelling. The differential diagnosis of parotid swelling is broad, ranging from mumps, to sialadenitis, to neoplasms. The initial diagnosis will relate to presenting symptoms. Acute-onset fever, redness, parotid swelling, and elevated white blood cell count (WBC) usually signifies an infectious process (ie, sialadenitis) or obstructive process (ie, salivary stones). Although rare, benign and malignant tumors may present acutely via tumor obstruction of a drainage duct, which may get infected and expand rapidly.

Benign tumors may be asymptomatic for months to even decades. However, parotid cancers also lack symptoms 50% to 70% of the time.[24] With the increasing utilization of imaging (eg, computed tomography [CT], ultrasound, MRI, PET) for unrelated indications, there has been an increasing incidence of parotid incidentalomas, tumors that would not have been found otherwise. This increasing incidence results in needle biopsy and/or surgery due to the risk of malignancy or growth of the tumor. A recent review of parotidectomies at the University of Wisconsin found an increase in the number of incidentalomas, up to 10.2% in the 2004 to 2013 period, from 4% in 1994 to 2003. The investigators also noted a significant decrease in the rate of malignancy found within incidentalomas versus clinically apparent masses.[25]

Rapid growth or pain in a parotid mass may herald a malignant transformation (eg, in a known PA). Red flags, such as pain, facial paresis, soft tissue fixation, trismus, skin ulceration, lymphadenopathy, numbness, and weight loss, should heighten suspicion for malignancy.[26] Facial paresis from Bell palsy has a fast onset and eventual resolution. A slow and worsening progression of facial nerve involvement with facial tics or spasms should raise concern for malignancy, although benign cases with facial paresis have been reported.[27] Bilateral parotid involvement is more likely an inflammatory process (eg, mumps, Sjögren disease) than a synchronous neoplastic process. Because of the intraparotid and periparotid lymph nodes, a parotid mass may be metastatic from malignancies of the face, scalp, or even a distant site.

Grossly, benign superficial tumors are typically solid, mobile, and well circumscribed within the parotid gland. These tumors should be easily palpable. Deep tumors within the parapharyngeal space that medialize the oropharynx may be obvious with a deviated tonsil or soft palate.

DIAGNOSTIC WORK-UP

This section focuses on the noninfected parotid mass or swelling.

Clinical evaluation should begin with obtaining a full history and physical examination. The location, size, extent, and features of the mass should be characterized. Visual intraoral examination should be performed in every suspected parotid mass. Fiberoptic examination and assessment for mucosal lesions is necessary if malignancy is suspected or deep lobe extension is evident. Additional imaging studies, such as CT, MRI and/or ultrasound, are often warranted.[26] Ruling out malignancy—ideally in the preoperative setting—in each case of parotid mass is paramount.

Historically, surgery was considered for every parotid tumor. Advances in fine-needle aspiration biopsy (FNAB), radiographic imaging, and the well-described nature of tumors have trended evaluation toward preoperative imaging and needle biopsy. Diagnoses of cysts, stones, and lymphoma may preclude surgery; thus, accurate diagnosis and appropriate planning are essential. Usually, any parotid mass can be considered for CT or MRI. CT provides excellent resolution for evaluating tumor location, size, extent, and lymph nodes if malignancy is suspected. CT and MRI provide excellent anatomic information because of the gland's high fat content. However, they are poor on their own for determining individual histologies and benign versus malignant features.[28] Vascular lesions may necessitate imaging before biopsy or surgery. Ultrasound is another cheap and effective tool that is useful for delineating cystic versus solid masses and characterizing anatomy of superficial lobe tumors. Its primary shortcomings include poor visualization of the deep lobe (obscured by mandibular ramus) and poor visualization of the facial nerve. For tumors with benign clinical and cytologic features, no obvious deep lobe involvement, and benign features on ultrasound, additional imaging with MRI or CT may not be necessary.[29] Otherwise, diagnosis is typically confirmed with surgery and histologic analysis.

FNAB is an accurate and inexpensive method with low complication rates for differentiating benign versus malignant lesions. It has a sensitivity and specificity of 80% and 97% and a positive predictive value (PPV) and negative predictive value (NPV) of 90% and 94%, respectively.[30] For benign disease, Tryggvason and colleagues[28] found a PPV and NPV for FNAB of 94.3% and 98.6%. Carcinoma ex-pleomorphic adenoma caused the most false negatives (n = 6). FNA's pitfall is its nondiagnostic rate, estimated at 8%.[30] However, given its ease and accuracy in benign disease, FNAB should be considered for every parotid mass before resection. Contraindications to FNAB include bleeding disorders and acute sialadenitis.

Image-guided FNAB may be necessary for deep, clinically nonpalpable tumors or those close to vital structures. Ultrasound or CT-guided core-needle biopsy (CNB) is a proposed alternative for tumors with a prior FNA that was nondiagnostic or could not be reached with other techniques. Compared to FNAB, it involves a larger needle and can be more painful. Because it extracts more tissue, it may be diagnostic for lesions such as lymphoma. Previously, clinicians avoided it out of fears for safety and tumor seeding. Recent studies suggest otherwise, citing it as a safe and more accurate preoperative alternative to the FNAB, especially for malignant tumors.[31] A recent meta-analysis reported a sensitivity of 96% and specificity of 100% when comparing benign versus malignant lesions, with a nondiagnostic rate of 1.6% (versus 8.0% for FNAB). There were no reports of tumor seeding; the most significant adverse event was hematoma formation, at 1.6% per procedure. The investigators concluded CNB may be a reasonable alternative, especially at institutions with a high rate of FNAB inadequacy (up to 30%).[31]

Sonoelastography is a newer technique using ultrasound that measures deformation of tissues after a mechanical force is applied (with the probe). It is under investigation as a diagnostic tool to distinguish between varying histologies of parotid tumors and even to look at malignancy versus benign tissue. PAs and malignant tumors tend to be stiffer than other benign pathologies, but larger studies are needed to validate this as a useful clinical tool.[32] Nevertheless, a thorough history, examination, and work-up are necessary for all parotid masses.

A more detailed discussion of head and neck imaging for parotid lesions and the evaluation of parotid masses is discussed in chapters 2 and 3.

BENIGN PAROTID NEOPLASMS

The following sections are dedicated to the specific benign neoplasms by cell type. Special attention is given to PAs and WTs because they represent up to 93% of all benign parotid tumors. Very rare histologies are not discussed, but a summary is provided in **Table 2**.

Pleomorphic Adenoma (Benign Mixed Tumor)

PA or benign mixed tumor is the most common benign parotid tumor (53.3%–68.6% of benign parotid tumors).[1,21] Its namesake comes from its mixture of both epithelial and mesenchymal components, with variation in stromal and epithelial morphology as well as microscopic architecture (**Figs. 4** and **5**).[39] The subtypes of myxoid, cellular, or classic (balanced epithelial-mesenchyme ratio) refer to the ratio of the two tissue components within the tumor. Epithelial cells form duct structures and may vary in morphologic appearance. These tumors present more often in women and middle-aged individuals (mean age 52.8 years)[7] as a slow, unilateral, asymptomatic swelling. Very rarely, multifocal and/or bilateral PAs in previously untreated patients have been reported.[40]

Eighty percent to 87% of PAs originate superficial to the facial nerve, 80% of which are in the parotid tail region. Grossly, typical PAs are firm, mobile, demarcated, and tan-white in appearance. FNAB diagnosis is more straightforward given the stromal and epithelial elements, but a small carcinoma ex-PA can be easily missed.[33] Given that most tumors occur in the superficial lobe, a superficial parotidectomy or

Table 2
Summary of benign parotid gland tumors

Histopathology	Sex Preference[33]	Relative Incidence	FNA Findings[33]	Malignant Potential	Considerations
PA	Female	53%–69%[1,2,21]	Characteristic mix of epithelial & stromal features	3%–15%[34]	Recurrence is challenging to treat and may require adjuvant radiotherapy.
WT	Male	25%–32%[7,21,35]	Oncocytic epithelial cells with lymphocytes	1%[17]	There is a strong association with smoking.
Basal cell adenoma	—	2%–7%[2,3,36]	Overlapping features with other benign & malignant tumors; small hyperchromatic oval cells	Rare	The membranous subtype is more common in men and may have a higher malignant transformation rate.
Myoepithelioma	—	1%–3%[2,3]	Bundles of epithelioid/plasmacytoid cells and stellate cells	Rare	Tumors with spindled or clear cell predominance may have more malignant potential.
Oncocytoma	—	1%[2,3]	Numerous oncocytic cells with granular cytoplasm	Rare	The clear cell variant requires ruling out metastatic renal cell carcinoma or thyroid carcinoma.
Cystadenoma	Female	<1%[2,3]	Cystic spaces may drain eosinophilic fluid	Rare	Malignant transformation is reported in the mucinous variant.
Canalicular adenoma	—	<10 cases ever reported in parotid[37]	—	—	It is usually found in the upper lip and oral cavity.
Sebaceous adenoma	Male	<1%[38]	—	—	—
Ductal papillomas	—	<1%[38]	—	Rare	It is mostly found in minor salivary glands.
Hemangioma	Female	50% of pediatric parotid tumors	—	—	It typically regresses after 7 y; segmental variant requires work-up for PHACE syndrome. Active treatment is preferred to watchful waiting.

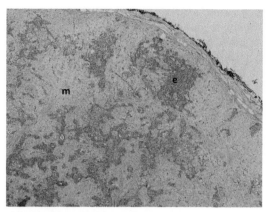

Fig. 4. PAs have highly variable amounts of epithelial cells (e) and mesenchymal tissue (m) (hematoxylin-eosin, original magnification ×20).

extracapsular dissection is sufficient, though optimal technique is still debated. Superficial tumors that encroach on the facial nerve demand more extensive dissection.[41]

Parotid PAs are usually encapsulated; but more than half will demonstrate focal absences of capsule, particularly in the myxoid (71%) or stroma-rich subtype. Capsules can have a variable thickness that varies by subtype. PAs recurred frequently following intracapsular enucleation, thought to be due to tumor pseudopodia encroaching beyond the tumor capsule. Changes in management, namely, from taking wider margins outside of the tumor capsule, have reduced recurrence rates to 0% to 2.5%.[42] A second theory of recurrence involves tumor spillage, whereby violation of a tumor may seed tumor cells into the surgical wound and may contribute to the multifocality often seen, sometimes tracking along a surgical scar. Witt[43] reported a significant 5% increase in recurrence rate with tumor spillage. Even with modified surgical techniques, tumor size, younger age at initial surgery, female sex, and tumor location are associated with more frequent recurrence.

Recurrent PAs (RPAs) typically appear 7 to 10 years after initial surgery and can be challenging to manage. Imaging with MRI is preferred to evaluate the extent, as RPAs

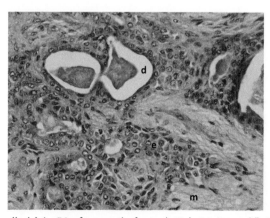

Fig. 5. Epithelial cells (e) in PAs frequently form ductal structures (d). The mesenchymal component (m) is often myxoid, with a blue-gray appearance (hematoxylin-eosin, original magnification ×400).

are often multifocal. Once recurred, re-recurrence is common as Wittekindt and colleagues[44] found a re-recurrence rate of 75% after 15 years despite extensive parotidectomy (without radiotherapy). The surgical management of an RPA is typically total parotidectomy, and multiple surgeries may be necessary. Adjuvant radiation may be necessary for recalcitrant disease, as many investigators have reported significantly better locoregional control in this manner.[45]

Malignant transformation can occur in 3% to 15%, and the risk increases with continued observation; thus, surgical treatment at the time of PA diagnosis is ideal.[34] Despite its benign nature, metastatic PA with distant spread to bone, regional lymph nodes, and lungs have been reported in the literature, usually after a local recurrence has already occurred.[46]

MONOMORPHIC ADENOMA

Monomorphic adenoma refers to a category of benign parotid tumors that lack the stromal cell line found in PAs, composed solely of either epithelial or myoepithelial components.

Warthin Tumor (Papillary Cystadenoma Lymphomatosum, Adenolymphoma)

WTs compose 25% to 32%[7,21,35] of benign parotid tumors as the second most common histopathology. They almost exclusively occur in the parotid gland (98.3%), Caucasians (94% vs 4% in African Americans),[7] and smokers (92.3% smokers).[47] They are bilateral 5% to 12% of the time, with a 2:1 male predominance. Reports of multicentricity range from 2% to up to 20% in an Asian study.[35] Relative to other benign tumors, WTs appear in an older demographic (mean age 59.5 years).[7] Anatomically, WTs have a predilection for the parotid tail, near the angle of the mandible, and may present as an upper neck swelling.

Histologically, WTs contains both lymphoid tissue and an epithelium that is arranged in papillary and cystic structures (**Figs. 6** and **7**). The papillary, or cystic, lining is a bilayered eosinophilic epithelium. The cyst lumens may contain thick secretions or cellular debris.[48] Given its characteristic appearance, histologic diagnosis is typically not challenging. Grossly, tumors have a smooth or lobulated surface and are

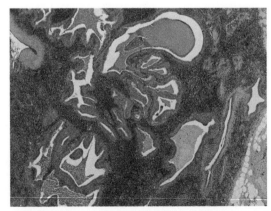

Fig. 6. WTs have an eosinophilic epithelial component, arranged in tubules and papillary projections, and a prominent lymphoid component (hematoxylin-eosin, original magnification ×20).

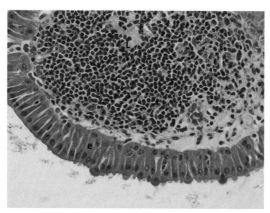

Fig. 7. The epithelium (e) of a WT contains a double layer of eosinophilic cells. The lymphoid component (L) contains predominantly mature lymphocytes (hematoxylin-eosin, original magnification ×400).

encapsulated. FNAB shows a mixture of oncocytic-appearing epithelial cells and mature lymphocytes, often clustered.[33]

Pathogenesis is traditionally thought to be a neoplastic growth of trapped salivary tissues within the parotid lymph nodes, but little is known about the mechanism of tumor formation. A subset of WTs is linked to a t(11:19) translocation forming a CRTC1-MAML fusion protein also shared by some mucoepidermoid carcinomas. Some investigators speculate that there may be a predilection toward malignant transformation in this subset of WTs.[49] Hormones, radiation, viruses (Epstein-Barr virus and Human Herpesvirus-8), and comorbidity with autoimmune diseases (eg, Hashimoto thyroiditis, Sjögren syndrome) have been associated with WT. Recently, there has been emerging evidence to suggest that autoimmune processes, combined with a toxic insult from smoking and viruses, may be key in driving WT formation.[50]

The treatment is surgery; like PAs, the extent of surgery is debated. A large case series at Johns Hopkins found a recurrence rate of 4.2% with superficial parotidectomies. Malignant transformation (1%) is very rare.[17]

Oncocytoma (Oxyphilic Adenoma, Oncocytic Adenoma)

Oncocytomas compose 0.6% to 1.1%[2,3] of benign parotid tumors and are completely composed of oncocytic cells. Oncocytes are large, granular eosinophilic cells with hyperplastic mitochondria that have undergone metaplasia from epithelial cells and are the predominant finding on FNAB. However, oncocytic cells can also be seen in other benign and malignant salivary pathologies. The pathogenesis and stimulus for oncocytic change are unclear, though a possible connection to head and neck radiation has been suggested.[51] Clear cell oncocytoma (a clear cell appearance) is a histologic variant that necessitates evaluation for metastatic renal cell carcinoma or thyroid carcinoma. Grossly, oncocytomas are lobulated, encapsulated, and may have an orange or red hue.[52] Transformation to oncocytic carcinoma is rare; the treatment is surgical removal, with a good prognosis. Despite its benign classification, oncocytomas can be locally destructive.[33]

Basal Cell Adenoma

Basal cell adenomas compose approximately 2.4% to 7.1%[2,3,36] of benign parotid tumors and more commonly occur in women, between the fourth to ninth decades of life. They follow PA and WT as the third most common benign parotid tumor. Histologically, these tumors are characterized by basaloid-appearing epithelial cells and have 4 morphologic subtypes: trabecular, tubular, solid (most common), and membranous. The distinctive membranous subtype (also known as dermal analogue tumor because of its similar appearance to cylindromas in the skin) occurs mostly in men, frequently lacks a capsule, and has the highest risk of malignant transformation (up to 28%).[53] Histologically, the solid type is characterized by peripheral nuclear palisading and solid collections of small, hyperchromatic basal cells. Diagnosis on FNAB is more difficult because of its overlapping features with adenoid cystic carcinoma, basal cell adenocarcinoma, and PA.[54] Treatment is surgical excision with a good prognosis.

Myoepithelioma (Myoepithelial Adenoma, Benign Myoepithelial Tumor)

Myoepitheliomas are 0.8% to 3.4%[2,3] of benign parotid tumors. Histologically, they show predominantly from myoepithelial differentiation, mostly composed of spindle cells and other cell types, including clear cells, plasmacytoid (hyaline) cells, and epithelioid cells. Tumors with spindled or clear cell predominance have more malignant potential.[33] Immunohistochemistry with markers, such as p63 and calponin, will demonstrate myoepithelial differentiation in tumor cells. Grossly, they are smooth, white, encapsulated tumors with numerous protuberances. FNAB shows characteristic bundles of spindle cells, epithelioid, stellate, and plasmacytoid cells arranged in sheets. Treatment is surgical excision, and malignant transformation is rare. Although myoepitheliomas are typically solid tumors, a benign cystic variant has been reported[55] (**Fig. 8**).

Hemangioma (Cellular Hemangioma, Immature Capillary Hemangioma, Juvenile Hemangioma, Congenital Hemangioma)

Hemangiomas are benign lesions composed of endothelial cells that form blood vessels in various stages of maturation. The most common form is the capillary hemangioma, also known as infantile or juvenile hemangioma. They are the most common benign tumors in children (4%–10% of infants, 50% of pediatric parotid tumors) and typically do not appear at birth. They are more common in Caucasians, females, and premature children.[56] They are dark-red tumors that may discolor the overlying skin with a bluish hue, sometimes accentuated by crying. Histologically, these

Fig. 8. Myoepitheliomas have a similar appearance to PAs but lack ductal structures and myxoid stroma (hematoxylin-eosin, original magnification ×100).

unencapsulated tumors are characterized by endothelial cell hyperplasia surrounding small capillaries, with variability in vessel size and shape. Mitoses are frequently seen but are not atypical and bear no impact on prognosis. These tumors have 2 rapid proliferation phases: 1 to 2 months after birth and 4 to 5 months after birth. Fortunately, 75% to 90% involute by 7 years[57] of age and are replaced with fibrofatty tissue. Infantile hemangiomas present either focally or diffusely (segmental) in the V3 mandibular distribution.[58] The latter behaves aggressively and can grow for up to 2 years. Very large tumors may ulcerate, bleed, and cause complications, such as high-output heart failure (from excessive shunting), airway involvement (up to 29% of diffuse cases and may require tracheostomy), soft tissue destruction, and even death. Those with segmental disease require an evaluation for the neurocutaneous PHACE syndrome, characterized by hemangiomas and structural anomalies of the eyes, sternum, cerebral vasculature, and/or aorta.[59] An equivocal diagnosis of hemangioma should be evaluated with MRI to determine the extent. Direct laryngoscopy is needed if airway involvement is suspected.

Early and active treatment should be sought not only to prevent additional tumor proliferation but also to diminish psychosocial impact. Treatment options include oral propranolol (first-line pharmacotherapy), topical beta-blockers, oral or topical corticosteroids, bleomycin injection, laser therapy (superficial lesions only), endovascular sclerotherapy, vincristine, interferon-α2a, and surgery; a multimodality approach is usually necessary for more advanced tumors.[60]

MANAGEMENT

For most benign parotid tumors, complete surgical excision is sufficient. Adequate preoperative planning is vital to performing safe and oncologically adequate parotidectomy without submitting patients to excessive morbidity. Intracapsular enucleation should be avoided. Large superficial lobe tumors may necessitate a complete superficial parotidectomy, whereas more conservative techniques (partial superficial parotidectomy, extracapsular dissection) may be sufficient for smaller tumors with adequate oncologic and safer outcomes. Tumors involving the superficial and deep lobes may require total parotidectomy with meticulous facial nerve dissection. Endoscope-assisted and minimally invasive approaches to the parotid gland have also been described. However, further follow-up is needed to verify locoregional control.[61]

For a more detailed discussion of parotidectomy for benign lesions, see chapter 7.

REFERENCES

1. Spiro RH. Salivary neoplasms: overview of a 35-year experience with 2,807 patients. Head Neck Surg 1986;8(3):177–84.
2. Bradley PJ, McGurk M. Incidence of salivary gland neoplasms in a defined UK population. Br J Oral Maxillofac Surg 2013;51(5):399–403.
3. Tian Z, Li L, Wang L, et al. Salivary gland neoplasms in oral and maxillofacial regions: a 23-year retrospective study of 6982 cases in an eastern Chinese population. Int J Oral Maxillofac Surg 2010;39(3):235–42.
4. Thompson L. World Health Organization classification of tumours: pathology and genetics of head and neck tumours. Ear Nose Throat J 2006;85(2):74.
5. Przewoźny T, Stankiewicz C. Neoplasms of the parotid gland in northern Poland, 1991–2000: an epidemiologic study. Eur Arch Otorhinolaryngol 2004;261(7): 369–75.

6. Vuhahula EA. Salivary gland tumors in Uganda: clinical pathological study. Afr Health Sci 2004;4(1):15–23.

7. Pinkston JA, Cole P. Incidence rates of salivary gland tumors: results from a population-based study. Otolaryngol Head Neck Surg 1999;120(6):834–40.

8. Carlson GW. The salivary glands. Embryology, anatomy, and surgical applications. Surg Clin North Am 2000;80(1):261–73, xii.

9. Som PM, Smoker W, Reidenberg JS, et al. Embryology and anatomy of the neck. In: Som PM, Curtin HD, editors. Head and neck imaging. St. Louis, Missouri: Mosby, Inc; 2011. p. 2117–79.

10. Regezi JA, Batsakis JG. Histogenesis of salivary gland neoplasms. Otolaryngol Clin North Am 1977;10(2):297–307.

11. Dardick I, Burford-Mason AP. Current status of histogenetic and morphogenetic concepts of salivary gland tumorigenesis. Crit Rev Oral Biol Med 1993;4(5):639–77.

12. Bell D, Hanna E. Salivary gland cancers: biology and molecular targets for therapy. Curr Oncol Rep 2012;14(2):166–74.

13. Xu L, Tang H, Chen DW, et al. Genome-wide association study identifies common genetic variants associated with salivary gland carcinoma and its subtypes. Cancer 2015;121(14):2367–74.

14. Takeichi N, Hirose F, Yamamoto H, et al. Salivary gland tumors in atomic bomb survivors, Hiroshima, Japan. II. Pathologic study and supplementary epidemiologic observations. Cancer 1983;52(2):377–85.

15. Modan B, Chetrit A, Alfandary E, et al. Increased risk of salivary gland tumors after low-dose irradiation. Laryngoscope 1998;108(7):1095–7.

16. Sadetzki S, Chetrit A, Jarus-Hakak A, et al. Cellular phone use and risk of benign and malignant parotid gland tumors—a nationwide case-control study. Am J Epidemiol 2008;167(4):457–67.

17. Yoo GH, Eisele DW, Driben JS, et al. Warthin's tumor: a 40-year experience at the Johns Hopkins hospital. Laryngoscope 1994;104(7):799–803.

18. Zheng W, Shu X-O, Ji B-T, et al. Diet and other risk factors for cancer of the salivary glands: a population-based case-control study. Int J Cancer 1996;67(2):194–8.

19. Horn-Ross PL, Morrow M, Ljung B-M. Menstrual and reproductive factors for salivary gland cancer risk in women. Epidemiology 1999;10(5):528–30.

20. Weinreb I. Translocation-associated salivary gland tumors: a review and update. Adv Anat Pathol 2013;20(6):367–77.

21. Ichihara T, Kawata R, Higashino M, et al. A more appropriate clinical classification of benign parotid tumors: investigation of 425 cases. Acta Otolaryngol 2014;134(11):1185–91.

22. Bron LP, O'Brien CJ. Facial nerve function after parotidectomy. Arch Otolaryngol Head Neck Surg 1997;123(10):1091–6.

23. Newberry TR, Kaufmann CR, Miller FR. Review of accessory parotid gland tumors: pathologic incidence and surgical management. Am J Otol 2014;35(1):48–52.

24. Zbären P, Vander Poorten V, Witt RL, et al. Pleomorphic adenoma of the parotid: formal parotidectomy or limited surgery? Am J Surg 2013;205(1):109–18.

25. Britt CJ, Stein AP, Patel PN, et al. Incidental parotid neoplasms: pathology and prevalence. Otolaryngol Head Neck Surg 2015;153(4):566–8.

26. Day TA, Deveikis J, Gillespie MB, et al. Salivary gland neoplasms. Curr Treat Options Oncol 2004;5(1):11–26.

27. Wilkie TF, White RA. Benign parotid tumor with facial nerve paralysis. Plast Reconstr Surg 1969;43(5):528–30.

28. Tryggvason G, Gailey MP, Hulstein SL, et al. Accuracy of fine-needle aspiration and imaging in the preoperative workup of salivary gland mass lesions treated surgically. Laryngoscope 2013;123(1):158–63.

29. Brennan PA, Herd MK, Howlett DC, et al. Is ultrasound alone sufficient for imaging superficial lobe benign parotid tumours before surgery? Br J Oral Maxillofac Surg 2012;50(4):333–7.

30. Schmidt RL, Hall BJ, Wilson AR, et al. A systematic review and meta-analysis of the diagnostic accuracy of fine-needle aspiration cytology for parotid gland lesions. Am J Clin Pathol 2011;136(1):45–59.

31. Witt BL, Schmidt RL. Ultrasound-guided core needle biopsy of salivary gland lesions: a systematic review and meta-analysis. Laryngoscope 2014;124(3): 695–700.

32. Klintworth N, Mantsopoulos K, Zenk J, et al. Sonoelastography of parotid gland tumours: initial experience and identification of characteristic patterns. Eur Radiol 2012;22(5):947–56.

33. Wenig BM. Atlas of head and neck pathology. Philadelphia, PA: Elsevier Health Sciences; 2008.

34. Lüers J-C, Wittekindt C, Streppel M, et al. Carcinoma ex pleomorphic adenoma of the parotid gland. Study and implications for diagnostics and therapy. Acta Oncol 2009;48(1):132–6.

35. Chung YFA, Khoo MLC, Heng MKD, et al. Epidemiology of Warthin's tumour of the parotid gland in an Asian population. Br J Surg 1999;86(5):661–4.

36. IKawata R, Yoshimura K, Lee K, et al. Basal cell adenoma of the parotid gland: a clinicopathological study of nine cases—basal cell adenoma versus pleomorphic adenoma and Warthin's tumor. Eur Arch Otorhinolaryngol 2010;267(5):779–83.

37. Philpott CM, Kendall C, Murty GE. Canalicular adenoma of the parotid gland. J Laryngol Otol 2005;119(01):59–60.

38. Maffini F, Fasani R, Petrella D, et al. Sebaceous lymphadenoma of salivary gland: a case report and a review of the literature. Acta Otorhinolaryngol Ital 2007;27(3): 147–50.

39. Fujita Y, Yoshida T, Sakakura Y, et al. Reconstruction of pleomorphic adenoma of the salivary glands in three-dimensional collagen gel matrix culture. Virchows Arch 1999;434(2):137–43.

40. van Egmond SL, de Leng WWJ, Morsink FHM, et al. Monoclonal origin of primary unilateral multifocal pleomorphic adenoma of the parotid gland. Hum Pathol 2013;44(5):923–6.

41. Iro H, Zenk J, Koch M, et al. Follow-up of parotid pleomorphic adenomas treated by extracapsular dissection. Head Neck 2013;35(6):788–93.

42. Stennert E, Guntinas-Lichius O, Klussmann JP, et al. Histopathology of pleomorphic adenoma in the parotid gland: a prospective unselected series of 100 cases. Laryngoscope 2001;111(12):2195–200.

43. Witt RL. The significance of the margin in parotid surgery for pleomorphic adenoma. Laryngoscope 2002;112(12):2141–54.

44. Wittekindt C, Streubel K, Arnold G, et al. Recurrent pleomorphic adenoma of the parotid gland: analysis of 108 consecutive patients. Head Neck 2007;29(9): 822–8.

45. Witt RL, Eisele DW, Morton RP, et al. Etiology and management of recurrent parotid pleomorphic adenoma. Laryngoscope 2015;125(4):888–93.

46. Wenig BM, Hitchcock CL, Ellis GL, et al. Metastasizing mixed tumor of salivary glands: a clinicopathologic and flow cytometric analysis. Am J Surg Pathol 1992;16(9):845–8.

47. Pinkston JA, Cole P. Cigarette smoking and Warthin's tumor. Am J Epidemiol 1996;144(2):183–7.
48. Önder T, Tiwari RM, van der Waal I, et al. Malignant adenolymphoma of the parotid gland: report of carcinomatous transformation. J Laryngol Otol 1990; 104(08):656–61.
49. O'Neill ID. New insights into the nature of Warthin's tumour. J Oral Pathol Med 2009;38(1):145–9.
50. Dell' Aversana Orabona G, Abbate V, Piombino P, et al. Warthin's tumour: aetiopathogenesis dilemma, ten years of our experience. J Craniomaxillofac Surg 2015;43(4):427–31.
51. Brandwein MS, Huvos AG. Oncocytic tumors of major salivary glands: a study of 68 cases with follow-up of 44 patients. Am J Surg Pathol 1991;15(6):514–28.
52. Zhou C-X, Gao Y. Oncocytoma of the salivary glands: a clinicopathologic and immunohistochemical study. Oral Oncol 2009;45(12):e232–8.
53. Yu GY, Ubmüller J, Donath K. Membranous basal cell adenoma of the salivary gland: a clinicopathologic study of 12 cases. Acta Otolaryngol 1998;118(4): 588–93.
54. Kawahara A, Harada H, Akiba J, et al. Fine-needle aspiration cytology of basal cell adenoma of the parotid gland: characteristic cytological features and diagnostic pitfalls. Diagn Cytopathol 2007;35(2):85–90.
55. Astarci H, Celik A, Sungu N, et al. Cystic clear cell myoepithelioma of the parotid gland. A case report. Oral Maxillofac Surg 2009;13(1):45–8.
56. Haggstrom AN, Drolet BA, Baselga E, et al. Prospective study of infantile hemangiomas: demographic, prenatal, and perinatal characteristics. J Pediatr 2007; 150(3):291–4.
57. Buckmiller LM, Richter GT, Suen JY. Diagnosis and management of hemangiomas and vascular malformations of the head and neck. Oral Dis 2010;16(5): 405–18.
58. Waner M, North PE, Scherer KA, et al. The nonrandom distribution of facial hemangiomas. Arch Dermatol 2003;139(7):869–75.
59. Metry D, Heyer G, Hess C, et al. Consensus statement on diagnostic criteria for PHACE syndrome. Pediatrics 2009;124(5):1447–56.
60. Zheng JW, Zhou Q, Yang XJ, et al. Treatment guideline for hemangiomas and vascular malformations of the head and neck. Head Neck 2010;32(8):1088–98.
61. Woo SH, Kim JP, Baek C-H. Endoscope-assisted extracapsular dissection of benign parotid tumors using hairline incision. Head Neck 2016;38(3):375–9.

Diagnosis and Management of Malignant Salivary Gland Tumors of the Parotid Gland

 CrossMark

Aaron G. Lewis, MD[a], Tommy Tong, MD[b], Ellie Maghami, MD[c],*

KEYWORDS

- Parotid cancer • Malignant salivary cancers • Surgery for parotid salivary cancer
- Radiation therapy for parotid cancers • Chemotherapy for parotid tumors
- Molecular diagnostics • Genetic translocations of parotid tumors
- Molecular targeted therapies

KEY POINTS

- Histology, immunohistochemistry, and identification of gene translocations are important for parotid tumor diagnosis.
- Parotid cancers have diverse histopathology and clinical behavior.
- Treatment requires a multidisciplinary approach and surgery to negative margins is a mainstay, supplemented by radiation for better locoregional control and chemotherapy, usually in the palliative recurrent or metastatic setting.
- Targeted therapies are under active investigation; however, they are not yet proven in the clinical setting.

INTRODUCTION

Salivary gland cancers are rare with an annual incidence of approximately 3.0 cases per 100,000 in the United States accounting for less than 3% of all head and neck cancers. They are the most heterogeneous of any group of cancers and pose diagnostic challenges due to their rarity of occurrence, diversity of types, and the limited

Disclosure Statement: The authors have nothing to disclose.
[a] Department of Surgery, City of Hope National Medical Center, 1500 East Duarte Road, Duarte, CA 91010, USA; [b] Department of Pathology, City of Hope National Medical Center, 1500 East Duarte Road, Duarte, CA 91010, USA; [c] Division of Head and Neck Surgery, City of Hope National Medical Center, 1500 East Duarte Road, Duarte, CA 91010, USA
* Corresponding author.
E-mail address: emaghami@coh.org

Otolaryngol Clin N Am 49 (2016) 343–380
http://dx.doi.org/10.1016/j.otc.2015.11.001
0030-6665/16/$ – see front matter © 2016 Elsevier Inc. All rights reserved.

oto.theclinics.com

experience of most cytopathologists. New molecular tests are being identified and may add to the diagnostic accuracy.[1]

Approximately 70% of salivary cancers occur in the parotid gland. This article discusses primary salivary cancers with emphasis on the parotid gland. It provides an overview of select parotid cancers and up-to-date trends in management.

CAUSES

The causes of salivary gland tumors are not well understood. Radiation exposure has been clearly established as a risk factor for parotid malignancies. This association was first observed in atomic bomb survivors[2] but has also been seen in cancer survivors who were treated with radiation.[3] Even patients with exposure to low-dose radiation[4] or those treated with radioactive iodine[5] may be at risk. A possible dose–response relationship of cellular telephone use with epithelial parotid gland malignancy has also been described.[6] Despite parotid communication with the oral cavity, human papilloma virus has no proven role in parotid carcinogenesis.[7] Benign tumors, if untreated, can transform into malignant forms over time. There is generally no ethnic propensity for salivary cancers, although a higher incidence of malignant oncocytoma has been reported in Eskimos.[8]

HISTOLOGY AND IMMUNOHISTOCHEMISTRY

An understanding of the normal architecture and histology of the salivary gland aids in tumor categorization. The glandular structure is composed of 2 types of cells: luminal (acinar and ductal) and abluminal (myoepithelial and basal). The gland is further organized into lobules containing several acini, which then connect into intercalated followed by striated ducts. Cuboidal cells line the acini and may produce serous, mucoserous, or mucous secretions. Parotid acini secretions are predominantly serous. Intercalated and striated ducts are lined with cuboidal and simple columnar epithelium, respectively. Each cell type expresses a variety of markers that allows for identification and characterization (**Table 1**).

TRANSLOCATIONS AND FUSION GENES

Although salivary cancers are uncommon, growing understanding of their unique biologic characteristics is paving the way toward specific and personalized treatment. It is now known that most mucoepidermoid carcinoma (MEC) harbors the MECT1-MAML2 gene rearrangement. The MYB-NFIB translocation has recently been identified in adenoid cystic carcinoma (ACCa). Finally, the newly described mammary analogue secretory carcinoma harbors the ETV6-NTRK3 translocation. Although these translocations are mainly of diagnostic value, they may evolve as potential therapeutic targets in the future (**Table 2**).[9]

CLASSIFICATION OF MALIGNANT PAROTID TUMORS

The last formal histologic classification of salivary cancers was published by the World Health Organization (WHO) in 2005 and included 24 separate entities. Since then, new subtypes have been described and are included in a modified WHO list of 28 separate entities (**Box 1**). This classification helps facilitate accurate and consistent diagnoses.

Histology and grade are important determinants of local, regional, and distant disease control.[10] For the purpose of study and reporting, each cancer can be categorized into low-grade, intermediate-grade, or high-grade categories (**Table 3**).[11]

Table 1
Important immunohistochemical markers of the salivary gland

| Antigen | Luminal Cells | | Abluminal Cells | |
	Acinar	Ductal	Myoepithelial	Basal
CK (AE1/AE3)	+	+	+	+
EMA	+	+	−	−
CEA	+	+	−	−
CK14	−	−	+	
p63	−	−	+	+
α-Smooth muscle actin	−	−	+	−
Muscle-specific actin	−	−	+	−
Calponin	−	−	+	−
Podoplanin	−	−	+	−
Vimentin	−	−	+	−
S-100	Variable	Variable	Variable	Variable

Immunohistochemical markers are important for identification of cell types. These markers help breakdown the complex architecture of the salivary gland and supplement the H&E staining in obtaining a diagnosis.

Data from Namboodiripad PC. A review: immunological markers for malignant salivary gland tumors. J Oral Biol Craniofac Res 2014;4:127–34.

A detailed discussion of each cancer type is beyond the scope of this article. Nonetheless, a select group of parotid cancers is highlighted.

MUCOEPIDERMOID CARCINOMA

MEC is the most common salivary cancer affecting the parotid gland and comprising approximately 30% of malignant tumors. It occurs uniformly across

Table 2
Common translocations within malignant salivary gland tumors

Tumor Type	Chromosomal Translocation	Fusion Oncogenes
MEC	t(11;19) (q21;p13)	CRTC1[a]-MAML2; CRTC3-MAML2
	t(6;22) (p21;q12)	EWSR1-POU5F1
ACCa	t(6;9) (q22–23;p23–24)	MYB-NFIB
Carcinoma ex pleomorphic adenoma[b]	t(3;8) (p21;q12) or t(5;8) (p13;q12)	PLAG1
	t(3;12) (p14.2;q14–15)	HMGA2[b]
Mammary analogue secretory carcinoma	t(12;15) (p13q25)	ETV6-NTRK3
Hyalinizing clear cell carcinoma	t(12;22) (q13;q12)	EWSR1-ATF1

Several translocations and fusion gene products are unique to individual histologic subtypes and aid in the diagnosis.

[a] Formerly MECT1.

[b] Translocations are found in benign pleomorphic adenoma and carry over into carcinoma ex pleomorphic adenoma.

Box 1
World Health Organization (WHO) classification of malignant salivary gland tumors of the parotid gland

Acinic cell carcinoma

Mucoepidermoid carcinoma

Adenoid cystic carcinoma

Polymorphous low-grade adenocarcinoma

Epithelial-myoepithelial carcinoma

Clear cell carcinoma, not otherwise specified, and hyalinizing variant

Basal cell adenocarcinoma

Malignant sebaceous tumors

Cystadenocarcinoma

Low-grade cribriform cystadenocarcinoma

Mucinous adenocarcinoma

Oncocytic carcinoma

Salivary duct carcinoma

Adenocarcinoma, not otherwise specified

Myoepithelial carcinoma

Carcinoma ex pleomorphic adenoma

Carcinosarcoma

Metastasizing pleomorphic adenoma

Squamous cell carcinoma

Small cell carcinoma

Large cell carcinoma

Lymphoepithelial carcinoma

Sialoblastoma

Carcinoma arising in Warthin tumor

Sebaceous carcinoma

Sebaceous lymphadenocarcinoma

Malignant transformation of ductal papilloma

Signet ring cell adenocarcinoma

Adapted from Barnes L, Eveson JW, Reichart P, et al. 2005 World Health Organization classification of tumours. Pathology and genetics of head and neck tumours. Lyon: IARC Press;2005.

all ages. It is composed of mucus-secreting, intermediate, and epidermoid (squamous) cells in varying proportion with low-grade MEC containing more cystic spaces lined with mucous cells and high-grade MEC containing more squamous cells (**Figs. 1–10**).

Table 3
Tumor behavior by histologic subtype. Malignancies that mainly affect minor salivary glands are in italics

Malignant Salivary Tumors	
Low-grade to intermediate-grade	**High-grade**
Low-grade MEC[a]	High-grade MEC[a]
Tubular or cribriform ACCa[a]	Solid ACCa[a]
Low-grade adenocarcinoma, NOS[a]	High-grade adenocarcinoma, NOS[a]
Acinic cell carcinoma	Salivary duct carcinoma
Polymorphic low-grade adenocarcinoma	Carcinoma ex pleomorphic adenoma
Mucinous adenocarcinoma	Metastasizing pleomorphic adenoma
Clear cell carcinoma, NOS	Squamous cell carcinoma
Epithelial-myoepithelial carcinoma	Undifferentiated carcinoma
Myoepithelial carcinoma	Mucinous adenocarcinoma
Basal cell adenocarcinoma	Oncocytic carcinoma
Cystadenocarcinoma	Carcinosarcoma
Sialoblastoma	Small cell carcinoma
Sebaceous carcinoma	Large cell carcinoma
Sebaceous lymph adenocarcinoma	—
Mammary analogue secretory carcinoma	—
Signet ring cell adenocarcinoma	—
Carcinoma arising in Warthin	—
Malignant transformation of ductal papilloma	—
Low-grade cribriform cystadenocarcinoma (intraductal carcinoma)	—

Abbreviation: NOS, not otherwise specified.
[a] Histologic subtypes that range in behavior by grade.

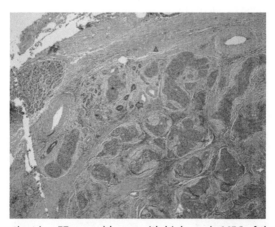

Fig. 1. MEC. The patient is a 57-year-old man with high-grade MEC of the deep lobe of his left parotid gland. This tumor is partially encapsulated (*arrowhead*). Small tumor islands are present at the invasive front and entrapping benign salivary gland (*arrow*). Hematoxylin-eosin stain (H&E) 40×.

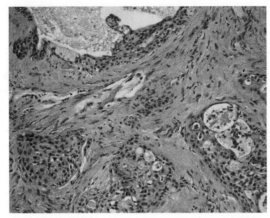

Fig. 2. MEC. Same case as **Fig. 1**. A low-grade cystic component is present in the upper field, amounting to less than 10% of the tumor. Mucous (goblet) cells are depicted with *arrowhead*. There are neutrophils infiltrating the high-grade component, not to be misconstrued as tumor necrosis (*arrow*). H&E 200×.

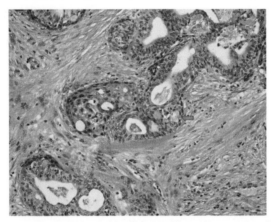

Fig. 3. MEC. Same case as **Fig. 1**. Epidermoid cells (*center*) have dense eosinophilic cytoplasm, well defined cell borders, central nuclei, and intercellular bridges. Surrounding this epidermoid nest are glandular spaces lined by tall columnar cells with several goblet cells (*arrow*). H&E 200×.

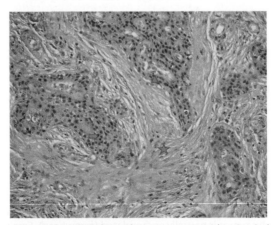

Fig. 4. MEC. Same case as **Fig. 1**. High-grade component with mitosis (*arrow*), prominent neovascularization within tumor islands (*arrowhead*), and desmoplastic stroma (*star*). There is moderate nuclear atypia but no anaplasia. H&E 200×.

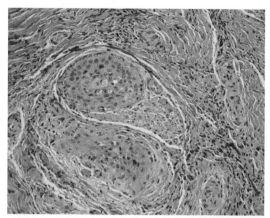

Fig. 5. MEC. Same case as **Fig. 1**. The nerve in the center is invaded by a big nest of MEC. This case also has facial nerve invasion (not illustrated). H&E 200×.

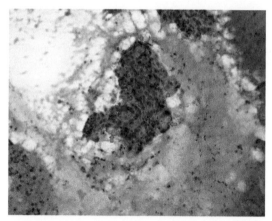

Fig. 6. MEC, fine-needle aspiration (FNA) cytology. Same case as **Fig. 1**. This Papanicolaou (PAP) stained smear shows a 3-dimensional group of mildly atypical cells containing goblet cells with eccentric nuclei (*arrows*), and epidermoid cell with abundant cytoplasm and centrally placed nucleus (*arrowhead*). Mucin is not evident in the background, as is often the case in high-grade MEC. Mucinous metaplasia can occur in several neoplastic and benign conditions and, by itself, is not diagnostic of MEC. PAP stain 200×.

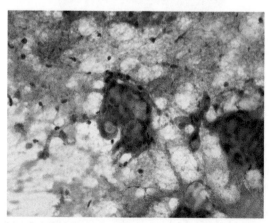

Fig. 7. MEC, FNA cytology. Same case as **Fig. 1**. Close up of mucous cells with large intracytoplasmic goblet of mucin. PAP stain 400×.

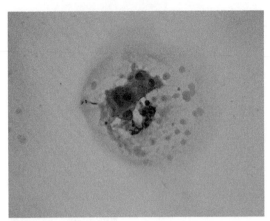

Fig. 8. MEC, FNA cytology. Same case as **Fig. 1**. Close-up of epidermoid cells with voluminous cytoplasm; keratohyaline granules; and centrally placed, moderately atypical nuclei. No cytoplasmic keratinization is seen. Similar to mucous cells, metaplastic squamous cells can also be seen in several benign and neoplastic conditions. PAP stain 400×.

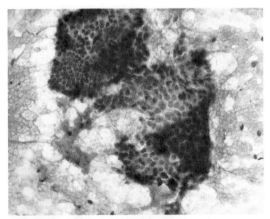

Fig. 9. MEC, FNA cytology. Same case as **Fig. 1**. A relatively flat sheet of intermediate cells (neither epidermoid nor mucous) showing mild nuclear atypia (compare with honeycombed benign ductal epithelial cells in the upper left field). Notice the lack of anaplasia in this case. There is also no mitotic activity or necrosis, cytologic parameters associated with malignancy, seen in the limited sample. Because grading of MEC depends on the evaluation of 8 histologic parameters (see **Table 4**), FNA can only give a narrative diagnosis and not a histologic grade. The morphologic findings in this case overlaps considerably with non-neoplastic conditions. PAP stain 400×.

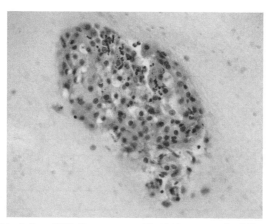

Fig. 10. MEC, cell block from FNA. Same case as **Fig. 1**. A group of mildly atypical tumor cells with neutrophils (compare with right lower area of **Fig. 2**). Ancillary techniques, such as histochemical stain for mucin (mucicarmine) and immunohistochemical stains for proliferation index (Ki-67), MUC5AC, MUC4, MUC1, and CK7, may be applied. H&E stain 400×.

Several molecular markers have both diagnostic and prognostic value in MEC. These include a variety of membrane-bound secretory mucins. For example, MUC1 is associated with a high histologic grade, high rate of recurrence, metastasis, and short disease-free interval.[12] MUC4, on the other hand, is expressed in low-grade MEC and is associated with a low recurrence rate and a long disease-free interval. In addition, the t(11;19) chromosomal translocation seems to be specific to MEC and predicts a better prognosis. The translocation results in CRTC1 (formerly MECT1)-MAML2 and CRTC3-MAML2 fusion proteins that disrupt the NOTCH signaling pathway. MAML2 rearrangements occur in up to 80% of MEC tumors[13] and are more common in low-grade tumors.[14] CRTC1/MAML2 translocation imparts a better prognosis even when found in high-grade MEC tumors. Epidermal growth factor receptor (EGFR) is also expressed in approximately two-thirds of MECs[15] and may be associated with higher grade irrespective of MAML2 fusion status.[16]

Prognosis is largely based on age, clinical stage, and grade. A lack of consistency among grading systems has led to a discrepancy in reports on prognosis for intermediate-grade MEC. This discrepancy can be explained by the use of multiple grading systems, including the Armed Forces Institute of Pathology (AFIP) system, Brandwein system, and the Modified-Healy classification.[17] Chen and colleagues[18] found that the Brandwein grading system (**Table 4**) predicted low-grade behavior in intermediate-grade MEC; however, Aro and colleagues[19] used the AFIP grading system and suggested intermediate-grade MEC be treated like high-grade tumors.

Higher grade is associated with male sex, older age, larger tumors, locally aggressive tumors, and higher rates of nodal and distal metastases.[18] A review of the Surveillance, Epidemiology, and End Results (SEER) database reveals a significant increase in nodal level I-III metastases with increasing grade (3.3%, 8.1%, and 34.0% in low-grade, intermediate-grade, and high-grade MEC, respectively).[18] Furthermore, 8.9% of patients with high-grade MEC have level IV-V nodes. These findings suggest that treatment should be tailored to the grade and predicted behavior. Overall prognosis is favorable with a 5-year overall survival of 79% but depends upon grade.[20]

Table 4 The Brandwein grading system for mucoepidermoid cancer	
Parameter	**Points**
Intracystic component<25%	+2
Neural invasion	+3
Necrosis	+3
4 or more mitoses/10 high-power field	+3
Anaplasia	+2
Lymphovascular invasion	+3
Invasive front: small nest and islands	+2
Bone invasion	+3
Grade (G)	**Sum of Points (Score)**
Low (G1)	0
Intermediate (G2)	2–3
High (G3)	4 or more

Adapted from Brandwein MS, Ivanov K, Wallace DI, et al. Mucoepidermoid carcinoma: a clinico-pathologic study of 80 patients with special reference to histologic grading. Am J Surg Pathol 2001;25:838; with permission.

ADENOID CYSTIC CARCINOMA

ACCa is the second-most common cancer of the parotid gland; however, the incidence seems to be decreasing over time.[21] ACCa typically occurs in between the fourth and sixth decade of life with a slight predisposition toward women. The behavior of ACCa is unique in that it is indolent, yet often highly fatal, with a propensity for neural and occult bony invasion. Neurotropism is a hallmark of ACCa. ACCa presents with pain and facial nerve dysfunction more often than other types of malignant salivary gland tumors. There is a strong correlation between pain and perineural invasion.[22] Perineural invasion occurs in 29.2% to 62.5% of patients with ACCa and is associated with local tumor recurrence but not distant failure.[23]

ACCa is a biphasic salivary gland tumor containing myoepithelial or basal cells with a minor population of epithelial or luminal cells growing in gland-like cystic architecture (**Figs. 11–13**). Histologically, ACCa may easily be confused with low-grade adenocarcinoma, basal cell adenoma, basal cell adenocarcinoma, or cellular pleomorphic adenoma (PA). Three histologic growth types are appreciated in varying patterns: tubular, cribriform, and solid. A grading system was developed based on the percent solid component ranging from no solid component in grade 1 to less than 30% solid component in grade 2 and a predominantly solid component in grade 3. A solid pattern is associated with aggressive behavior and a higher rate of distant metastasis.[22] The aggressive nature of the solid growth subtype is observed even in early stage I or II ACCa.[24] Transformation of ACCa into poorly differentiated cribriform adenocarcinoma or solid, undifferentiated carcinoma has been described and portends much worse prognosis. The reported median survival in such cases is only 12 months.[25]

Immunohistochemical markers for ACCa include nonspecific markers for basal cells and ductal cells (see **Table 1**) as well as CD43, a sialoglycoprotein that may assist in narrowing down the differential diagnosis.[26] Ki-67 is both a diagnostic and prognostic marker found in ACCa.[27] Neural cell adhesion molecule (NCAM) expression suggests ACCa and is associated with a higher incidence of perineural invasion.[3] A unique tumor-specific translocation, t(6;9) (q22–23;p23–24), has been described.[28]

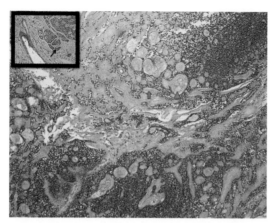

Fig. 11. ACCa of palate, grade 2. Patient is a 42-year-old man. This tumor has characteristic (although not diagnostic) feature of Swiss cheese-like (cribriform) areas containing mucoid ground substance (*arrowhead*) or eosinophilic basement membrane-like material (*arrow*). Also present are solid areas (<30%; *right upper, middle lower*) and tubules (*center*), some of which appear strangulated by abundant basement membrane-like material. Tumor cells are basaloid with angulated, relatively uniform nuclei and scanty cytoplasm. H&E 100×. Inset (*left upper*) shows a case of submandibular ACCa with perineural invasion (*black arrow*), a frequent finding in ACCa.

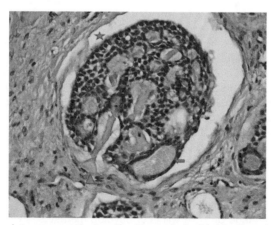

Fig. 12. ACCa of palate, same patient as **Fig. 11**, grade 2 with bland nuclear features. Some grade 3 adenoid cystic carcinoma may also lack overt nuclear anaplasia, although mitoses and necrosis may become identifiable. Luminal cells lining true glands are few (*arrow*, note granular eosinophilic intraluminal secretion). Most spaces are pseudoglands lined by basal or myoepithelial cells and contains pink basement membrane-like material (continuous with the stroma, *arrowhead*) and bluish mucoid material. There is no nuclear palisading at the epithelial-stromal interface (*star*), helping to distinguish ACCa from basal cell adenoma and adenocarcinoma. The stroma is not desmoplastic and without bluish hyaline chondroid appearance, featured in some carcinomas and pleomorphic adenoma, respectively.

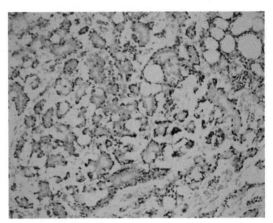

Fig. 13. ACCa, immunohistochemical stain for p63. This metastatic ACCa to the lung in a different patient shows strong nuclear staining (brown) of basal or myoepithelial cells. The luminal epithelial cells are negative and stained with the blue nuclear counterstain. The opposite pattern (cytoplasmic and membranous) would be evident for epithelial markers (CK7, CEA, EMA) and c-kit, respectively (not illustrated here).

This translocation fuses the MYB oncogene to the transcription factor gene NFIB, leading to the potential activation of MYB targets, including genes associated with apoptosis, cell cycle control, and cell growth. The MYB-NFIB gene fusion is identified by fluorescence in situ hybridization (FISH) in 52.9% of tumors, although there is not always a chimeric transcript. MYB overexpression is correlated with poor survival.[29]

Several growth factor receptor proteins and ligands have been identified within ACCa; however, none are specific to this particular disease.[23] A significant number of cases have abnormalities in receptor tyrosine kinases (c-kit, EGFR, HER2/neu).[12] C-kit is expressed in 80% to 90% of tumors but is not pathognomonic of ACCa.[30] Although c-kit expression is common, gene mutations are rare, resulting in a poor response to tyrosine kinase inhibitors.[31] There is no predictive value of c-kit mutation in terms of prognosis.[32] In addition, phase II trials using imatinib in ACCa have been disappointing with significant toxicity.[33] Similarly, phase II clinical trials with sunitinib, a multityrosine kinase inhibitor that includes vascular endothelial growth factor (VEGF), have failed to show any objective response.[34]

The overall prognosis of ACCa varies but is generally poor due to late distant failures. Nodal metastases are rare, ranging between 3% and 10% in most studies.[23] Conversely, distant metastases are common even after treatment with surgery and locoregional radiation, and usually occur in the lungs (80%) or bones (15%).[23,35] Distant metastases occur in 31% of patients, and at least 20% of patients with early-stage disease will later develop metastases without local recurrence.[36] Distant failures in early-stage ACCa present within a median of 31.5 months.

The indolent course is usually drawn out over 10 to 15 years. A review of the SEER database from 1973 to 2007 showed optimistic 5, 10, and 15 years overall survival rates of 90.3%, 79.9%, and 69.2%, respectively.[21] Another study reports overall survival rates of 5, 10, and 20 years at 85.6%, 67.4%, and 50.4%, respectively, for patients without distant metastasis at presentation; and 69.1%, 45.7%, and 14.3%, respectively, for patients who presented with distant metastasis.

Median survival after detection of metastasis is 36 months (range 1–112 months). Treatment of distant metastatic recurrences does not seem to offer any survival benefit based on historical data.[36] Survival seems to be better for women and married persons.[36] Older age (age>60 years), advanced stage, positive resection margin, high histologic grade, and high expression of Ki-67 were significantly correlated with poor prognosis.[37]

ACINIC CELL CARCINOMA

Acinic cell carcinoma (AcCC) is a low-grade malignancy that accounts for 10% to 15% of parotid tumors. In the past, this was regarded as a benign tumor; however, late recurrences and metastases led to reclassification as a malignancy. AcCC may occur at any age; however, the mean age of occurrence tends to be younger than other parotid malignancies. Bilateral tumors are unusual but may occur.

The hallmark of AcCC is serous acinar cell differentiation; however, multiple cell types and histologic growth patterns are recognized (**Figs. 14–20**). Thus, AcCC can present as several variants, which may confound the diagnosis. Cytologic diagnosis by fine-needle aspiration (FNA) hinges on the identification of acinar cells, which are more apparent in better differentiated AcCC, and the elimination of other histologies. DOG1 was recently described as a marker for acinar tissue and may aid in the diagnosis of AcCC.[38] The rarity and indolent nature of AcCC has made it difficult to develop a grading system. Although AcCC generally follows an indolent course, it tends to be more aggressive when found in the parotid gland in comparison to the minor salivary glands.

AcCC is unpredictable in behavior. Prognosis is determined by recurrence and cervical lymph node metastases with some recurrences occurring late. Historically, recurrence was reported as high as 44%.[39] In more recent studies, recurrence occurs in approximately one-third of patients with a disease-associated death rate of about 15%.[40] This may reflect the difficulty in following patients out far enough to capture the late recurrences or, possibly, better surgical techniques. Stage, positive margins, local and neural invasion, high Ki-67 expression, desmoplasia, anaplasia, and a paucity of inflammation are also markers for worse prognosis.[39]

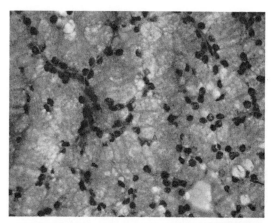

Fig. 14. AcCC of parotid in a 52-year-old man. Carcinoma has defining acinar cell differentiation, seen here as basophilic cytoplasmic granules (*arrowhead*). H&E 600×.

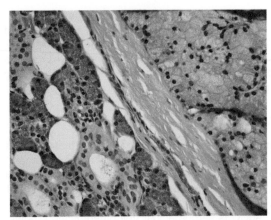

Fig. 15. AcCC of parotid. Tumor cells (*right*) are less granular than normal parotid acini (*left*).

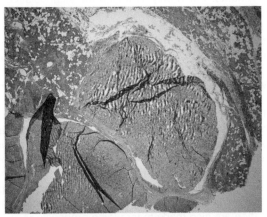

Fig. 16. AcCC of parotid. Tumor is multinodular and invasive of the normal parotid (*right* and *upper left*) with a pushing edge. H&E 20×.

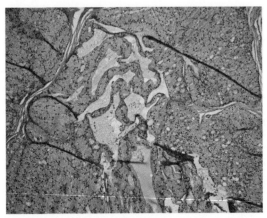

Fig. 17. AcCC of parotid. Most of this tumor is solid. Focal microcystic change is seen (*center*) and may be predominant in other cases. H&E 100×.

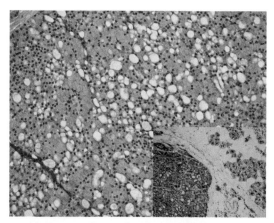

Fig. 18. AcCC of parotid. Tumor cells are focally vacuolated. Inset: Immunohistochemical stain for DOG.1, showing diffuse strong staining in tumor (*left*) and canalicular staining in benign acinus-intercalated duct units (*right*).

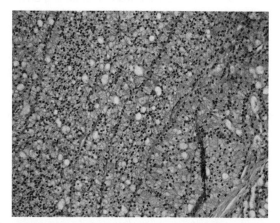

Fig. 19. AcCC of parotid. Tumor has an abundance of delicate capillary-sized neovasculature, here highlighted by regimented tumor cell nuclei.

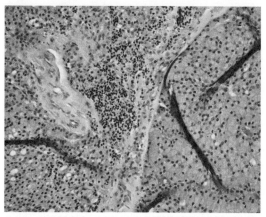

Fig. 20. AcCC of parotid. Focal lymphocytic infiltration is present in the stroma (*center*). An abundance of these cells, along with germinal centers and a pure microcystic appearance is associated with excellent prognosis.

MAMMARY ANALOGUE SECRETORY CARCINOMA

Mammary analogue secretory carcinoma is a newly described salivary cancer that, as it sounds, is an analogue of AcCC but lacks acinar differentiation.[41] More than 100 cases have been reported in the literature since its original description in 2010.[41–44] Microscopically, the tumors have a lobulated growth pattern and are composed of microcystic and glandular spaces with abundant eosinophilic homogenous or bubbly secretory material positive for periodic acid-Schiff, mucicarmine, MUC1, MUC4, and mammaglobin. The neoplasms also show strong vimentin, S-100 protein, and STAT5a positivity.[41] This tumor is unique for the chromosomal translocation, t(12;15) (p13;q25), which leads to a fusion gene between the ETV6 gene on chromosome 12 and the NTRK3 gene on chromosome 15. Data are limited on prognosis but suggests that these tumors are indolent similar to AcCC with a risk for late recurrences.[41]

SALIVARY DUCTAL CARCINOMA

Salivary ductal carcinoma (SDC) is rare but worth mentioning because it is notorious for its rapid and locally aggressive growth, most commonly in the parotid gland. SDC most commonly occurs in older men and is associated with poor prognosis. Histologically, SDC seems reminiscent of high-grade ductal carcinoma of the breast composed of pleomorphic, epithelioid cells with a cribiform growth pattern. In the authors' institution, most cases seem to have arisen from a pre-existing PA, although de novo cases undoubtedly occur. Generally, cases arising in a PA may remain confined by the original capsule. Frequently, however, the tumor has extended beyond the capsule and is grossly infiltrative (**Fig. 21**). The cut surfaces are solid and remarkable

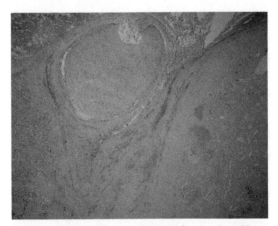

Fig. 21. Salivary duct carcinoma. This is a 3.3 cm parotid tumor in a 62-year-old man who has facial palsy and regional lymphadenopathy. Preoperative FNA performed outside was reviewed, changing the diagnosis from favor MEC to favor salivary duct carcinoma (see **Figs. 22** and **23**). Radical parotidectomy with sacrifice of facial nerve and neck dissection was performed. This image shows salivary duct carcinoma colonizing residual PA (*right*), extending beyond the capsule by greater than 5.5 mm (*left*) and invading the facial nerve branch (*upper field*). Benign parotid parenchyma is visible on the left upper corner. H&E 20×. Extension of carcinoma for more than 5 mm beyond the capsule of the parent PA is considered frank invasion, and is associated with worse prognosis. This patient has multiple involved lymph nodes (16/35) with extranodal extension. Tumor is positive for HER2 gene amplification by interphase FISH analysis, which is also an adverse prognostic indicator.

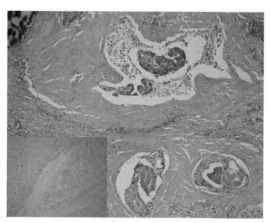

Fig. 22. Salivary duct carcinoma. Close-up showing marked nuclear atypia; abundant eosin-ophilic cytoplasm; central comedo-like necrosis; and hyalinized, focally calcified (*upper left*) stroma of residual PA (*upper field*). H&E 100×. Inset (*left lower*) illustrates absence of p63-staining myoepithelial nuclei around invasive carcinoma (*upper left*) as well as around intraductal-like tumor (*lower right*).

for foci of necrosis. Microscopically, marked pleomorphism and necrosis is the rule (**Fig. 22**), rendering a rather straightforward cytologic diagnosis, provided the diagnosis is entertained (**Figs. 23–25**).

Salivary duct carcinoma exhibits rapid growth, pain, facial palsy, and nodal metastasis in a significant proportion of patients at presentation. Despite resection, there is a high incidence of locoregional recurrence and/or distant metastasis. Perineural spread is a hallmark of SDC occurring in most patients. In a recent series of SDC cases, up to a third of patients presented with paralysis of at least 1 branch of the facial nerve and more than half required facial nerve sacrifice.[49]

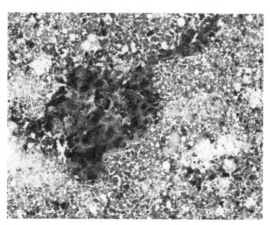

Fig. 23. Salivary duct carcinoma. FNA, showing disorganized, overlapping, markedly pleo-morphic tumor cells in a background of abundant necrotic material. Air-dried smear stained with Romanowksy stain, 200×.

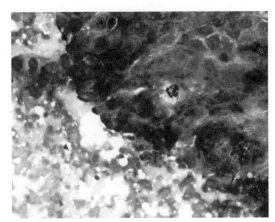

Fig. 24. Salivary duct carcinoma. An atypical mitotic figure is seen in this cluster of tumor cells. Air-dried smear stained with Romanowksy stain, 400×.

The prognosis is poor with a 5-year overall survival of 43%[49] and a mean 5-year recurrence-free survival of 34%.[50] Only patients with intracapsular and microinvasive salivary duct CXPA have a favorable prognosis. Thus, careful pathologic evaluation is crucial. Interestingly, 20% of tumors overexpress HER2, which is associated with a poor prognosis. Overexpression is less common in other types of salivary cancer.[51] SDC is also the only histologic subtype that expresses androgen receptor, which provides an opportunity for molecular targeted therapy or androgen deprivation therapy (see later discussion).[52]

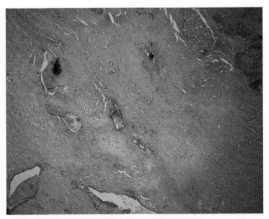

Fig. 25. Salivary duct carcinoma confined to the capsule of a sublingual PA (different case, 55 yo F). Tumor measures 2.2 cm. Note residual PA (*upper right*) with hyalinized, calcified stroma and gaping spaces lined by markedly pleomorphic tumor cells with central comedo-like necrosis. H&E 20×. The tumor is considered an intracapsular carcinoma (ie, noninvasive), which is associated with excellent prognosis.

CARCINOMA EX PLEOMORPHIC ADENOMA (MALIGNANT MIXED TUMOR)

Carcinoma ex pleomorphic adenoma (CXPA) is a rare tumor that contains both a benign and malignant component. It arises from a long-standing or recurrent pleomorphic adenoma (PA) with the incidence increasing from 1.5% at 5 years to 10% after 15 years.[45] Diagnosis is usually made based on the presence of an infiltrative and destructive growth pattern. Frank malignancy is manifested clinically as sudden rapid growth, fixation, ulceration, facial palsy, and regional lymphadenopathy. The existence of CXPA reflects the importance of adequate resection of benign PAs to negative margins.

The transformation of PA goes through phases recognized morphologically as carcinoma in situ (retained myoepithelial layer, see **Fig. 26**), intracapsular carcinoma (see **Figs. 27–29**), microinvasive carcinoma (<5 mm extracapsular invasion), and invasive carcinoma. The malignant component is often a high-grade carcinoma such as adenocarcinoma not otherwise specified (ANOS) or salivary duct carcinoma (see **Figs. 21–25**). Occasionally, it is adenosquamous, undifferentiated, small cell, or sarcomatoid carcinoma. Low-grade carcinoma may also occur. Residual PA is represented by chondroid stroma, residual hyalinized or calcified areas, thick fluffy elastic fibers (elastic stain), and immunohistochemical demonstration of S100, actin or p63-positive spindle cells in the hyalinized areas. Most PAs (70%), including those in skin and soft tissues, have diagnostic chromosomal aberrations and overexpression of PLAG1 and HMGA2 (see **Table 2**).[46,47] In addition, HER2, MIB-1, and p53 are involved in the early changes of PA.[45]

Reported survival rates vary significantly. This is explained by the various phases of transformation, tumor type, and degree of extracapsular invasion. Prognosis of CXPA may be predicted based on a noninvasive, minimally invasive, or invasive classification. Up to 70% of patients will develop locoregional recurrence and/or distant metastases, including sites such as lung, bone, abdomen, and central nervous system, in descending order of frequency.[45] Historical studies show a 5-year overall survival ranging from 22% to 65%.[48] A more recent population study found a 5-year overall survival of 49.1%, consistent with previous studies.[40]

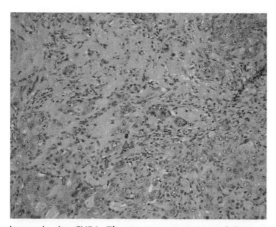

Fig. 26. Adenocarcinoma in situ CXPA. The tumor presents as a 2.5 cm parotid mass in a 68-year-old man. There is diffuse atypia involving the ductal lining cells, with frequent mitoses (*arrowhead*). The myoepithelial layer (*arrows*) is preserved and without atypia. There is no intracapsular carcinoma. The patient is alive and free of disease at 2-year follow-up. H&E 200×.

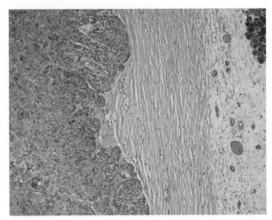

Fig. 27. Intracapsular squamous CXPA. This is a 2.2 cm submandibular tumor in a 77-year-old woman, composed of pure keratinizing squamous carcinoma confined within the capsule of the parent PA. The tumor is to the left and benign parotid is seen in the upper right. The thick capsule is seen in the center. Keratin pearls are readily identified in the carcinoma. H&E 100×.

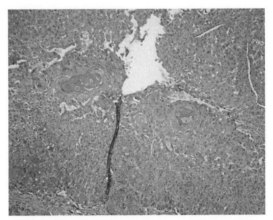

Fig. 28. Intracapsular squamous CXPA. Same tumor as **Fig. 27**, showing sheets of squamous carcinoma without glandular formations or goblet cells. H&E 100×.

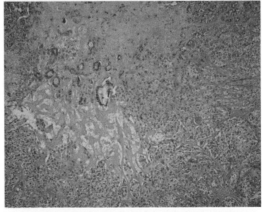

Fig. 29. Intracapsular squamous CXPA. Same tumor as **Fig. 27**, showing residual PA, which is nearly completely overrun by the carcinoma. These residual tubules and stromal mucin justifiably raise the differential diagnoses of adenosquamous carcinoma and high-grade MEC, respectively. H&E 100×.

ADENOCARCINOMA NOT OTHERWISE SPECIFIED

Many of the parotid malignancies are by definition adenocarcinoma. ANOS is a waste-basket diagnosis for malignant salivary tumors that by definition exhibit ductal differentiation but lack resemblance to other well-defined salivary gland malignancies (**Figs. 26–29**). The exact definition of ANOS is vague; therefore, the reported incidence of ANOS is quite variable, making it a more common parotid tumor in some series and less common in others.[53] This raises the question of whether these tumors may represent dedifferentiated tumors that no longer express their typical markers. ANOS is often lumped together with SDC. As with SDC, patients with ANOS will typically behave like a high-grade tumor. A grading system based on the extent of gland formation is proposed: high-grade ANOS should be distinguished from low-grade ANOS based on nuclear atypia, high mitotic rate, atypical mitotic figures, necrosis, perineural invasion, bony invasion, angiolymphatic invasion, and an aggressive pattern of invasion.[53,54]

PRESENTATION AND WORK-UP OF A PAROTID MASS

The most common presentation of a parotid tumor is an asymptomatic preauricular mass. The following features increase concern for malignancy: rapid growth rate, pain, facial tics or weakness, trismus, local soft tissue or bone invasion, and enlarged cervical lymph nodes. Pain occurs in up to 40% of malignant tumors and may be associated with perineural invasion. Facial nerve dysfunction can be seen in up to 25% of malignant parotid tumors and predicts a worse disease outcome.[55]

Imaging supplements physical findings, especially for larger and deeper tumors. Imaging is especially useful when there is limited tumor mobility, deep lobe disease, and/or suspected malignancy. Both computed tomography (CT) and magnetic resonance imaging (MRI) play an important role in evaluating parotid tumors. CT scans are ideal for ruling out lymphadenopathy and bony involvement; whereas MRI is better at assessing parapharyngeal space (PPS) involvement and perineural invasion. In dynamic contrast enhancement MRI, malignant salivary gland tumors typically show rapid enhancement and slow washout of the contrast agent. In diffusion-weighted MRI, the apparent diffusion coefficient of malignant tumors is generally lower than that of benign tumors. Ultrasound is not as informative as CT or MRI scans; it is most useful in assisting image-guided needle biopsies. There is an increasing use of PET; however, PET lacks specificity for malignancy because benign tumors may also have fluorodeoxyglucose (FDG) avidity. PET-CT may be useful in assessing regional and distant metastases in the patient with a biopsy-proven malignancy. A retrospective review of 55 patients with salivary gland cancer found that PET-CT scan contributed to disease management in 47% of patients, often identifying the need for additional surgery.[56]

Current imaging technologies are limited diagnostically; therefore, needle biopsy becomes useful when malignancy is suspected. FNA is most useful in distinguishing between primary salivary tumors and non-neoplastic inflammatory or infectious processes, lymphoma, and metastases from other nonsalivary primary sites. FNA is performed with a 21-gauge needle and has a 79% accuracy in discriminating between benign and malignant histology.[57] Judicious use of immunohistochemical stains assists in differentiating between benign and malignant tumors; however, there is still a high false-negative rate such that cancer cannot ever be adequately ruled out with needle biopsy.[58] Even so, an incisional biopsy should never be performed on an indeterminate FNA because this may place the facial nerve at risk and increase the risk of recurrence. An ultrasound-guided core needle biopsy is an alternative safe option for tissue sampling and enhanced diagnostic accuracy.[59,60]

A complete preoperative workup allows for formulation of a working American Joint Commission on Cancer (AJCC) clinical stage (**Table 5**). The clinical stage and other patient and tumor-related factors are then integrated into a treatment plan. There are some concerns regarding the latest staging system for parotid cancers. In a Japanese study of parotid cancers, only 0.8% (9/1074) of patients had stage III designation, which begs validation on whether this is a balanced enough staging system.[57]

SURGICAL MANAGEMENT

Surgery is the mainstay of treatment for malignant salivary gland tumors. Surgery should be pursued when negative surgical margins can be achieved. Most parotid tumors are confined to the superficial lobe and require a superficial parotidectomy with only 10% to 20% of tumors involving the deep lobe. Only 1% of parotid tumors involve the accessory lobe.

Careful planning should precede any operation to assure negative margins and, in parotid tumors, preservation of the facial nerve when preoperative imaging and physical examination do not suggest invasion. Intraoperative assessment of the nerve is required to identify early nerve invasion not detected on preoperative imaging. The authors recommend facial nerve monitoring during parotid surgery, especially for large, possibly malignant tumors and/or when facial nerve resection and grafting may be necessary. Every effort is spent to preserve this nerve when it is not directly invaded by cancer; however, the surgeon should be prepared to perform a total parotidectomy with nerve resection and facial reanimation in cases of preoperative facial nerve palsy. The operation may extend into the temporal bone to allow for a proximal negative margin resection of the facial nerve. Intraoperative frozen section helps define histology and guides surgical execution.[61] Locoregional control of disease remains the most important predictor of long-term outcome and disease-specific survival.

Adequate exposure is essential to allow for safe facial nerve identification. The parotid is exposed by either the modified Blair incision or the facelift incision.[62] The modified Blair incision is preferable for larger anterior tumors and can be extended into the neck to allow for a same-stage node dissection as necessary. A subplatysmal flap is created in the neck and connected to a facial skin flap elevated above the superficial musculoaponeurotic system (SMAS). The flap can be thinned as necessary to obtain negative margins. The overlying skin and soft tissues should be resected in continuity with the tumor if invaded.

The dissection begins in the preauricular region adjacent to the tragal cartilage dissecting in a broad fashion for best exposure. Bipolar cautery offers precision, hemostasis, and minimizes heat injury to the facial nerve. The facial nerve main trunk is usually reliably identified using the following landmarks: the tympanomastoid suture, the tragal cartilaginous pointer, and the digastric muscle ridge on the mastoid bone. The nerve is in a plane superficial to the styloid process.

Large tumors may prevent the usual preauricular approach to facial nerve identification, in which case two alternative approaches exist: antegrade and retrograde. The antegrade approach involves identifying the nerve at the stylomastoid foramen by removal of the mastoid process with large rongeurs. This may require a formal mastoidectomy when the cancer invades the temporal bone or facial nerve at the stylomastoid foramen. A lateral or subtotal temporal bone resection[63] via an infratemporal fossa approach[64] may be necessary to clear tumors that invade the ear canal and temporal bone. An otologic surgeon should be involved with these advanced tumors.

Table 5
Tumor-nodes-metastasis classification for malignant salivary gland tumors (parotid, submandibular, and sublingual)

Primary Tumor (T)

Tx	Primary tumor cannot be assessed
T0	No evidence of primary tumor
Tis	Carcinoma in situ
T1	Tumor = 2 cm in greatest dimension without extraparenchymal extension (clinical or macroscopic evidence of invasion of the soft tissues, not microscopic evidence)
T2	Tumor>2 cm but not more than 4 cm in greatest dimension without extraparenchymal extension
T3	Tumor>4 cm and/or tumor has extraparenchymal extension
T4a	Moderately advanced disease Tumor invades the skin, mandible, and/or facial nerve
T4b	Very advanced disease Tumor invades skull base and/or pterygoid plates and/or encases carotid artery

Regional lymph nodes (N)

Nx	Regional nodes cannot be assessed
N0	No regional lymph node metastasis
N1	Metastasis in a single ipsilateral lymph node = 3 cm in greatest dimension
N2	Metastasis in a single ipsilateral lymph node>3 cm but not more than 6 cm in greatest dimension; or in multiple ipsilateral lymph nodes, none>6 cm in greatest dimension; or in bilateral or contralateral lymph nodes, none>6 cm in greatest dimension
N2a	Metastasis in a single ipsilateral lymph node>3 cm but not more than 6 cm in greatest dimension
N2b	Metastasis in multiple ipsilateral lymph nodes, none>6 cm in greatest dimension
N2c	Metastasis in bilateral or contralateral lymph nodes, none>6 cm in greatest dimension
N3	Metastasis in a lymph node>6 cm in greatest dimension

Distant metastasis (M)

M0	No distant metastasis
M1	Distant metastasis

Stage	T	N	M
Anatomic stage or prognostic groups			
0	Tis	N0	M0
I	T1	N0	M0
II	T2	N0	M0
III	T3	N0	M0
	T1–T3	N1	M0
IVA	T4a	N0–N1	M0
	T1–T4a	N2	M0
IVB	T Any	N3	M0
	T4b	any N	M0
IVC	T Any	N Any	M1

Adapted from Edge SB, Byrd DR, Compton CC, et al. AJCC cancer staging manual. 7th edition. New York: Springer; 2010; with permission.

The retrograde approach finds the distal branches first. The buccal branch adjacent to Stenson duct and superficial to the masseter is identified and followed back toward the main trunk.[65] Alternatively the marginal nerve is identified at the inferior border of the mandible and followed proximally. There is tremendous variability in the extratemporal branching patterns of the facial nerve. The tumor is elevated off the uninvaded nerve branches in progression until gross tumor clearance is achieved.

Most patients (83%) will present with a clinically negative neck (N0).[66] The role of elective neck dissection in this setting has not been well established but should be considered in the high-stage, high-grade cancers. Alternatively, elective neck radiation may be given; however, the performance of elective neck radiation versus elective neck dissection in management of the N0 neck remains controversial. Either approach is supported by a 20% rate of occult neck metastases and with a 5% locoregional failure rate after treatment; however, the risk varies significantly by histology. SDC, ANOS, and high-grade MEC carry the highest risk of lymph node involvement.[67]

The optimal extent of a neck dissection in N0 cases is unclear. Supraomohyoid neck dissection addresses the most at-risk nodes in levels II and III. Routine sampling of the level II and III lymph nodes improves staging and helps decide the extent of neck dissection to perform. Inclusion of level IV nodes is supported by published reports of skip metastases.[68] The rate of recurrence in level V nodes is low enough in clinically N0 necks such that a routine level V neck dissection is not warranted. The role of lymphoscintigraphy and sentinel node biopsy in the setting of N0 neck is yet to be defined.[69]

The overall distribution of cervical disease in primary parotid carcinoma with N+ disease is broad. A pooled analysis of 3 published topographic nodal distribution reports found that 28% of N+ cases had involvement of level I, 59% of level II, 52% of level III, 38% of level IV, and 41% of level V. Ipsilateral skip metastases to level V were frequent.[70] The investigators make a strong case for a comprehensive neck dissection of all ipsilateral nodal levels in all parotid cancers with clinical evidence of nodal metastasis.

RECONSTRUCTIVE CONSIDERATIONS

Reconstruction aims to restore facial contour, improve facial nerve function, and prevent Frey syndrome. A variety of techniques have been described to restore parotidectomy-associated contour deformities. These techniques include acellular dermal implants (AlloDerm [Lifecell] and DermaMatrix [Synthes]), nonvascularized fat grafts, dermal-fat grafts, and autologous regional vascularized flaps (platysma, SMAS, temporoparietal fascia, sternocleidomastoid muscle, pectoralis major muscle with or without skin, and supraclavicular island flap).[71] For larger volume defects, microvascular free-flaps are used, such as rectus abdominis myocutaneous flap, lateral arm flap, radial forearm flap, gracilis or latissimus dorsi neurovascular free-muscle transfer, deep inferior epigastric perforator flap, and anterolateral thigh flap.[72]

The anterolateral thigh flap is a favored flap for the large total parotidectomy defect because it allows for simultaneous 2-team surgery, minimal donor site morbidity, and the ability to sculpt and match tissue type. The tensor fascia lata is exposed while harvesting which can be then used for facial static suspension procedures. Patients with anticipated postoperative radiation are reconstructed with an estimated overcorrection of free flap tissue bulk to account for future radiation-induced tissue contracture. This allows for desirable long-term soft tissue volume and facial symmetry despite radiation therapy. Placement of healthy vascularized soft tissue in the parotidectomy bed is thought to be a necessary prerequisite to facial nerve grafting and reanimation procedures.[73] In addition, placement of soft tissue may reduce the risk and severity of Frey Syndrome (see later discussion).[69,74,75]

Facial nerve repair is best done at the time of the extirpative surgery. Earlier repair leads to better outcomes. Brachytherapy and radiation do not affect results attainable with facial nerve grafts.[76] Reconstruction of the facial nerve is usually done with an interposition graft, using the sural nerve or cervical nerves identified during neck dissection. Other techniques include hypoglossal to facial nerve (XII-VII) jump graft versus crossover. XII-VII jump graft is thought to be superior to direct XII-VII crossover because it prevents tongue disability. A hybrid method of interposition graft for the upper division and XII-VII jump graft for the lower division is preferable because it avoids upper and lower face synkinesis.[77] The greater auricular nerve may be used for both the upper and lower reanimation. Nerve regeneration occurs within 12 to 16 months.

A gold weight may be inserted into the upper eyelid in the same surgery to improve eye closure and decrease dryness.[77] Furthermore, facial reanimation may include plastic surgical techniques such as rhytidectomy, blepharoplasty, brow lift, canthopexy, and lid-tightening procedures. Midface suspension with AlloDerm, temporalis tendon, or tensor fascia lata is another adjunctive restoration technique.[78]

COMPLICATIONS

Most reports on postoperative complications are in the context of parotidectomy predominately for benign disease and cases without adjuvant radiation therapy.[79] Complications of radiation are discussed separately with radiation treatment. Surgical complications are presented here.

Sialocele

Sialocele, or drainage of saliva into the tissues, is a known complication following surgery of the salivary glands and can cause significant problems for the patient and surgeon when it occurs. They often are self-limited but can be associated with delayed wound healing, increased utilization of clinic resources and frustration. The use of products such as Surgicel [Ethicon], AlloDerm, and DermaMatrix increases the risk of postoperative sialocele formation.[80]

Facial Nerve Palsy

Facial nerve palsy is not uncommon after parotidectomy. The reported rate of facial nerve palsy is 0.7% in a series of both benign and malignant tumors.[79] This increases to 16% for malignant disease in which the nerve or branches were not intentionally sacrificed. Temporary facial nerve palsy can occur in 42% of surgeries with 38% of these resolving within one month and 78% resolving within three months. Palsy is significantly higher in patients undergoing deep lobe or total parotidectomy (90%) but does not seem to be affected by radiation.[79] Use of the nerve stimulator does not affect the incidence of facial nerve palsy. Large tumors (>4 cm) and nerve infiltration are associated with higher rates of postoperative palsy.

Frey Syndrome

Frey syndrome was first described in 1923 by Lucia Frey, a Polish neurologist. After parotid surgery, traumatized auriculotemporal postganglionic parasympathetic nerve fibers reinnervate the sweat glands and subcutaneous vessels, resulting in gustatory sweating and facial flushing. Few patients report symptoms despite objective testing indicating an extremely high prevalence. The objective and subjective rates of Frey syndrome may vary greatly with reported rates of 79% and 40%, respectively, in a review of 7 studies.[81] Furthermore, positive starch-iodine tests may reach as high as 95% with a correlating survey rate of 35% and unsolicited rate of 10%.[81]

Preventive and treatment strategies are wide ranging. Preventive strategies with some potential efficacy include sub-SMAS elevation of the skin flap,[82] interposition of fat grafts,[10] or acellular dermal matrix,[83] and/or vascularized autologous flaps.[74] Treatment strategies include topical antiperspirants, anticholinergic creams, tympanic neurectomy, Botulinum toxin, radiation therapy, and revision surgery with soft tissue interposition. The results are variable and are beyond the scope of this review.

First Bite Syndrome

First bite syndrome (FBS) refers to facial pain characterized by a severe cramping or spasm in the parotid region with the first bite of each meal that diminishes during the next several bites. Most cases have been described in the postoperative setting; there are reports of this syndrome in the preoperative setting in patients with deep lobe parotid or PPS tumors.[84,85] It is a potential sequela of surgery involving the infratemporal fossa, PPS, and/or deep lobe of the parotid gland. FBS developed in 48.6% of patients undergoing sympathetic chain sacrifice, 22.4% of patients undergoing PPS dissection, 38.4% of patients undergoing isolated deep lobe parotid resection, and 0.8% of patients undergoing total parotidectomy. Partial resolution of FBS symptoms occurred in 69% and complete resolution in 12%. Of 45 FBS patients, 15 (33%) underwent at least one type of treatment for symptomatic relief.[86] No treatment was consistently effective. Patients undergoing surgery with dissection and/or manipulation of the deep lobe or PPS structures should be thoroughly counseled about the risk of developing FBS.

RADIATION THERAPY

Low-stage, low-grade tumors can generally be cured by surgery alone. Postoperative radiotherapy improves locoregional control and is usually reserved in the adjuvant setting for cancers with high-risk features, including close or positive surgical margins, nodal metastases, extracapsular spread (ECS), perineural invasion, lymphovascular invasion, advanced tumor (T) stage, and high-grade histopathology (see **Table 3**). All patients with ACCa should receive adjuvant radiation.[87] Radiation may also be considered for deep lobe and/or recurrent cancers. High doses (>60 Gy) are necessary to achieve maximal local tumor control in the adjuvant setting.

The benefit of adjuvant radiation is derived from retrospective reviews. Selection bias aside, patients with poor prognostic features who are selected for combined therapy have improved locoregional control.[88,89] The benefit holds true even for low-grade tumors with positive margins or ECS.[10] The Dutch Head and Neck Oncology Cooperative Group showed a relative risk of local recurrence in surgery-alone patients that was 9.7 times higher than patients treated with surgery and radiation together.[90] A SEER database analysis of 2170 patients treated between 1988 and 2005 showed improved survival for high-grade and/or locally advanced malignant major salivary gland tumors treated with adjuvant radiation therapy (hazard ratio [HR] 0.76, 95% CI: 0.65–0.89, $P<.001$).[91]

Radiation therapy either alone or in combination with chemotherapy may be used in the definitive management of medically or technically unresectable tumors at a higher dose of 66 Gy or more. Clinical complete response is not uncommon in this setting and may be seen in nearly two-thirds of cases, half of which are treated with radiation alone.[92] Furthermore, there was a significant opportunity for facial nerve preservation in those rendered resectable after upfront therapeutic radiation. Factors predictive of a partial response to definitive radiation include size greater than 4 cm, T4 stage cancer, and stage IV disease.

Options for radiation therapy include electron beam, photon beam, and particle beam (proton, neutron, carbon ion) therapies.[93,94] Particle beam therapy has shown the highest local control rates in ACCa.[95] Electron beam therapy may be used for superficial parotid lesions. Photon beam radiotherapy is most commonly used through modern techniques such as intensity modulated radiation therapy (IMRT). IMRT allows precise dose escalation to the primary tumor site with significant reductions in dose exposure to normal tissues; however, it is subject to significant interobserver variability in segmentation of the postoperative clinical target volumes and organs at risk.[96] Inaccuracies may unnecessarily treat the healthy surrounding tissue or risk marginal tumor recurrence.[97] A novel mixed-beam therapy is currently being investigated in the COSMIC (combined treatment of malignant salivary gland tumors with intensity modulated radiation therapy and carbon ions) trial[98] in which potential advantages include homogeneity in target dose distribution and maximal sparing of normal tissues. Preliminary results are promising and show 3-year local control, PFS, and OS of 81.9%, 57.9%, and 78.4%, respectively.[99]

The acute toxicities of radiation therapy include mucositis, dysphagia, xerostomia, dermatitis, and pain.[96] The late radiation-induced toxicities include xerostomia (60%–90%), grade 3 dysphagia (15%–30%), osteoradionecrosis of the jaw and/or temporal bone (5%–15%), permanent sensorineural hearing loss (40%–60%), skin fibrosis, and laryngeal chondronecrosis. These late effects are permanent and considerably reduce quality of life for the patient. Radiation induced secondary malignancy such as radiation-induced sarcoma is another reported late complication of radiation therapy for malignant parotid tumors.[100]

CHEMOTHERAPY

Chemotherapy trials frequently include a heterogeneous group of parotid cancers and as such are difficult to interpret. Systemic therapy in malignant parotid tumors is mainly used in the palliative setting in patients with metastatic or recurrent disease.[101] Multiple agents and regimens have been studied. The most active single agents include cisplatin, cyclophosphamide, doxorubicin, and 5-fluorouracil.[101] A study of combination therapy with cyclophosphamide, doxorubicin, and cisplatin showed a response rate of 60%, effective for ANOS but not ACCa.[102] In general, combination chemotherapy response rates are between 15% to 70% with a median response duration of 6 to 7 months. In general, multiagent chemotherapy does not seem to offer a survival advantage compared with single-agent chemotherapy. Polychemotherapy with cisplatin or carboplatin may offer higher response rates compared with monochemotherapy but at the expense of increased toxicity and with no proven survival advantage. The decision to use platinum alone or as combination chemotherapy should be individualized based on patient specific considerations. Further research is needed in this area.

Other agents, including taxol, have been studied but show minimum effect. Evaluation of paclitaxel in a phase II ECOG trial (E1394) for metastatic or recurrent salivary gland tumors found a partial response rate of 25% among patients with adenocarcinoma or MEC but no responses among those patients with ACCa. No survival benefit was appreciated either overall or among histologic subtypes.[103] Treatment with paclitaxel is currently not standard treatment.

Chemoradiotherapy may be considered in the postoperative adjuvant setting for indicators of locoregional failure, including perineural invasion, positive margins, nodal involvement, or T3 or T4 stage tumors.[82] Multiple regimens have been evaluated in the adjuvant setting. All were limited by poor overall accrual, heterogeneity of tumor histology, and the long latency period of ACCa recurrence, which skews the results.[104] In the high-risk adjuvant setting, postoperative platinum-based concurrent chemoradiation was demonstrated superior to radiation alone with 3-year overall survival rates of 83% versus 44% ($P = .05$).[105] This potential advantage is further queried in the radiation therapy oncology group (RTOG) 1008 randomized phase II/III study of adjuvant concurrent radiation and weekly cisplatin versus radiation alone in resected high-risk malignant salivary gland tumors, including high-grade MEC, SDC, and high-grade adenocarcinoma. ACCa is not included. This study is currently accruing patients (clinicaltrials.gov). Again, adjuvant treatment with concurrent chemoradiation should be decided on a case-by-case basis at this point.

ACCa often behaves differently than other high-grade tumors. The indolent course makes it less likely to exhibit an objective response to chemotherapy. Evaluation of clinical trials exclusively for ACCa was undertaken by Laurie and colleagues.[106] Only modest gains were appreciated at best from cytotoxic, hormonal, or targeted agents. The routine use of chemotherapy in ACCa is not supported outside of clinical trials.

MOLECULAR TARGETED THERAPIES

The development of novel drugs against molecular targets in epithelial malignancies have led to intensive investigations on molecular profiling of salivary cancers for both prognostication and targeting. Overexpression rates of hormone receptors, EGFR, HER2, and c-kit vary according to published series that highlight the remarkable diversity of these tumors and lack of standardized methodology. Expression rates of various markers are listed in **Table 6**. So far, the results of various phase II trials of targeted therapies directed against one or several of these targets in the management of patients with advanced disease have been disappointing.[33]

Despite high rate of c-kit positivity in ACCa, several phase II trials of tyrosine kinase inhibitors in ACCa fail to demonstrate a significant benefit. Four trials using imatinib in 75 subjects have found only 5 partial responses; 2 with imatinib alone, and 3 in combination with cisplatin.[34] Only one study reported stable disease in more than 50% of subjects over 6 months.[109] There have been similar lackluster response rates for sunitinib, lapatinib, and dasatinib.[34,110,111] The disappointing results may again be explained by the indolent nature of ACCa and the long periods of stable disease appreciated without any therapeutic intervention.

EGFR protein expression is common in salivary gland tumors but is not associated with gene-activating mutations. EGFR expression does not correlate with outcome or prognosis. Nonetheless, a select but currently unknown group of patients with salivary

Table 6
Hormonal and molecular marker expression in salivary cancers

	EGFR	HER2	c-kit	VEGF	Estrogen Receptor or Progesterone Receptor	Androgen Receptor
MEC	Moderate	Moderate[a]	Rare	Moderate	Rare	Rare
ANOS	Moderate	Moderate	Rare	High	Rare	Rare
SDC	Moderate	High	Rare	High	Rare	Very high
ACC	Low	Rare	Very high	Very high	Rare	Rare

Hormonal and molecular marker expression varies by histologic subtype. Their relative expression is listed as rare, low, moderate, high, or very high expressing tumors.
[a] Usually in high-grade tumors.
Data from Refs.[33,107,108]

gland carcinomas might potentially benefit from anti-EGFR therapy. So far, anti-EGFR therapies have also failed to show measurable tumor responses in phase II studies; however, studies of cetuximab and gefitinib show significant long-term disease stabilization in ACCa.[112,113] Such results are encouraging.

Trastuzumab in combination with taxanes has changed the way HER2-positive breast cancers are treated. Similar studies are being attempted in certain salivary gland cancers. A phase II study of trastuzumab in salivary cancer difficulty accruing due to a limited number of cases and showed only one partial response with trastuzumab in a patient with metastatic MEC out of 14 evaluable subjects.[114] Approximately 80% of SDCs expressed HER2, and a few case studies report good responses with trastuzumab in the treatment of metastatic SDC.[115,116] Expression of HER2 in ACCa does not play a major role in the management of ACCa (<5% expression), although solid variants of ACCa show a significantly greater expression of HER2 compared with tubular or cribriform variants.

Androgen receptor-positive SDC is a distinct disease entity within salivary gland tumors. Androgen deprivation therapy with bicalutamide has shown efficacy in small case series of SDC.[117] Clinical benefit was seen in 50% of cases of androgen receptor-positive SDC. Jaspers and colleagues[117] propose antiandrogen therapy be used as first line of defense against metastasized SDC, followed by trastuzumab with chemotherapy for progressive disease. This strategy warrants further investigation.

Vander Poorten and colleagues[57] provide a detailed review on advances in molecular biology of parotid cancers. The details provided are beyond the scope of this article. More sophisticated approaches to identification of putative molecular targets will be required before any standard application of molecular targeting drugs in clinical applications can be recommended. International collaborations in designing histopathology-specific clinical trials with integrated translational components are necessary to further the understanding of these cancers.

PROGNOSIS

Prognostic factors relating to the patient, histology, stage, and management account for variability in cure rates. Vander Poorten and colleagues[22] developed a prognostic model for disease-free survival in parotid cancer based on both pretherapeutic and post-therapeutic factors. Pretherapeutic factors include pain on presentation, age at diagnosis, T stage, nodal (N) stage, skin invasion, and facial nerve dysfunction. Post-therapeutic factors include age at diagnosis, T stage, N stage, skin invasion, facial nerve dysfunction, perineural invasion, and positive margins. A higher score is associated with a lower survival. A broader model for overall survival for salivary cancers was proposed by van der Schroeff and colleagues.[118] They found the following factors predictive in their multivariate analysis: sex, tumor size, N stage and metastasis (M) stage, localization, comorbidity, skin involvement, and pain. Histology did not seem to have a major additive value in either model proposed.

These models are supported in the literature, which suggest worse prognosis with trismus, bone invasion, facial nerve weakness, size greater than 4 cm, nodal metastasis, and recurrence. Facial nerve impairment before resection is a strong predictor of shorter disease-free survival as is associated with larger tumors and a higher histologic grade of malignancy.[55] Furthermore, microscopic findings, such as high-grade, advanced nodal metastasis, perineural invasion, ECS, and close or positive margins are negative prognostic factors.[10] ECS and margin status substantially improved the prediction of disease recurrence compared with cancer grade alone, supporting postoperative radiotherapy even for low-risk histologies in the presence of positive margins or ECS.[10] Advanced nodal disease predicts worse relapse-free (N2 vs N0-1, HR 3.05, $P = .002$) and overall survival (N2 vs N0-1, HR 3.11, $P = .001$).[119] The median overall survival for patients with N0 to N1 stage was 6.6 years compared with 2.8 years for patients with N2 stage, even with the addition of adjuvant radiation therapy ($P = .003$).

PEDIATRIC PATIENTS

With an annual incidence of less than 1 per million, salivary gland malignancies in children are rare, constituting less than 10% of pediatric head and neck cancers. Fewer histologic subtypes are generally encountered in children. MEC is the most common histologic type, followed by AcCC. The overall prognosis is often favorable with complete surgical resection. Sultan and colleagues[120] reported that children and adolescents had more favorable tumors with well to moderately well differentiated histology (88% vs 49% in adults, $P<.001$) and no extension to adjacent tissues or lymphatic spread (76% vs 50% in adults, $P<.001$). Furthermore, children and adolescents enjoyed superior 5-year overall survival (95% +/−1.5% vs 59% +/− 0.5% for adults, $P<.001$).

A French multicenter retrospective study of 38 children and adolescents treated for MEC between 1980 and 2010 was conducted. Parotid subsite, low-grade, and early primary-stage tumors were encountered in 81%, 82%, and 68% of cases, respectively. All except 1 patient were treated by primary site surgery, and 53% by neck dissection (80% of high-grade cases). Postoperative radiation therapy and chemotherapy were performed in 29% and 11% of cases. With a median 62-month follow-up, overall survival and local control rates were 95% and 84%, respectively. There was 1 nodal relapse. Like adults, neck dissection is recommended in high-grade tumors. Radiation therapy should be proposed for high-grade and/or advanced primary-stage MEC. For high-grade tumors without massive neck involvement, irradiation volumes may be limited to the primary area, given the risk of long-term side effects of radiation therapy in children.[121]

The MD Anderson Cancer Center study of 61 pediatric patients showed that most tumors arose in the parotid gland (83%), and the most common pathologic condition was MEC (46%). Lymphatic metastasis was identified in 37% of patients, nearly all with MEC. Although 65% of patients had prior treatment elsewhere, more than 75% of patients underwent surgical resection. External beam radiation was used in 45% of patients for (1) close or positive surgical margins, (2) gross residual disease, (3) high-grade lesions, and (4) for those with ACCa or adenocarcinoma, with an average dose of 58.6 Gy. Average patient follow-up was 153 months. The overall survival rate was 93% at 5 years, and 26% developed a recurrence. Particular to salivary gland cancers, recurrences beyond 5 years were common, with the locoregional recurrences presenting at a median of 8 years after treatment.[122]

The addition of radiotherapy in the treatment of pediatric cancers is fraught with risks, including facial dysmorphism, growth disruption, dental complications, hearing loss, endocrine dysfunction, cataracts, cognitive dysfunction, and the development of radiation-associated neoplasms. There are some reports in the literature that 5% to 10% of children treated for first malignancy have developed subsequent second tumors with long-term follow-up. The important radiation-induced second malignant tumors are central nervous system tumors, thyroid tumors, osteosarcoma, soft tissue sarcomas, and nonmelanoma skin cancer. Long-term follow-up of pediatric patients treated with radiation therapy is necessary with particular attention to development and survivorship issues.

To date, no prospective or retrospective data comparing outcomes of surgery alone versus multimodality therapy in the management of salivary gland malignancies in the pediatric population exists. Consequently, management decisions are made on a case-by-case basis, taking prognosis, treatment-related morbidity, and long-term sequelae into account.[123]

SURVEILLANCE

Lifetime surveillance is recommended to detect disease relapse,[95] address survivorship issues, and diagnose potential second primary cancers.[124]

Risk factors for disease recurrence after treatment include advanced local disease, incomplete surgical resection with positive margins, bone invasion, named nerve involvement, nodal involvement, and high histopathologic grading. Surgery, irradiation or reirradiation with or without chemotherapy and/or targeted therapy are treatment options for locoregional relapse (see previous discussion).[125] Unfortunately treatment options are limited and frequently ineffective.

Distant metastasis is the most common cause for treatment failure. The lungs are the most common site of distant metastasis (65%), followed by bone (13%), and then liver and brain (4% each). ACCa is the most common histology (47%), followed by ANOS (20%).[126] Although regional treatment failure can be a predictive factor for distant metastasis, distant metastasis can occur irrespective of locoregional control. The risk of developing distant metastasis remains for life for all histologic subtypes; therefore, it is recommended that all patients undergoing treatment of malignant salivary gland tumor be clinically assessed at least once annually for life.[126,127] Even low-risk tumors may recur. Of those that recur, 90% will recur within the first 5 years, supporting follow-up for at least 5 years in this group.[10,127]

Management of metastatic disease depends on histology, number of metastases, site of metastasis, and presence of symptoms; and may include radiotherapy, chemotherapy, targeted therapy, or a combination thereof. Oligometastasis resection may offer a benefit in a select few patients.[128–130]

Patients with major salivary gland cancers are also at a risk for certain second primary cancers, even 10 years out from the diagnosis and treatment of the primary cancer. This highlights the need for long-term surveillance in these patients, not only for recurrence but also for second primary cancers.[124]

SUMMARY

Salivary gland tumors are a heterogeneous group of tumors that behave quite differently based on the histology. Immunohistochemistry and the discovery of unique translocations and gene fusions have allowed for better characterization as well as the discovery of new histologic subtypes. Management of salivary cancers should be considered in a multidisciplinary fashion with attention to prognostic features. Surgery remains the mainstay of therapy and occasionally warrants more radical operations to achieve complete resection. Reconstructive techniques have evolved to improve cosmetic and functional outcomes. Adjuvant radiation therapy plays a major role in locoregional disease control in high-risk cases. Chemotherapy is mainly used for inoperable, recurrent, or metastatic disease, with a modest response at best. The role of molecular targeted therapies is being actively investigated. Lifetime surveillance is recommended to detect disease relapse, address survivorship issues, and identify and treat potential second primary cancers. Enrollment of patients with salivary cancer onto carefully designed clinical trials is critical for better understanding of these cancers and progress in management.

REFERENCES

1. Namboodiripad PC. A review: Immunological markers for malignant salivary gland tumors. J Oral Biol Craniofac Res 2014;4:127–34.
2. Saku T, Hayashi Y, Takahara O, et al. Salivary gland tumors among atomic bomb survivors, 1950-1987. Cancer 1997;79:1465–75.
3. Shang J, Sheng L, Wang K, et al. Expression of neural cell adhesion molecule in salivary adenoid cystic carcinoma and its correlation with perineural invasion. Oncol Rep 2007;18:1413–6.
4. Fortson JK, Rosenthal M, Patel V, et al. Atypical presentation of mucoepidermoid carcinoma after radiation therapy for the treatment of keloids. Ear Nose Throat J 2012;91:286–8.
5. Klubo-Gwiezdzinska J, Van Nostrand D, Burman KD, et al. Salivary gland malignancy and radioiodine therapy for thyroid cancer. Thyroid 2010;20:647–51.
6. Duan Y, Zhang HZ, Bu RF. Correlation between cellular phone use and epithelial parotid gland malignancies. Int J Oral Maxillofac Surg 2011;40:966–72.
7. Descamps G, Duray A, Rodriguez A, et al. Detection and quantification of human papillomavirus in benign and malignant parotid lesions. Anticancer Res 2012;32:3929–32.
8. Donaldson CD, Jack RH, Moller H, et al. Oral cavity, pharyngeal and salivary gland cancer: disparities in ethnicity-specific incidence among the London population. Oral Oncol 2012;48:799–802.
9. Hunt JL. An update on molecular diagnostics of squamous and salivary gland tumors of the head and neck. Arch Pathol Lab Med 2011;135:602–9.
10. Walvekar RR, Andrade Filho PA, Seethala RR, et al. Clinicopathologic features as stronger prognostic factors than histology or grade in risk stratification of primary parotid malignancies. Head Neck 2011;33:225–31.
11. Stenner M, Klussmann JP. Current update on established and novel biomarkers in salivary gland carcinoma pathology and the molecular pathways involved. Eur Arch Otorhinolaryngol 2009;266:333–41.
12. Andreadis D, Epivatianos A, Poulopoulos A, et al. Detection of C-KIT (CD117) molecule in benign and malignant salivary gland tumours. Oral Oncol 2006;42:57–65.
13. Bishop JA, Yonescu R, Batista D, et al. Mucoepidermoid carcinoma does not harbor transcriptionally active high risk human papillomavirus even in the absence of the MAML2 translocation. Head Neck Pathol 2014;8:298–302.
14. Kimihide K, Tomoko M, Takashi N. Adenosquamous carcinoma of the parotid gland. Histopathology 2013;63:593–5.
15. Shang J, Shui Y, Sheng L, et al. Epidermal growth factor receptor and human epidermal growth receptor 2 expression in parotid mucoepidermoid carcinoma: possible implications for targeted therapy. Oncol Rep 2008;19:435–40.
16. Nakano T, Yamamoto H, Hashimoto K, et al. HER2 and EGFR gene copy number alterations are predominant in high-grade salivary mucoepidermoid carcinoma irrespective of MAML2 fusion status. Histopathology 2013;63:378–92.
17. Seethala RR. An update on grading of salivary gland carcinomas. Head Neck Pathol 2009;3:69–77.
18. Chen MM, Roman SA, Sosa JA, et al. Histologic grade as prognostic indicator for mucoepidermoid carcinoma: a population-level analysis of 2400 patients. Head Neck 2014;36:158–63.
19. Aro K, Leivo I, Makitie AA. Management and outcome of patients with mucoepidermoid carcinoma of major salivary gland origin: a single institution's 30-year experience. Laryngoscope 2008;118:258–62.

20. McHugh CH, Roberts DB, El-Naggar AK, et al. Prognostic factors in mucoepi-dermoid carcinoma of the salivary glands. Cancer 2012;118:3928–36.

21. Ellington CL, Goodman M, Kono SA, et al. Adenoid cystic carcinoma of the head and neck: Incidence and survival trends based on 1973-2007 Surveillance, Epidemiology, and End Results data. Cancer 2012;118:4444–51.

22. Vander Poorten VL, Balm AJ, Hilgers FJ, et al. The development of a prognostic score for patients with parotid carcinoma. Cancer 1999;85:2057–67.

23. Dantas AN, de Morais EF, Macedo RA, et al. Clinicopathological characteristics and perineural invasion in adenoid cystic carcinoma: a systematic review. Braz J Otorhinolaryngol 2015;81:329–35.

24. Bhayani MK, Yener M, El-Naggar A, et al. Prognosis and risk factors for early-stage adenoid cystic carcinoma of the major salivary glands. Cancer 2012; 118:2872–8.

25. Seethala RR, Hunt JL, Baloch ZW, et al. Adenoid cystic carcinoma with high-grade transformation: a report of 11 cases and a review of the literature. Am J Surg Pathol 2007;31:1683–94.

26. Woo VL, Bhuiya T, Kelsch R. Assessment of CD43 expression in adenoid cystic carcinomas, polymorphous low-grade adenocarcinomas, and monomorphic adenomas. Oral Surg Oral Med Oral Pathol Oral Radiol Endod 2006;102: 495–500.

27. Nordgard S, Franzen G, Boysen M, et al. Ki-67 as a prognostic marker in adenoid cystic carcinoma assessed with the monoclonal antibody MIB1 in paraffin sections. Laryngoscope 1997;107:531–6.

28. Persson M, Andren Y, Mark J, et al. Recurrent fusion of MYB and NFIB transcription factor genes in carcinomas of the breast and head and neck. Proc Natl Acad Sci U S A 2009;106:18740–4.

29. Mitani Y, Rao PH, Futreal PA, et al. Novel chromosomal rearrangements and break points at the t(6;9) in salivary adenoid cystic carcinoma: association with MYB-NFIB chimeric fusion, MYB expression, and clinical outcome. Clin Cancer Res 2011;17:7003–14.

30. Epivatianos A, Poulopoulos A, Dimitrakopoulos I, et al. Application of alpha-smooth muscle actin and c-kit in the differential diagnosis of adenoid cystic carcinoma from polymorphous low-grade adenocarcinoma. Oral Oncol 2007;43: 67–76.

31. Moskaluk CA, Frierson HF Jr, El-Naggar AK, et al. C-kit gene mutations in adenoid cystic carcinoma are rare. Mod Pathol 2010;23:905–6 [author reply: 906–7].

32. Lee SK, Kwon MS, Lee YS, et al. Prognostic value of expression of molecular markers in adenoid cystic cancer of the salivary glands compared with lymph node metastasis: a retrospective study. World J Surg Oncol 2012;10:266.

33. Adelstein DJ, Rodriguez CP. What is new in the management of salivary gland cancers? Curr Opin Oncol 2011;23:249–53.

34. Chau NG, Hotte SJ, Chen EX, et al. A phase II study of sunitinib in recurrent and/or metastatic adenoid cystic carcinoma (ACC) of the salivary glands: current progress and challenges in evaluating molecularly targeted agents in ACC. Ann Oncol 2012;23:1562–70.

35. Al-Mamgani A, van Rooij P, Sewnaik A, et al. Adenoid cystic carcinoma of parotid gland treated with surgery and radiotherapy: long-term outcomes, QoL assessment and review of the literature. Oral Oncol 2012;48:278–83.

36. Gao M, Hao Y, Huang MX, et al. Clinicopathological study of distant metastases of salivary adenoid cystic carcinoma. Int J Oral Maxillofac Surg 2013;42:923–8.

37. Lin YC, Chen KC, Lin CH, et al. Clinicopathological features of salivary and non-salivary adenoid cystic carcinomas. Int J Oral Maxillofac Surg 2012;41:354–60.

38. Chenevert J, Duvvuri U, Chiosea S, et al. DOG1: a novel marker of salivary acinar and intercalated duct differentiation. Mod Pathol 2012;25:919–29.

39. Lewis JE, Olsen KD, Weiland LH. Acinic cell carcinoma. Clinicopathologic review. Cancer 1991;67:172–9.

40. Guntinas-Lichius O, Wendt TG, Buentzel J, et al. Incidence, treatment, and outcome of parotid carcinoma, 1996-2011: a population-based study in Thuringia, Germany. J Cancer Res Clin Oncol 2015;141(9):1679–88.

41. Skalova A, Vanecek T, Sima R, et al. Mammary analogue secretory carcinoma of salivary glands, containing the ETV6-NTRK3 fusion gene: a hitherto undescribed salivary gland tumor entity. Am J Surg Pathol 2010;34:599–608.

42. Woo J, Seethala RR, Sirintrapun SJ. Mammary analogue secretory carcinoma of the parotid gland as a secondary malignancy in a childhood survivor of atypical teratoid rhabdoid tumor. Head Neck Pathol 2014;8:194–7.

43. Pisharodi L. Mammary analog secretory carcinoma of salivary gland: cytologic diagnosis and differential diagnosis of an unreported entity. Diagn Cytopathol 2013;41:239–41.

44. Ito S, Ishida E, Skalova A, et al. Case report of Mammary Analog Secretory Carcinoma of the parotid gland. Pathol Int 2012;62:149–52.

45. Gnepp DR, B-GM, El-Naggar AK, et al. World health organization classification of tumours: pathology and genetics of head and neck tumours. Lyon, France: IARC Press; 2005.

46. Bahrami A, Dalton JD, Shivakumar B, et al. PLAG1 alteration in carcinoma ex pleomorphic adenoma: immunohistochemical and fluorescence in situ hybridization studies of 22 cases. Head Neck Pathol 2012;6:328–35.

47. El-Naggar AK, Callender D, Coombes MM, et al. Molecular genetic alterations in carcinoma ex-pleomorphic adenoma: a putative progression model? Genes Chromosomes Cancer 2000;27:162–8.

48. Gnepp DR. Malignant mixed tumors of the salivary glands: a review. Pathol Annu 1993;28(Pt 1):279–328.

49. Johnston ML, Huang SH, Waldron JN, et al. Salivary duct carcinoma: treatment, outcomes, and patterns of failure. Head Neck 2015. [Epub ahead of print].

50. Pons Y, Alves A, Clement P, et al. Salivary duct carcinoma of the parotid. Eur Ann Otorhinolaryngol Head Neck Dis 2011;128:194–6.

51. Clauditz TS, Reiff M, Gravert L, et al. Human epidermal growth factor receptor 2 (HER2) in salivary gland carcinomas. Pathology 2011;43:459–64.

52. Fan CY, Melhem MF, Hosal AS, et al. Expression of androgen receptor, epidermal growth factor receptor, and transforming growth factor alpha in salivary duct carcinoma. Arch Otolaryngol Head Neck Surg 2001;127:1075–9.

53. Li J, Wang BY, Nelson M, et al. Salivary adenocarcinoma, not otherwise specified: a collection of orphans. Arch Pathol Lab Med 2004;128:1385–94.

54. Matsuba HM, Mauney M, Simpson JR, et al. Adenocarcinomas of major and minor salivary gland origin: a histopathologic review of treatment failure patterns. Laryngoscope 1988;98:784–8.

55. Wierzbicka M, Kopec T, Szyfter W, et al. The presence of facial nerve weakness on diagnosis of a parotid gland malignant process. Eur Arch Otorhinolaryngol 2012;269:1177–82.

56. Razfar A, Heron DE, Branstetter BF 4th, et al. Positron emission tomography-computed tomography adds to the management of salivary gland malignancies. Laryngoscope 2010;120:734–8.

57. Vander Poorten V, Bradley PJ, Takes RP, et al. Diagnosis and management of parotid carcinoma with a special focus on recent advances in molecular biology. Head Neck 2012;34:429–40.
58. Moore FR, Bergman S, Geisinger KR. Metastatic hepatocellular carcinoma mimicking acinic cell carcinoma of the parotid gland: a case report. Acta Cytol 2010;54:889–92.
59. Schmidt RL, Hall BJ, Layfield LJ. A systematic review and meta-analysis of the diagnostic accuracy of ultrasound-guided core needle biopsy for salivary gland lesions. Am J Clin Pathol 2011;136:516–26.
60. Pfeiffer J, Ridder GJ. Diagnostic value of ultrasound-guided core needle biopsy in patients with salivary gland masses. Int J Oral Maxillofac Surg 2012;41: 437–43.
61. Olsen KD, Moore EJ, Lewis JE. Frozen section pathology for decision making in parotid surgery. JAMA Otolaryngol Head Neck Surg 2013;139:1275–8.
62. Upile T, Jerjes WK, Nouraei SA, et al. Further anatomical approaches to parotid surgery. Eur Arch Otorhinolaryngol 2010;267:793–800.
63. Gidley PW, Thompson CR, Roberts DB, et al. The results of temporal bone surgery for advanced or recurrent tumors of the parotid gland. Laryngoscope 2011; 121:1702–7.
64. Leonetti JP, Benscoter BJ, Marzo SJ, et al. Preauricular infratemporal fossa approach for advanced malignant parotid tumors. Laryngoscope 2012;122: 1949–53.
65. Mahmmood VH. Buccal branch as a guide for superficial parotidectomy. J Craniofac Surg 2012;23:e447–9.
66. Valstar MH, van den Brekel MW, Smeele LE. Interpretation of treatment outcome in the clinically node-negative neck in primary parotid carcinoma: a systematic review of the literature. Head Neck 2010;32:1402–11.
67. Ettl T, Gosau M, Brockhoff G, et al. Predictors of cervical lymph node metastasis in salivary gland cancer. Head Neck 2014;36:517–23.
68. Armstrong JG, Harrison LB, Thaler HT, et al. The indications for elective treatment of the neck in cancer of the major salivary glands. Cancer 1992;69:615–9.
69. Coca-Pelaz A, Rodrigo JP, Bradley PJ, et al. Adenoid cystic carcinoma of the head and neck—An update. Oral Oncol 2015;51:652–61.
70. Chisholm EJ, Elmiyeh B, Dwivedi RC, et al. Anatomic distribution of cervical lymph node spread in parotid carcinoma. Head Neck 2011;33:513–5.
71. Epps MT, Cannon CL, Wright MJ, et al. Aesthetic restoration of parotidectomy contour deformity using the supraclavicular artery island flap. Plast Reconstr Surg 2011;127:1925–31.
72. Cannady SB, Seth R, Fritz MA, et al. Total parotidectomy defect reconstruction using the buried free flap. Otolaryngol Head Neck Surg 2010;143:637–43.
73. Motomura H, Yamanaka K, Maruyama Y, et al. Facial nerve reconstruction using a muscle flap following resection of parotid gland tumours with thorough recipient bed preparation. J Plast Reconstr Aesthet Surg 2011;64:595–601.
74. Liu DY, Tian XJ, Li C, et al. The sternocleidomastoid muscle flap for the prevention of Frey syndrome and cosmetic deformity following parotidectomy: a systematic review and meta-analysis. Oncol Lett 2013;5:1335–42.
75. Krishnamurthy A, Vaidhyanathan A, Majhi U. Polymorphous low-grade adenocarcinoma of the parotid gland. J Cancer Res Ther 2011;7:84–7.
76. Hontanilla B, Qiu SS, Marre D. Effect of postoperative brachytherapy and external beam radiotherapy on functional outcomes of immediate facial nerve repair after radical parotidectomy. Head Neck 2014;36:113–9.

77. Volk GF, Pantel M, Streppel M, et al. Reconstruction of complex peripheral facial nerve defects by a combined approach using facial nerve interpositional graft and hypoglossal-facial jump nerve suture. Laryngoscope 2011;121:2402–5.

78. Griffin GR, Abuzeid W, Vainshtein J, et al. Outcomes following temporalis tendon transfer in irradiated patients. Arch Facial Plast Surg 2012;14:395–402.

79. Henney SE, Brown R, Phillips D. Parotidectomy: the timing of post-operative complications. Eur Arch Otorhinolaryngol 2010;267:131–5.

80. Herbert HA, Morton RP. Sialocele after parotid surgery: assessing the risk factors. Otolaryngol Head Neck Surg 2012;147:489–92.

81. Shuman AG, Bradford CR. Ethics of Frey syndrome: ensuring that consent is truly informed. Head Neck 2010;32:1125–8.

82. Pederson AW, Salama JK, Haraf DJ, et al. Adjuvant chemoradiotherapy for locoregionally advanced and high-risk salivary gland malignancies. Head Neck Oncol 2011;3:31.

83. Waldron CA, el-Mofty SK, Gnepp DR. Tumors of the intraoral minor salivary glands: a demographic and histologic study of 426 cases. Oral Surg Oral Med Oral Pathol 1988;66:323–33.

84. Diercks GR, Rosow DE, Prasad M, et al. A case of preoperative "first-bite syndrome" associated with mucoepidermoid carcinoma of the parotid gland. Laryngoscope 2011;121:760–2.

85. Deganello A, Meccariello G, Busoni M, et al. First bite syndrome as presenting symptom of parapharyngeal adenoid cystic carcinoma. J Laryngol Otol 2011; 125:428–31.

86. Linkov G, Morris LG, Shah JP, et al. First bite syndrome: incidence, risk factors, treatment, and outcomes. Laryngoscope 2012;122:1773–8.

87. Terhaard CH, van der Schroeff MP, van Schie K, et al. The prognostic role of comorbidity in salivary gland carcinoma. Cancer 2008;113:1572–9.

88. Terhaard CH. Postoperative and primary radiotherapy for salivary gland carcinomas: indications, techniques, and results. Int J Radiat Oncol Biol Phys 2007;69:S52–5.

89. Terhaard CH, Lubsen H, Rasch CR, et al. The role of radiotherapy in the treatment of malignant salivary gland tumors. Int J Radiat Oncol Biol Phys 2005;61:103–11.

90. Terhaard CH, Lubsen H, Van der Tweel I, et al. Salivary gland carcinoma: independent prognostic factors for locoregional control, distant metastases, and overall survival: results of the Dutch head and neck oncology cooperative group. Head Neck 2004;26:681–92 [discussion: 692–3].

91. Mahmood U, Koshy M, Goloubeva O, et al. Adjuvant radiation therapy for high-grade and/or locally advanced major salivary gland tumors. Arch Otolaryngol Head Neck Surg 2011;137:1025–30.

92. Matthiesen C, Thompson S, Steele A, et al. Radiotherapy in treatment of carcinoma of the parotid gland, an approach for the medically or technically inoperable patient. J Med Imaging Radiat Oncol 2010;54:490–6.

93. Rieken S, Habermehl D, Nikoghosyan A, et al. Assessment of early toxicity and response in patients treated with proton and carbon ion therapy at the Heidelberg ion therapy center using the raster scanning technique. Int J Radiat Oncol Biol Phys 2011;81:e793–801.

94. Stannard C, Vernimmen F, Carrara H, et al. Malignant salivary gland tumours: can fast neutron therapy results point the way to carbon ion therapy? Radiother Oncol 2013;109:262–8.

95. Gillespie MB, Albergotti WG, Eisele DW. Recurrent salivary gland cancer. Curr Treat Options Oncol 2012;13:58–70.

96. Bhide SA, Newbold KL, Harrington KJ, et al. Clinical evaluation of intensity-modulated radiotherapy for head and neck cancers. Br J Radiol 2012;85:487–94.

97. Mukesh M, Benson R, Jena R, et al. Interobserver variation in clinical target volume and organs at risk segmentation in post-parotidectomy radiotherapy: can segmentation protocols help? Br J Radiol 2012;85:e530–6.

98. Jensen AD, Nikoghosyan A, Windemuth-Kieselbach C, et al. Combined treatment of malignant salivary gland tumours with intensity-modulated radiation therapy (IMRT) and carbon ions: COSMIC. BMC Cancer 2010;10:546.

99. Jensen AD, Nikoghosyan AV, Lossner K, et al. COSMIC: A Regimen of Intensity Modulated Radiation Therapy Plus Dose-Escalated, Raster-Scanned Carbon Ion Boost for Malignant Salivary Gland Tumors: Results of the Prospective Phase 2 Trial. Int J Radiat Oncol Biol Phys 2015;93(1):37–46.

100. Brusic SK, Pusic M, Cvjetkovic N, et al. Osteosarcoma of the mastoid process following radiation therapy of mucoepidermoid carcinoma of the parotid gland—a case report. Coll Antropol 2012;36(Suppl 2):223–5.

101. Rizk S, Robert A, Vandenhooft A, et al. Activity of chemotherapy in the palliative treatment of salivary gland tumors: review of the literature. Eur Arch Otorhinolaryngol 2007;264:587–94.

102. Debaere D, Vander Poorten V, Nuyts S, et al. Cyclophosphamide, doxorubicin, and cisplatin in advanced salivary gland cancer. B-ENT 2011;7:1–6.

103. Gilbert J, Li Y, Pinto HA, et al. Phase II trial of taxol in salivary gland malignancies (E1394): a trial of the Eastern Cooperative Oncology Group. Head Neck 2006;28:197–204.

104. Triozzi PL, Brantley A, Fisher S, et al. 5-Fluorouracil, cyclophosphamide, and vincristine for adenoid cystic carcinoma of the head and neck. Cancer 1987;59:887–90.

105. Tanvetyanon T, Qin D, Padhya T, et al. Outcomes of postoperative concurrent chemoradiotherapy for locally advanced major salivary gland carcinoma. Arch Otolaryngol Head Neck Surg 2009;135:687–92.

106. Laurie SA, Ho AL, Fury MG, et al. Systemic therapy in the management of metastatic or locally recurrent adenoid cystic carcinoma of the salivary glands: a systematic review. Lancet Oncol 2011;12:815–24.

107. Nasser SM, Faquin WC, Dayal Y. Expression of androgen, estrogen, and progesterone receptors in salivary gland tumors. Frequent expression of androgen receptor in a subset of malignant salivary gland tumors. Am J Clin Pathol 2003;119:801–6.

108. Alotaibi AM, Alqarni MA, Alnobi A, et al. Human epidermal growth factor receptor 2 (HER2/neu) in salivary gland carcinomas: a review of literature. J Clin Diagn Res 2015;9:ZE04–8.

109. Ghosal N, Mais K, Shenjere P, et al. Phase II study of cisplatin and imatinib in advanced salivary adenoid cystic carcinoma. Br J Oral Maxillofac Surg 2011;49:510–5.

110. Stuart J, Wong EEWC, Karrison T, et al. A phase II study of dasatinib (BMS 354825) in recurrent or metastatic ckit-expressing adenoid cystic (ACC) and non-ACC malignant salivary glands tumors (MSGT). J Clin Oncol 2013;(Suppl) [abstract: 6022]. Available at: http://meetinglibrary.asco.org/content/109918-132.

111. Agulnik M, Cohen EW, Cohen RB, et al. Phase II study of lapatinib in recurrent or metastatic epidermal growth factor receptor and/or erbB2 expressing adenoid cystic carcinoma and non adenoid cystic carcinoma malignant tumors of the salivary glands. J Clin Oncol 2007;25:3978–84.

112. Jakob JA, Kies MS, Glisson BS, et al. Phase II study of gefitinib in patients with advanced salivary gland cancers. Head Neck 2015;37:644–9.
113. Locati LD, Bossi P, Perrone F, et al. Cetuximab in recurrent and/or metastatic salivary gland carcinomas: A phase II study. Oral Oncol 2009;45:574–8.
114. Haddad R, Colevas AD, Krane JF, et al. Herceptin in patients with advanced or metastatic salivary gland carcinomas. A phase II study. Oral Oncol 2003;39:724–7.
115. Kaidar-Person O, Billan S, Kuten A. Targeted therapy with trastuzumab for advanced salivary ductal carcinoma: case report and literature review. Med Oncol 2012;29:704–6.
116. Limaye SA, Posner MR, Krane JF, et al. Trastuzumab for the treatment of salivary duct carcinoma. Oncologist 2013;18:294–300.
117. Jaspers HC, Verbist BM, Schoffelen R, et al. Androgen receptor-positive salivary duct carcinoma: a disease entity with promising new treatment options. J Clin Oncol 2011;29:e473–6.
118. van der Schroeff MP, Terhaard CH, Wieringa MH, et al. Cytology and histology have limited added value in prognostic models for salivary gland carcinomas. Oral Oncol 2010;46:662–6.
119. Feinstein TM, Lai SY, Lenzner D, et al. Prognostic factors in patients with high-risk locally advanced salivary gland cancers treated with surgery and postoperative radiotherapy. Head Neck 2011;33:318–23.
120. Sultan I, Rodriguez-Galindo C, Al-Sharabati S, et al. Salivary gland carcinomas in children and adolescents: a population-based study, with comparison to adult cases. Head Neck 2011;33:1476–81.
121. Thariat J, Vedrine PO, Temam S, et al. The role of radiation therapy in pediatric mucoepidermoid carcinomas of the salivary glands. J Pediatr 2013;162:839–43.
122. Kupferman ME, de la Garza GO, Santillan AA, et al. Outcomes of pediatric patients with malignancies of the major salivary glands. Ann Surg Oncol 2010;17:3301–7.
123. Yoshida EJ, Garcia J, Eisele DW, et al. Salivary gland malignancies in children. Int J Pediatr Otorhinolaryngol 2014;78:174–8.
124. Megwalu UC, Shin EJ. Second primaries after major salivary gland cancer. Otolaryngol Head Neck Surg 2011;145:254–8.
125. Pederson AW, Haraf DJ, Blair EA, et al. Chemoreirradiation for recurrent salivary gland malignancies. Radiother Oncol 2010;95:308–11.
126. Mariano FV, da Silva SD, Chulan TC, et al. Clinicopathological factors are predictors of distant metastasis from major salivary gland carcinomas. Int J Oral Maxillofac Surg 2011;40:504–9.
127. National Comprehensive Cancer Network Guidelines. Head and Neck Cancers, Version 1;2015. Available at: http://www.nccn.org/professionals/physician_gls/pdf/head-and-neck.pdf. Accessed December 9, 2015.
128. Liu D, Labow DM, Dang N, et al. Pulmonary metastasectomy for head and neck cancers. Ann Surg Oncol 1999;6:572–8.
129. Locati LD, Guzzo M, Bossi P, et al. Lung metastasectomy in adenoid cystic carcinoma (ACC) of salivary gland. Oral Oncol 2005;41:890–4.
130. Qureshi SS, Nadkarni MS, Shrikhande SV, et al. Hepatic resection for metastasis from adenoid cystic carcinoma of parotid gland. Indian J Gastroenterol 2005;24:29–30.

Parotitis and Sialendoscopy of the Parotid Gland

Stephen Hernandez, MD, Carlos Busso, PhD, Rohan R. Walvekar, MD*

KEYWORDS

- Parotitis • Acute sialadenitis • Chronic sialadenitis • Sialolithiasis
- Salivary duct stricture • Sialendoscopy • Salivary endoscopy

KEY POINTS

- Chronic inflammatory disorders of the parotid gland can usually be related to salivary stasis, ductal obstruction, or reduced salivary flow rates from any etiology.
- Traditional management of nonneoplastic disorders of the parotid gland include conservative measures, with surgical management (parotidectomy) reserved for treatment failure.
- Sialendoscopy is a relatively new, gland-sparing, minimally invasive technique offering diagnostic capabilities and interventional modalities for management of nonneoplastic disorders of the salivary glands.

 Video content accompanies this article at http://www.oto.theclinics.com

INTRODUCTION

The great majority of nonneoplastic disorders of the salivary glands involve inflammatory processes related to a multitude of underlying etiologies. Historically, these disorders have been managed with conservative measures, including antibiotics, warm compresses, massage, sialogogues, and adequate hydration. Although beneficial for some patients, it has been reported that up to 40% of patients may have an inadequate response or persistent symptoms despite appropriate first steps in management.[1] Traditionally, when conservative techniques fail, the next step is

Funding Source: None.
Department of Otolaryngology – Head and Neck Surgery, Louisiana State University-Health Science Center, 533 Bolivar Street, Suite 566, New Orleans, LA 70112, USA
* Corresponding author. Department of Otolaryngology – Head and Neck Surgery, Louisiana State University-Health Science Center, 533 Bolivar Street, Suite 566, New Orleans, LA 70112.
E-mail address: rwalve@lsuhsc.edu

Otolaryngol Clin N Am 49 (2016) 381–393
http://dx.doi.org/10.1016/j.otc.2015.12.003
0030-6665/16/$ – see front matter © 2016 Elsevier Inc. All rights reserved.

oto.theclinics.com

operative intervention. In the case of nonneoplastic disorders of the parotid gland, this would involve superficial or total parotidectomy with all of its potential complications, including facial nerve paresis or paralysis. In 1988, salivary endoscopy techniques were introduced in Europe. Salivary endoscopy is now being practiced widely globally and in the United States. Sialendoscopy offers a minimally invasive option for the diagnosis and management of chronic inflammatory disorders of the salivary glands and offers the option of gland and function preservation. In this article, we review some of the more common nonneoplastic disorders of the parotid gland, indications for diagnostic and interventional sialendoscopy, and operative techniques.

RELEVANT ANATOMY AND PHYSIOLOGY

The parotid gland is the largest of the 3 major salivary glands. It is located anterior to the external auditory canal and lateral to the mandibular ramus and masseter muscle. It is encapsulated by a very dense connective tissue that is continuous with the investing layer of deep cervical fascia in the neck. Histologically, the parotid gland differs from the other salivary glands in that the acinar cells purely secrete a protein-rich serous fluid and there are no mucinous secreting acinar cells. Salivary flow is then mediated through the intercalated ducts, the striated ducts, and ultimately the excretory ducts. The main excretory duct of the parotid gland is known as the parotid duct, or Stenson's duct. This projects from the anterior surface of the parotid gland where it courses over the masseter muscle and pierces the buccinator to enter the oral cavity at about the level of the second maxillary molar.[2] The anatomy of Stenson's duct is important when discussing operative techniques. In general, the duct can measure up to 6 cm in length with a diameter anywhere from 0.5 to 1.4 mm. The narrowest segment of the duct is located at the ostium.[3] Specifically pertaining to sialendoscopy, it is important to remember that the parotid papilla is easier to enter but more difficult to navigate compared with the submandibular papilla. The masseter muscle around which the parotid duct curves to enter the mouth can provide a bend to the duct that is endoscopically recognized as the "masseteric bend."

It is also important to understand the production and flow of saliva as stasis is thought to be a mediator of chronic sialadenitis. The autonomic nervous system plays a major role in regulation of salivary production and flow. The parotid gland receives its sympathetic innervation from postganglionic fibers as they travel with the vascular supply following their synapse in the superior cervical ganglion. The preganglionic parasympathetic fibers originate from the inferior salivatory nucleus associated with the glossopharyngeal nerve. The postganglionic fibers then leave the otic ganglion with the auriculotemporal nerve, where they ultimately find their way into the substance of the parotid gland. The neurotransmitter of the parasympathetic nervous system is acetylcholine, and when binding to muscarinic receptors, the end result is increased production of watery saliva with enhanced flow. This physiologic concept helps to explain why antimuscarinic and anticholinergic medications are implicated in the development of sialadenitis. It also explains why some clinicians prescribe muscarinic agonists, such as cevimeline, in an attempt to increase salivary production and flow in certain salivary gland disorders.

The average daily flow of saliva may range anywhere from 1 to 1.5 L. During rest, the submandibular gland is the main contributor to salivary flow but during stimulation, the parotid gland is thought to contribute to more than 50% of salivary production. Any process that may promote the disruption of anterograde salivary flow (sialolithiasis, stenosis, anatomic anomaly, or medications) can ultimately lead to problems with obstructive sialadenitis that lead to acute or chronic symptoms for patients.

ACUTE SUPPURATIVE PAROTITIS

As discussed, salivary stasis owing to any cause may be a precipitating factor for the development of acute bacterial sialadenitis. It is commonly encountered in the elderly population after an inciting event, although it can happen in any age group. Patients usually present with acute onset of pain, edema, and overlying skin changes at the level of the parotid gland. Physical examination may demonstrate induration, fluctuance, and trismus. On occasion, purulence can be expressed from Stenson's duct and, if present proximally, stones may be palpable. Computed tomography (CT) scan or ultrasound may be used to identify sites of potential obstruction or development of an abscess (**Fig. 1**). Ultrasound can not only be beneficial in the diagnosis of abscess formation, but can also be valuable intraoperatively to localize the abscess cavity.

When exudate can be expressed from the main excretory duct, it should be collected and sent for culture and sensitivity. While awaiting results, empiric intravenous antibiotic therapy should be initiated to address the most common etiologic organisms. Multiple microbes have been implicated in the development of acute bacterial sialadenitis, but *Staphylococcus aureus* accounts for the overwhelming majority of organisms cultured out.[4] In addition to antibiotic therapy, warm compresses, sialogogues, and massage should also be encouraged. Most patients respond with appropriate medical management, but some fail and go on to develop complications, including intraparotid abscess. Surgical management with incision and drainage is indicated in these cases. The use of ultrasound guidance may also be used for needle aspiration and drainage where appropriate. Currently, interventional sialendoscopy is contraindicated in the management of acute sialadenitis for fear of ductal injury, complications, and spread of infection. We have found salivary endoscopy to be valuable in the management of acute parotitis. In the senior author's experience, for patients not responding to medical management within 48 hours, we have performed dilation of the parotid duct and a conservative endoscopic washout of the parotid ductal

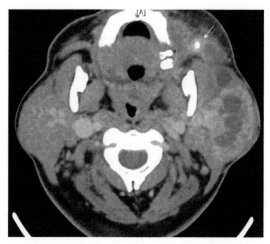

Fig. 1. An axial computed tomography scan showing a dilated left parotid duct with abscess formation secondary to an obstructing sialolith at the parotid papilla (*yellow arrow* points to the left parotid sialolith).

system. Although the endoscopic intervention does not decrease induration of the infected gland, patients who have undergone this intervention reported significant pain relief and benefit. Our work needs to be substantiated by larger numbers and is currently unpublished. Consequently, for practical purposes, until these results can be validated, endoscopic intervention for acute parotitis must be considered with caution.

Some patients may present with similar symptoms of acute parotid swelling, extreme tenderness, and xerostomia, but they may lack purulence or other signs of suppurative infection. It is important to consider other infectious causes for salivary gland enlargement, and these will primarily be viral in nature. Mumps is the most common viral cause of parotitis, but will commonly be seen with bilateral parotid gland enlargement.[5] The incidence of mumps has markedly been reduced after the advent of childhood immunization. Other viral etiologies to consider include Coxsackie virus, cytomegalovirus, influenza virus, and the human immunodeficiency virus. Diagnosis may be made with serology, although management is usually conservative and symptomatic in nature.

CHRONIC PAROTITIS

Chronic sialadenitis may develop as a consequence of repeated infections of the salivary glands, of which the parotid gland is the most likely to be affected. With the development of recurrent parotitis, the acini of the gland are destroyed and it becomes dysfunctional overtime resulting in xerostomia, among many other symptoms. As discussed, it is important to investigate why these patients are developing these recurrent inflammatory processes. History and physical examination may help to elicit underlying etiologies. Imaging will also play an important role in establishing a diagnosis. CT and ultrasonography are both good initial measures when considering salivary gland pathology. They can assist with identification of cysts, neoplasms, or calculi within the gland. Sialography is a valuable option when considering ductal pathology. More recently, MRI sialography, a unique technique using saliva as a contrast medium for the visualization of the salivary ductal system, has also been used to demonstrate ductal pathology at several institutions.[6,7]

Ultimately, chronic parotitis can be related to salivary stasis, physical obstruction, or reduced salivary flow rates. Common conditions encountered include sialolithiasis, salivary duct strictures or stenosis, juvenile recurrent parotitis (JRP), autoimmune processes such as Sjögren syndrome, and radioiodine-induced sialadenitis. We take some time to review some of these topics, in particular, those that may be amenable to management with sialendoscopy.

Sialolithiasis

Salivary stones are one of the most common nonneoplastic disorders of the salivary glands, and they represent a common cause of acute and chronic sialadenitis in the general population. It is estimated that annually, up to 60 people per million require treatment for acute sialadenitis related to sialolithiasis.[8] Although most commonly encountered in the submandibular gland, they can also be seen with moderate frequency in the parotid gland (20% of the time). Salivary calculi can be made of inorganic substances including calcium carbonate and calcium phosphate. There does not seem to be a predilection for the development of salivary calculi with other systemic diseases, other than gout.

Physical examination may reveal signs associated with generalized parotitis and occasionally, the salivary calculi may be palpable intraorally or overlying the masseter muscle. CT and ultrasonography are good imaging modalities for the assessment of sialolithiasis. CT essentially detects almost all salivary calculi, although if the stones are less than 2 mm, they may be missed. Sialography, including MRI sialography is another imaging modality that can identify obstruction within the parotid duct. At our institution, CT scan of the neck with and without contrast using 1 mm cuts is the standard radiologic study to detect size, location, shape, and orientation of the stone, all of which are relevant to predict success with sialendoscopy. Ultrasonography is extremely valuable when performed by the surgeon because it helps with real-time examination of the stone and assists in localization both in the office and intraoperatively.

Treatment for those patients with sialolithiasis is largely dependent on the size and location of the apparent calculus. Historically, conservative management with sialogogues, warm compresses, and massage may facilitate the spontaneous passage of very small stones (<2 mm). Sialendoscopy has become important for the management of sialolithiasis. For stones that are less than 3 mm in maximal dimension, interventional salivary endoscopy alone can often facilitate complete removal, (**Fig. 2**). For intermediate size stones, between 3 and 6 mm, endoscopy can be combined with techniques for fragmentation of the calculus. These include utilization of extracorporeal/intraductal lithotripsy (**Fig. 3**) or the holmium laser (Video 1; available online at http://www.oto.theclinics.com/) through the working port of the salivary endoscope.[9] Fragmentation of the calculus allows for piecemeal removal of the stone in select cases. Stones that are larger than 8 mm or those that extend far past the hilum may be best approached with combined techniques. These may include diagnostic sialendoscopy for stone localization and external or intraoral approaches for assisted removal. Combined techniques often obviate the need for parotidectomy and have resulted in a gland preservation rate of greater than 90%.[10] There are still some patients who ultimately may require parotidectomy for symptomatic relief.

Salivary Duct Strictures

Strictures or stenosis of Stenson's duct may be seen in many inflammatory etiologies involving the parotid gland. This may occur after recurrent parotitis or may even be a consequence of sialolithiasis. Similar to an intraductal stone, strictures inhibit the normal anterograde flow of saliva. As a consequence, salivary stasis can occur

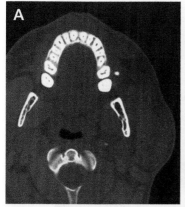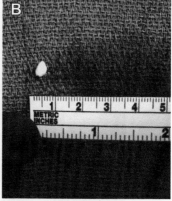

Fig. 2. (*A*) Axial computed tomography scan showing parotid stone in the left parotid duct distal segment. (*B*) Parotid stone, 3 mm, oval in shape, optimal for endoscopic removal.

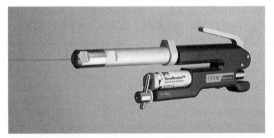

Fig. 3. Endoscopic "stone breaker"—an endoscopic CO_2 based lithotripter for a midsized stone. (*Courtesy of* Cook Medical, Bloomington, IN; with permission.)

resulting in chronic parotitis. Imaging studies may not reveal any obvious reason for recurrent parotitis, but sialography or MRI sialography may demonstrate ductal pathology (**Fig. 4**).

For patients who have failed medical and conservative management, sialendoscopy is the next step in assessing the ductal anatomy. Sialendoscopy is diagnostic and also therapeutic at the same time. Management of strictures includes endoscopic balloon dilation, steroid irrigation, and placement of a stent within the parotid duct (**Fig. 5**). Kopec and colleagues[11] reviewed 51 patients with ductal stenosis. After balloon dilation and stent placement for 2 to 3 weeks, a total of 47 patients (92%) reported improvement in symptoms. Similar to sialolithiasis, there are a select few who may fail endoscopic management, ultimately requiring parotidectomy for symptomatic control.

Juvenile Recurrent Parotitis

JRP, also commonly referred to as recurrent parotitis of childhood, is a commonly recognized salivary gland disorder in the pediatric population. These patients often present early on in life with recurrent inflammation of the parotid glands.

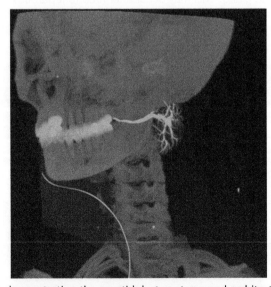

Fig. 4. Sialogram demonstrating the parotid duct anatomy and architecture.

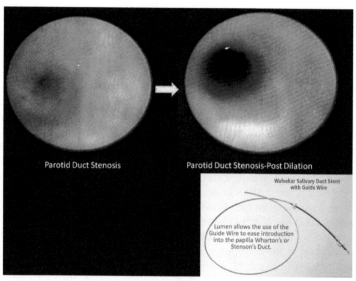

Fig. 5. Dilation of parotid stenosis using guide wire and dilators with stent placement. (*Courtesy of* Hood Laboratories, Pembroke, MA; with permission.)

Involvement can be unilateral or bilateral and the workup is the same as described elsewhere in this article. The diagnosis is essentially clinical. However, there are certain findings that can allude to the diagnosis. Ultrasonography may show scattered punctate sialectasis throughout the duct, but these patients may not have any identifiable pathology on ultrasound or even sialography. The etiology of this disorder remains unclear in nature. Many theories and suggestions have been made including genetic anomalies, congenital malformation of Stenson's duct, viral infection, and autoimmune disorders.[5] The diagnosis can be made clinically upon presentation, but it remains a diagnosis of exclusion after first ruling out other causes of chronic sialadenitis.

Traditionally, management has consisted of conservative measures during acute attacks. Although the disease itself has no clear etiology, it is usually self-remitting, usually subsiding by the time children enter their teens. Most recently, sialendoscopy has been advocated for the management of those with severe symptoms. Ramakrishna and colleagues[12] performed a systematic review and metaanalysis looking at sialendoscopy in the management of JRP. Seven studies were included in the review. Overall 73% of patients reported no further episodes of sialadenitis and 87% of patients required no further sialendoscopy. There were no complications reported, showing that sialendoscopy can be a safe and effective measure for select patients with JRP. The mechanism of benefit is still not well understood. However, endoscopic findings reveal what is commonly seen with most inflammatory disorders: debris, stenosis, and blanched ducts with the lack of vascular markings on the luminal walls. It is hypothesized that salivary endoscopy causes benefit by irrigating the debris and hydraulically dilating the ductal system giving the gland an opportunity to reboot and function more efficiently. The goal of endoscopic intervention ranges from complete symptom resolution to reducing the intensity and frequency of flareups until the child grows out of the disease. As a consequence, quality of life is improved and this may reduce long-term sequelae and the development of chronic parotid disease.

Sjögren Syndrome

Sjögren syndrome is a poorly understood autoimmune disorder that primarily affects exocrine gland function. As a result, patients will often present with lacrimal gland dysfunction and xerophthalmia or recurrent parotitis and xerostomia, the latter being the more common presenting symptom. Although the underlying pathophysiology is unclear, histopathologic findings always reveal both T- and B-cell infiltration with surrounding inflammation, presumably leading to the progressive destruction of the exocrine glands. Laboratory testing may reveal antibodies to the Ro/SS-A or La/SS-B protein complexes.

Major and/or minor salivary glands may be affected by this systemic process, but the parotid gland seems to be the most commonly involved (**Fig. 6**). Physical examination may often reveal significant xerostomia and a painful or painless swollen gland. The parotid gland is most often involved, but the submandibular gland or both glandular systems may be affected. Imaging with CT or MRI may aid in the diagnosis; patients with parotid involvement will sometimes have what is described as speckled calcifications within the glandular parenchyma. The European American Consensus Group Modification of the European Community Criteria for Sjögren Syndrome have developed a group of diagnostic criteria. These include symptoms of dry eye, signs of dry eye, symptoms of dry mouth, signs of abnormal salivary glandular function, minor salivary gland biopsy focus score of greater than 1, and presence of anti SS-A or anti SS-B antibodies.[13] A presumptive diagnosis of Sjögren syndrome can be made if 4 of the 6 criteria are met.

Management of Sjögren syndrome is focused primarily on symptomatic control and relief. Sialogogues, compresses, and artificial saliva exist as conservative options. Medical management can often be initiated and consists of muscarinic agonists to promote the production and flow of saliva. Pilocarpine does provide some symptomatic relief for patients, but it also has other systemic effects that can lead to poor tolerance. Cevimeline is another muscarinic agonist that is more selective for the receptors found in the salivary glands. Thus, it can provide symptomatic relief with far fewer side effects. In the presence of other systemic symptoms, these patients may require the

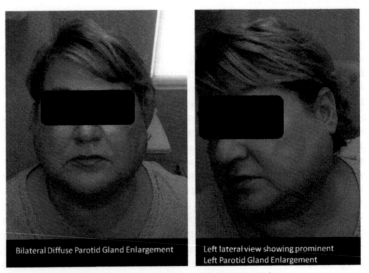

Bilateral Diffuse Parotid Gland Enlargement   Left lateral view showing prominent Left Parotid Gland Enlargement

Fig. 6. Diffuse parotid hypertrophy associated with sicca complex.

addition of steroids or immune modulators, such as hydroxychloroquine and rituximab, although they have not demonstrated distinct clinical efficacy.[14]

Sialendoscopy can be an adjunctive treatment option for those patients who have undergone medical management with no assistance in symptomatic relief. Intraductal pathology may exist, including inflammatory debris or stenosis, which may render conservative management ineffective. In this setting, sialendoscopy can provide diagnostic accuracy of intraductal pathology while at the same time providing steroid irrigation and relief of obstruction when present. It has proven to be a safe, repeatable, and effective alternative to parotidectomy in the management of Sjögren syndrome refractory to medical management.[15]

Radioactive Iodine–Induced Sialadenitis

Treatment with radioactive ^{131}I is recommended therapy as adjunctive treatment of well-differentiated thyroid carcinomas and for hyperfunctioning thyroid disease. In general, it is well-tolerated, but can have some associated side effects, of which sialadenitis is the most common.[16] Although mainly localizing to thyroid tissue, it also demonstrates some degree of uptake within the salivary glands. This is attributed to a sodium–iodine symporter located at the surface of acinar cells. It is estimated that up to 24% of an administered dose of ^{131}I can be lost through the saliva.[17] This seems to be a dose-dependent phenomenon because higher doses of ^{131}I have been associated with increased incidence of sialadenitis. Radioiodine primarily effects the acinar cells, resulting in alteration of salivary content and production of a more mucoid and viscous material. In addition, the ductal system can be affected resulting in strictures and stenosis. This leads to salivary stasis and ultimately, sialadenitis.

Preventative steps can be taken to decrease the incidence of radioiodine-induced sialadenitis. However, some patients may experience persistent symptoms, in particular those who have received high doses or those who have received multiple doses. These symptoms include chronic pain, xerostomia, and swelling and they can significantly impact quality of life. In 1 review, 21% of patients reported persistent symptoms beyond 12 months from the time of ^{131}I treatment.[18] It is unclear when and which patients receiving radioiodine will develop symptoms of sialadenitis. However, it can occur anywhere from weeks to a few years after therapy and symptoms can vary from being minimal to those causing day-to-day significant changes in quality of life. Patients with end-stage radioiodine-induced sialadenitis may require multiple gland excisions for symptom control.

Sialendoscopic management has become an important tool in the treatment of radioiodine-induced sialadenitis. Bomeli and colleagues[19] described a series of 12 patients, of which 75% reported some degree of symptomatic improvement in the short term after therapeutic sialendoscopy. Prendes and colleagues[20] demonstrated similar findings, with 91% of patients having some improvement and 55% of patients describing complete resolution of symptoms with a mean follow-up time of 18 months. For those patients recalcitrant to medical therapy, sialendoscopy has provided a safe and effective alternative to management. The operative intervention with salivary endoscopy mirrors that done with other inflammatory conditions, composed of ductal dilation, gland washout, and management of strictures with or without stenting. Irrigation can be done with and without steroid infusion with comparable results.

BASIC OPERATIVE TECHNIQUES IN SIALENDOSCOPY

The increase in popularity of sialendoscopy can be attributed mainly to the fact that it is a minimally invasive, gland-preserving alternative to the traditional option of gland resection. The rate-limiting step for successful endoscopic or combined approach techniques is access to the duct. Consequently, the first step in sialendoscopy is providing adequate exposure. This can be accomplished through a variety of mouth retractors and bite blocks, but maintaining this exposure will make subsequent steps easier. The next step, which is often the rate-limiting step, is accurate identification of the papilla. Magnification with surgical loupes and/or the operating microscope is helpful in accurate identification. Other described techniques and helpful tips include documentation of the location of the papilla in clinic notes to help localization in the operating room or on the day of the procedure, gland massage to facilitate salivary flow, or painting the site of the papilla with methylene blue to make the papilla more prominent.[21] This is followed by serial dilation of the papilla. There are multiple ways to accomplish dilation, including the use of metal dilator sets (Marchal dilator or Schaitkin dilator sets; **Fig. 7**), or using the Seldinger technique with guide wires and dilators (Cook Dilator System; **Fig. 8**). All of these sets begin with small dilators that gradually increase in diameter. If there is difficulty encountered when entering Stenson's duct, a papillotomy may be performed. Regardless of which technique is used, this will be the most important step. Adequate sialendoscopy cannot be performed without appropriately addressing the papilla. After serial dilation, success rates of sialendoscopy approach 98%.

Once the papilla is dilated, the sialendoscope can be introduced. Endoscopes range in size from 0.8 mm diagnostic (used in the pediatric population) to 1.6 mm "all-in-one" interventional endoscopes. The most commonly used dimensions are the 1.1 mm and the 1.3 mm "all-in-one" interventional salivary endoscopes. These are semirigid endoscopes with 3 channels for utility. There is an optic channel to transmit the image, an irrigation channel for the continuous infusion of saline for maintenance of ductal patency during endoscopy, and finally there is a working channel for the introduction of interventional instruments. There are multiple endoscopic tools to facilitate intervention. Stone baskets can facilitate removal of small and mid-sized stones (Video 2; available online at http://www.oto.theclinics.com/). Lithotripsy can be performed using a Holmium laser or the Stonebreaker device, an intraluminal lithotripsy device. The latter is still being assessed for safety and feasibility. Dilation of stenosis can be performed using a Seldinger technique or endoscopic balloons. In most cases, however, pure endoscopic tools are insufficient to tackle every clinical scenario. Consequently, external (parotid approach) or transoral combined (hybrid) techniques are often used to facilitate gland preservation (**Figs. 9** and **10**). These

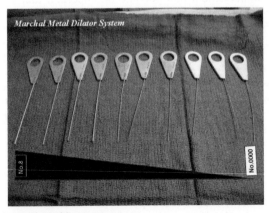

Fig. 7. Marchal salivary duct dilation system.

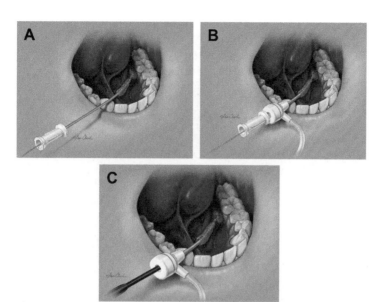

Fig. 8. Cook dilators and Kolenda introducer set: (*A*) Disposable dilators are passed over a guidewire for serial dilation of the salivary duct. (*B*) An indwelling sheath can then be placed to allow for placement of the sialendoscope (*C*) with a stable endoscopic surgical view. (*Courtesy of* Cook Medical, Bloomington, IN.)

techniques are most commonly used for the management of mid- and large-sized stones or stenosis. In the parotid gland, the use of salivary stents is of importance because, unlike the submandibular gland that drains into the floor mouth, salivary fistula and leak into the buccal space can cause sialoceles or the potential for abscess

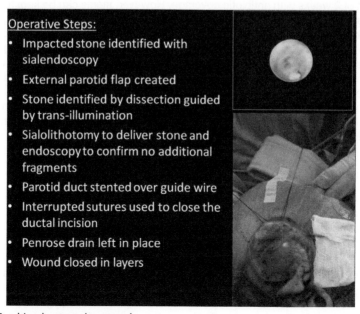

Operative Steps:
- Impacted stone identified with sialendoscopy
- External parotid flap created
- Stone identified by dissection guided by trans-illumination
- Sialolithotomy to deliver stone and endoscopy to confirm no additional fragments
- Parotid duct stented over guide wire
- Interrupted sutures used to close the ductal incision
- Penrose drain left in place
- Wound closed in layers

Fig. 9. Combined external approach.

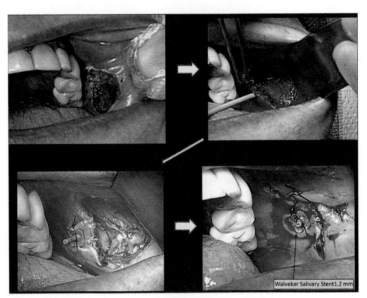

Fig. 10. Transoral combined approach technique. Figure demonstrates access for management of stones or strictures anterior to the masseter muscle. After sialolithotomy or repair of stenosis in the buccal space, reconstruction of the duct is performed after placement of salivary duct stent.

formation. The indications for stent placement include extensive trauma to the parotid papilla, combined approach techniques involving a sialodochotomy, an operative intervention using laser where there is endoluminal evidence of ductal trauma, ductal tear, or postdilation of strictures (**Fig. 10**). The author also advocates stenting for a minimum of 2 weeks with antibiotic coverage. However, stents can be kept for longer durations with close observation (range, 2–8 weeks).

As with any operative procedure, there is a learning curve to sialendoscopy and it can be technically challenging. After adequate experience and considering appropriate patient selection, salivary endoscopy can be very successful.[22] With improvement in techniques and continued evaluation of long-term outcomes, sialendoscopy has certainly expanded its indications, as seen throughout this article. It has proven to be a safe, effective, and gland-sparing alternative to those patients who have failed conservative management, and it will continue to be a very important treatment adjunct in the management of nonneoplastic disorders of the salivary glands.

SUPPLEMENTARY DATA

Supplementary data related to this article can be found online at http://dx.doi.org/10.1016/j.otc.2015.12.003.

REFERENCES

1. Motamed M, Laughame D, Bradley PJ. Management of chronic parotitis: a review. J Laryngol Otol 2003;117:521–6.
2. Walvekar RR, Loehn BC, Wilson MN. Anatomy and physiology of the salivary glands. In: Johnson JT, Rosen CA, editors. Bailey's head and neck

surgery – otolaryngology. 5th edition. Baltimore (MD): Lippincott Williams and Wilkins; 2014. p. 691–700.

3. Zenk J, Hosemann G, Iro H. Diameters of the main excretory ducts of the adult human submandibular and parotid gland: a histologic study. Oral Surg Oral Med Oral Pathol Oral Radiol Endod 1998;85(5):576–80.

4. Brook I, Frazier BH, Thompson DH. Aerobic and anaerobic microbiology of acute suppurative parotitis. Laryngoscope 1991;101:170–2.

5. Nahlieli O, Schacham R, Shlesinger M, et al. Juvenile recurrent parotitis: a new method of diagnosis and treatment. Pediatrics 2004;114:9–12.

6. Morimoto Y, Tanaka T, Tominaga K, et al. Clinical application of magnetic resonance sialographic 3-dimensional reconstruction imaging and magnetic resonance virtual endoscopy for salivary gland duct analysis. J Oral Maxillofac Surg 2004;62:1237–45.

7. Su YX, Liao GQ, Kang Z, et al. Application of magnetic resonance virtual endos-copy as a presurgical procedure before sialoendoscopy. Laryngoscope 2006; 116:1899–906.

8. Escudier MP, McGurk M. Symptomatic sialoadenitis and sialolithiasis in the English population, an estimate of the cost of hospital treatment. Br Dent J 1999;186:463–6.

9. Marchal F, Dulguerov P. Sialolithiasis management: the state of the art. Arch Otolaryngol Head Neck Surg 2003;129:951–6.

10. Carroll WW, Walvekar RR, Gillespie MB. Transfacial ultrasound-guided gland-preser-ving resection of parotid sialoliths. Otolaryngol Head Neck Surg 2013;148:229–34.

11. Kopec T, Szyfter W, Wierzbicka M, et al. Stenoses of the salivary ducts – sialen-doscopy based diagnosis and treatment. Br J Oral Maxillofac Surg 2013;51: 174–7.

12. Ramakrishna J, Strychowsky J, Gupta M, et al. Sialendoscopy for the manage-ment of juvenile recurrent parotitis: a systematic review and meta-analysis. Laryn-goscope 2015;125:1472–9.

13. Vitali C, Bombardieri S, Moutsopoulos HM, et al. Preliminary criteria for the classification of Sjogren's syndrome. Results of a prospective concerted action supported by the European Community. Arthritis Rheum 1993;36:340–7.

14. Ramos-Casals M, Tzioufas AG, Stone JH, et al. Treatment of primary Sjögren syn-drome: a systematic review. JAMA 2010;304:452–60.

15. Schacham R, Puterman MB, Ohana N, et al. Endoscopic treatment of salivary glands affected by autoimmune diseases. J Oral Maxillofac Surg 2011;69:476–81.

16. Allweiss P, Braunstein GD, Katz A, et al. Sialadenitis following I-131 therapy for thyroid carcinoma: concise communication. J Nucl Med 1984;25:755–8.

17. Mandel SJ, Mandel L. Persistent sialadenitis after radioactive iodine therapy: report of two cases. J Oral Maxillofac Surg 1999;57:738–41.

18. Hyer S, Kong A, Pratt B, et al. Salivary gland toxicity after radioiodine therapy for thyroid cancer. Clin Oncol (R Coll Radiol) 2007;19:83–6.

19. Bomeli SR, Schaitkin B, Carrau RL, et al. Interventional sialendoscopy for treat-ment of radioiodine-induced sialadenitis. Laryngoscope 2009;119:864–7.

20. Prendes BL, Orloff LA, Eisele DW. Therapeutic sialendoscopy for the management of radioiodine sialadenitis. Arch Otolaryngol Head Neck Surg 2012;138:15–9.

21. Luers JC, Vent J, Beutner D. Methylene blue for easy and safe detection of sali-vary duct papilla in sialendoscopy. Otolaryngol Head Neck Surg 2008;139:466–7.

22. Bowen MA, Tauzin M, Kluka EA, et al. Diagnostic and interventional sialendo-scopy: a preliminary experience. Laryngoscope 2011;121:299–303.

Parotidectomy for Benign Parotid Tumors

Babak Larian, MD[a,b,*]

KEYWORDS

- Pleomorphic adenoma • Recurrent pleomorphic adenoma
- Extracapsular dissection • Parotidectomy • Microparotidectomy
- Deep lobe parotid tumor • Frey's syndrome • Facial nerve paresis

KEY POINTS

- Facial nerve anatomy and variable risk of injury in different areas of the parotid gland.
- Pleomorphic adenoma's histologic characteristic leading to microscopic positive margins in most if not all cases, and its significance.
- Extracapsular dissection (limited parotid surgery) compares favorably with superficial parotidectomy in terms of outcomes but requires extensive experience to avoid morbidity.
- There are a great number of surgical approaches and incisions to access the parotid, and with greater experience less invasive approaches are appropriate.
- Recurrent pleomorphic adenomas are very difficult to cure, and the treatment plan needs to take into account the nature and extent of the primary surgery, and the role of adjuvant radiation therapy.
- Adjuvant radiation therapy plays a role in treatment of recurrent pleomorphic adenoma.

INTRODUCTION

Surgical treatment of benign parotid tumors in the early twentieth century was, as it is today, shaped by the significant risk to the facial nerve, and a lack of clear understanding of tumor biology. Surgery for benign tumors such as pleomorphic adenoma (PA) focused on intracapsular enucleation, in which the tumor capsule is opened and the contents removed.[1–3] Joseph McFarland from University of Pennsylvania in the 1940s is credited with recognizing a high rate of recurrence after parotidectomy.[4]

Disclosure: The author has nothing to disclose.
[a] Department of Head and Neck Surgery, David Geffen School of Medicine, University of California, Los Angeles, Los Angeles, CA, USA; [b] Center for Advanced Parotid & Facial Nerve Surgery, 9401 Wilshire Boulevard, Suite 650, Beverly Hills, CA 90212, USA
* Center for Advanced Head & Neck Surgery, 9401 Wilshire Boulevard, Suite 650, Beverly Hills, CA 90212.
E-mail address: dr@larianmd.com

Recurrence was observed in up to 45% of patients treated by intracapsular enucleation.[5,6]

As the reports for recurrence began to mount in the midcentury, and more in-depth pathologic studies were undertaken, the technique and philosophy of parotidectomy for benign parotid lesions were refined.[7] The resection of the tumor capsule and a margin of surrounding healthy tissue was advocated, as well as complete facial nerve dissection in an anterograde or retrograde direction.[8] This approach evolved into standard and obligatory dissection of the facial nerve and its branches and in most cases removal of the superficial parotid gland, and less frequently the totality of the gland, which is the philosophy of care in a great many centers around the world presently. Nevertheless, great controversy exists as to the appropriate extent of surgical treatment of benign disease.

Clinicians who support complete facial nerve dissection with superficial parotidectomy point to increased safety for the facial nerve and a decreased rate of recurrence in the long term. Other surgeons think that there is less risk and morbidity when meticulous dissection is done outside the tumor capsule without preidentification or exposure of the main trunk of the facial nerve (extracapsular dissection).[9,10] These surgeons also claim that dissection of the facial nerve increases the risk of intraoperative nerve damage, and causes scarring in the area of the nerve, which makes revision surgery much more difficult and risky.[11–15]

Just as in other fields of surgery, salivary gland surgery is moving toward minimally invasive techniques that reduce the length of incision and surgical dissection, thereby potentially decreasing the risk of short-term and long-term complications. However dealing with parotid tumors presents certain inherent complexities: (1) facial nerve anatomy is widely variable and unpredictable, and (2) fine-needle aspiration (FNA) diagnostic pathology carries a high false-negative rate (4%–7%).[16,17] These two factors demand that parotid surgeons have a high degree of expertise so that during the operation they can make decisions as to the appropriate extent and type of procedure, and how to address or avoid facial nerve injury. There is evidence to support both surgical philosophies in addressing benign parotid tumors, which means a nuanced approach must be considered.

CONSIDERATIONS IN PAROTID TUMORS

PAs represent the most challenging benign tumors to address because of their predominance, histologic characteristics, high recurrence rate, and potential for malignant transformation. The treatment that is appropriate for this type of tumor could be effectively used for other benign parotid tumors as well.

Facial Nerve Anatomy and Dysfunction

The facial nerve has widely variable branching anatomy that is akin to a tree; no two facial nerves are alike. During parotidectomy surgery, the facial nerve branches often abut the tumor. Most studies have indicated that risk factors for transient facial nerve dysfunction include size of tumor, inflammatory condition, patient's age, malignancy, and the type of surgical procedure.[18–23] However, the location of the tumor within the parotid is of utmost importance. Laws of real estate govern parotid tumor's involvement of the nerves as well; the areas that have more substance and allow a separation between the tumor and the branches of the facial nerve, such as the parotid tail or the posterior inferior parotid, are less likely to have nerve involvement. Areas of less substance, including superiorly where the superior division branching occurs or anteriorly over the masseter muscle, show a greater involvement with the nerve, and thus a higher incidence of temporary facial nerve dysfunction (see **Table 2**). This relationship holds true for the deep lobe of the parotid as well, in that tumors in the upper portion of the deep lobe tend to have closer association with the facial nerve, and require more manipulation of the nerve (circumferential dissection and transposition) and potential for injury.[24] Gaillerad and colleagues[20] suggested that manipulation of the facial nerve as it passed adjacent to the tumor was the cause of temporary facial nerve dysfunction (TFND) in most the cases. Cannon and colleagues[25] concluded that the length of facial nerve that is dissected and exposed correlated with TFND. Dulguerov and colleagues[19] reviewed the pathophysiology of TFND and reported nerve stretching as the cause of TFND.

In addition to the facial nerve, the greater auricular nerve (GAN), auriculotemporal nerve, and sympathetic fibers also innervate the parotid and adjacent tissue. The GAN courses behind the sternocleidomastoid muscle (SCM) and travels anteriorly and superiorly toward the parotid and the ear. Over the SCM it divides into anterior, posterior, and deep branches.[26] The anterior branches innervate the skin over the parotid, whereas the deep branch enters the gland. The posterior branching system gives sensation to the earlobe and the skin beneath the cartilaginous auricle. GAN sacrifice is routinely done at many centers when performing parotidectomy. Ryan and Fee[27] showed the following in patients who had GAN sacrificed during parotidectomy: 47% of the patients had anesthesia, 58% had paresthesia, and 26% had neither anesthesia nor paresthesia. None of their patients reported this deficit to be interfering with daily activities, which is echoed by other investigators. Although preservation of the GAN, specifically the posterior branch, does not prevent some degree of sensory loss, especially in the anterior distribution, it does minimize it. In addition, it can minimize other unwanted morbidity, including dysesthesia, discomfort on cold exposure, and traumatic neuroma.

The auriculotemporal nerve arises from deep in the parapharyngeal space and passes posterior to the temporomandibular joint to innervate the skin of the tragus and the temple. Along its course it gives secretomotor branches to the parotid gland as it passes posteromedial to the mandibular condyle. These nerve fibers are responsible for the development of Frey's syndrome. The sympathetic input into the gland comes from the fibers that travel on the superficial temporal artery and then branch out to innervate the gland.

Histology

One-fifth of the parenchyma of the parotid gland lies deep to the facial nerve (deep lobe).[28] Because most of the gland is superficial to the nerve, 90% of parotid tumors occur in the superficial lobe and 80% occur in the lower part of the gland.[29,30]

Parotid gland tumors represent 3% of tumors occurring in the head and neck area, and 80% of tumors of the salivary glands. Eighty percent of parotid gland tumors are benign.[31] Of these, the most common type is PA, which accounts for 65%, followed by cystadenoma lymphomatosum or Warthin tumor, which accounts for about 25%. Far less common, basal cell adenomas and oncocytomas are some of the other benign tumors. The remaining 20% of parotid tumors are cancers with varying degrees of aggressiveness and behavioral patterns. PA tumors occur in persons of all ages, with the highest incidence in the fourth to sixth decades.[31] PA is most often diagnosed when the tumor is located in the superficial lobe, small (<4 cm), and mobile.[32]

Most small cancers (T1/T2) of the parotid are clinically silent and appear demarcated on examination or even imaging.[13,33] FNA has a high sensitivity and specificity for PA, and has a notable false-negative rate (4%–7%).[16,17] However, FNA along with the imaging studies help guide clinicians as to whether the tumor is aggressive and requires more than limited surgery. Some clinicians advocate making a decision as to the aggressiveness of the tumor based on surgical findings and thus deciding to proceed with more involved surgery. However, this approach may be disappointing as well, because small cancers may have a normal appearance and feel soft, like benign tumors.

Zbären and colleagues[34] reviewed the histology of PAs and found that the capsule can be either thick or thin, and at times is absent in certain areas. Breaches in the capsule can allow the tumor to grow into the surrounding tissue and appear as finger-like projections or pseudopods. The capsule can be invaded and penetrated by tumor as well, again giving rise to pseudopods and, rarely, satellite lesions. In superficial parotid PAs, studies have shown there to be no satellite lesions in the deep lobe.[32] Deep lobe tumors seem to differ in that they have thicker capsules.[35]

Recurrent (or residual) pleomorphic adenomas

Recurrent (or residual) PAs (RPAs) are almost always multifocal.[36] Theories as to the increase of recurrence include capsular rupture, satellite lesions, pseudopods, and grossly positive margins. Enucleation procedure or incisional biopsy for suspected lymph nodes also leads to recurrence. Initial multicentricity of primary PAs seems to be an extremely rare phenomenon.[37,38] Biological and genetic factors may be at play as well, but are not well understood.[39] PA has a low rate of recurrence when treated by a nonenucleation procedure (1%–4%).[18] In the patient population that later develops RPA, the mean age at presentation is lower (33–35 years) than for those who remain free of disease (45–50 years).[36,40] Recurrences are typically observed 7 to 10 years after initial treatment, except in cases of enucleation of the PA, which recur after a much shorter interval.[41]

Although MRI can show the extent of disease, multinodularity, and deep lobe involvement, on histologic analysis of surgical specimens many more nodules are often found than imaging studies and clinical examination reveal.[42] MRI can also show the amount of residual parotid gland remaining and help determine the extent and appropriateness of further surgical intervention. The facial nerve is the main concern when deciding on the appropriate course of treatment of RPA. Trauma and scar tissue formation from the primary surgery can make it difficult to distinguish the nerve. The natural planes between salivary tissue, tumor, and nerve may be lost with surgery and thus recurrent tumors can be more adherent to the nerve. In addition, the normal course and anatomy of the nerve is distorted. Strategies to identify the facial nerve in RPA, therefore require significant preoperative planning. The authors typically identify the facial nerve in the vertical segment of the mastoid or peripherally in a retrograde fashion. If the tumor is located away from the area of the nerve, nerve stimulation and identification without exposure in the scar are also feasible.[43] It is also advisable to resect the incisional scar from the primary surgery, en bloc with the specimen if feasible. Recurrences are more common after treatment of recurrent tumors compared with primary surgery.

The widespread distribution of recurrent disease makes curative treatment difficult and often impossible, carrying with it a high risk of facial nerve complications and further recurrence, therefore the initial surgical approach must be sound and performed with expertise. PAs that are not surgically removed have the potential to undergo malignant transformation. The most common form of malignancy secondary to PAs is carcinoma ex PA.[44] The development of this malignancy has a direct relationship with duration of PA tumor presence, with rates being as high as 9.4% at 15 years. It is often unclear how long the tumor has been present at the time of diagnosis, to be able to assess the appropriate level of risk. Thackray and Lucas[45] estimated that 25%

of untreated PAs eventually undergo malignant transformation. The incidence of malignant transformation is even higher in recurrent PAs.[36,40]

In a landmark article by Witt and colleagues,[46] the significance of margins in parotid tumor surgery was assessed. Retrospective analysis of pathology specimens was done, comparing total parotidectomy, partial superficial parotidectomy (PSP), and extracapsular dissection (ECD). They concluded that:

1. The major outcomes (capsular exposure, tumor–facial nerve interface, capsular rupture, recurrence, and permanent facial nerve dysfunction) from surgical treatment of mobile, superficial PA smaller than 4 cm are not significantly altered by surgical approach (total parotidectomy, PSP, or ECD).
2. Greater parotid tissue sacrifice results in higher rates of transient facial nerve dysfunction and Frey's syndrome.
3. Focal capsular exposure is a near-universal finding for cases of small (<4 cm), mobile PA predominantly of the superficial lobe, regardless of the extent of parotid tissue sacrifice.
4. Dissecting PA from the facial nerve results in positive margins because of an incomplete capsule or perforating pseudopodia. Fewer separations of pseudopodia from the main tumor occur with expertly performed contemporary parotid surgery because most of the PA has a margin of normal parotid tissue.
5. Capsular rupture resulted in a significantly higher rate of recurrence but did not vary by extent of parotid tissue sacrifice for small PAs (excluding enucleation).
6. Hypocellular tumors did not result in a higher rate of capsular rupture or recurrence, and tumor multicentricity was not found in the clinically uninvolved deep lobe.
7. Recurrence now occurs in a small percentage of patients receiving the best care but happens most frequently because of the continued practice of enucleation.[46]

Other studies have shown little difference in recurrence rates between patients who had negative margins and those who had microscopic positive margins.[47]

Extracapsular Dissection Versus Superficial Parotidectomy

An ECD is defined as a partial parotid surgery that involves removal of the tumor with preservation of capsule without exposure of the main trunk of the facial nerve.[48] The incision to access the parotid varies between different centers, but most use the modified Blair incision. Once the incision is made and skin flaps are elevated, the tumor is localized and assessed. If the tumor is mobile and does not show suspicious physical findings, then ECD is performed. Neuromonitoring is used in all cases, assisted by nerve stimulation during the procedure. At first, a 5-mA current is used for nerve stimulation, and as soon as a branch is identified in the proximity of the tumor the current is reduced to 2 mA and the branch is exposed. If further exposure of the branch is deemed necessary for removal of the tumor, the current is reduced even further to 1 mA. A 2-mm to 3-mm margin of normal tissue is obtained when permissible by the facial nerve.[3] Theoretically, because of less exposure of the nerve and less manipulation, the incidence of nerve paresis should be fewer. Frey's syndrome should also occur with less frequency because the extent of parotid tissue exposure and thus secretomotor nerve reveal is much less.

Most studies with ECD come from European centers where this procedure is advocated for small, mobile, superficial lobe tumors.[9,10,49–53] McGurk[15] reported on one of the largest series comparing ECD with superficial parotidectomy, in which his group used a 4-cm cutoff for consideration for this technique as well as intraoperative determination of mobility of the tumor to decide which procedure was most appropriate.[9] Other studies show that the risk of facial nerve paresis after ECD of tumors 4 cm or greater was 21% compared with 4% for the smaller tumors.[49] European centers favor the use of ultrasonography for tumor assessment and thus as part of their decision making in terms of which technique to use preoperatively, and at times intraoperatively.

However, these concepts are not unique to European centers. Donovan and Conley[52] reported that 60% of the patients with PA surgery did not have clear margins on the capsule because of the facial nerve interface. None of these patients had a recurrence. These investigators challenged the popular belief that a wide margin of normal parotid tissue is necessary to prevent recurrence. The group at the Sydney Head and Neck Cancer Institute echoed these findings as well and advocated limited parotid surgery for PAs because of low morbidity and recurrence rates.[53]

In terms of outcomes, ECD shows similar recurrence rates with decreased surgical morbidity. Mehta and Nathan[54] reviewed the data and compared several of the larger studies, which overall showed similar recurrence rates and a much higher incidence of facial nerve paralysis or paresis and Frey's syndrome in the patient group that underwent superficial parotidectomy (**Table 1**).

The data from these large retrospective studies clearly favor ECD, but must be analyzed with caution, keeping in mind some key factors: the retrospective nature of these studies creates an issue with internal validity because it does not remove bias.[54] In addition, inherent within the ECD technique is the intraoperative decision making as to the extent of surgery, and thus more challenging or worrisome tumors are removed using more extensive parotidectomy techniques. These two factors create an inherent bias that skews the data. The data also come from large tertiary referral centers with high surgical volume and great technical experience, making application of this technique most appropriate for the more experienced surgeons.

Types of Incisions for Superficial Parotid Tumors

The modified Blair incision, initially described by Blair[55] in 1918 and later modified by Bailey[56] in 1941, has been the standard incision that most head and neck surgeons are trained to use for parotidectomy, and is most often used to treat benign parotid tumors. This technique is excellent in terms of offering a wide exposure that makes finding the facial nerve and its branches, as well as removing the tumor, effective and safe.[9] This technique is preferred in training programs because it allows excellent exposure and versatility to convert into more extensive surgery if needed (eg, neck dissection). The drawbacks include larger incision, greater area of dissection, and greater potential for asymmetry.[57-60]

Appiani[61] further modified the approach and described the use of a facelift incision to remove benign parotid tumors. By placing the incision behind the ear along the occipital hairline, the surgeon is able to reduce the visibility of the scar without

Table 1
Outcomes after extracapsular dissection versus superficial parotidectomy (SP)

Study	No. of Patients	Recurrence Rates (%)		Facial Nerve Paresis or Paralysis (%)		Frey's Syndrome (%)	
		ECD	SP	ECD	SP	ECD	SP
Albergotti et al,[9] 2012	1882	1.5	2.4	8	20.4	4.5	26.1
Barzan & Pin,[49] 2012	349	2.3	12	1.3	6	1.3	44
McGurk et al,[50] 2003	630	1.7	1.8	10	32	5	32

compromising on the exposure needed to perform nerve identification and dissection, as well as tumor removal.[62]

Both of these techniques were originally described without any reconstructive measures to prevent facial asymmetry and Frey's syndrome. A variety of techniques for such a reconstruction can be used. Any of the approaches can be modified to incorporate reconstructive measures for best functional and cosmetic outcome.

Martí-Pagès and colleagues[63] in Barcelona described an approach that included a more limited approach that involves an incision extending from the helical root, along the posterior aspect of the tragus, down under the earlobe, and up over the posterior aspect of conchal cartilage. There are no posterior occipital limbs extending to the hairline. We have been using this approach for the past 8 years with great success. We always combine this incision with a reconstructive technique to cover the exposed parotid gland, fill in the surgical defect, and create facial symmetry, and have termed it microparotidectomy (MIP) (**Figs. 1–12**). As with the group in Barcelona, we find this approach excellent in allowing wide access to the entire parotid gland and full visibility of the facial nerve. We have also been able to preserve the posterior branches of the GAN, dissect and transpose facial nerve branches to access the deep lobe tumors, as well as access the SCM muscle for local parotid reconstruction. When necessary, we make modifications to this incision to allow for mastoidectomy for facial nerve exposure, extending the incision to the hairline for larger or recurrent tumors, and even extending an inferior limb to perform more extensive surgery, including neck dissection. MIP serves as the primary approach in our practice for treatment of benign parotid tumors.

Types of Incisions for Deep Lobe Parotid Tumors

Deep lobe tumors present a special challenge in that the tumors are deep and adjacent to the nerve. Several approaches have been devised to access this limited space. They include the transparotid approach (TPA), transparotid approach with mandibulotomy, transcervical approach (TCA), or a combined transparotid transcervical approach (TPTCA).[64] TPA is best suited for tumors that appear to have involvement of the nerve, or tumors that go from the superficial lobe to the deeper lobe. It is also necessary in cases in which the tumor is high up in the parapharyngeal space, leaving little room between the top of the tumor and the skull base, which require an approach

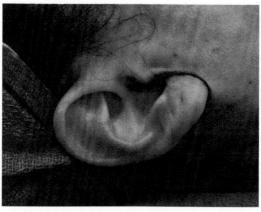

Fig. 1. Preauricular microparotidectomy incision marking.

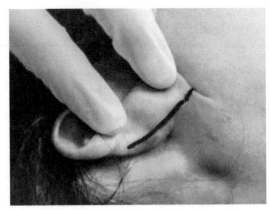

Fig. 2. Postauricular microparotidectomy incision marking.

from the side so that the tumor can be accessed on the top and cleared from the skull base and surrounding neurovascular structures. Although a mandibulotomy is an option, it is only used with extremely large tumors or malignancies.[65,66] TPA can be combined with reconstructive measures to minimize aesthetic and functional (Frey's syndrome) morbidity. TPA can be done through any of the parotidectomy incisions mentioned earlier for superficial parotidectomy, including the facelift and microparotidectomy incisions.

TCA is an excellent approach for selected cases. It is a less extensive surgery, and leaves patients with less morbidity and faster recovery. Small or medium-sized tumors in the lower aspect of the deep parotid lobe with an extraglandular pattern of growth into the parapharyngeal space are most appropriate for this approach. Casani and colleagues[64] describe the lateral pterygoid muscle (LPM) as a landmark for making the decision between TPA and TCA. If there is salivary tissue between the LPM and the tumor in the parapharyngeal space then they concluded that the craniocaudal and peripheral location of the tumor is such that it is safely accessible via TCA. When the tumors are extensive, or if there is a suspicion of malignancy, both incisions may be combined for better exposure.

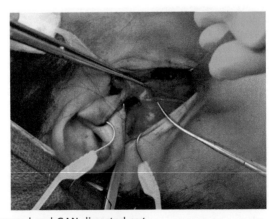

Fig. 3. Parotid exposed and GAN dissected out.

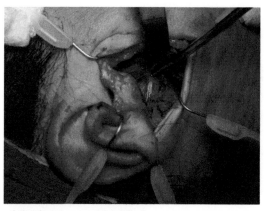

Fig. 4. Main trunk of the facial nerve identified.

DISCUSSION

All clinicians who perform parotid tumor surgery agree that parotidectomy is an intricate and elegant surgery. It is extremely challenging for a variety reasons: the facial nerve anatomy is variable and has an unpredictable branching pattern, the most common tumor type (PA) has an inconstant capsule and pseudopodia, as well as the inherent unreliability of preoperative testing (7% FNA false-negative rate) and the clinical similarity of early stage malignancies.[17] The high recurrence rate caused by enucleation procedures in the early years led to the more extensive parotid procedures combined with facial nerve dissection. Along with a more extensive surgery came greater morbidity, making it necessary for surgeons to have greater skill and be able to handle complications of facial nerve injury, as well as being able to reconstruct defects to prevent Frey's syndrome and facial asymmetry. All of this has led to the great divide between the 2 groups of surgeons: those who think that the facial nerve needs to be dissected and the superficial gland removed, and those who think that ECD is adequate to treat benign parotid tumors. The data indicate that both groups are correct to some extent.

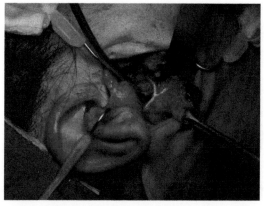

Fig. 5. Facial nerve: upper and lower division dissected and exposed.

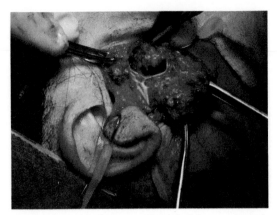

Fig. 6. Deep lobe tumor removed in between distal facial nerve branches.

Histologic studies indicate that complete removal of PAs is almost universally associated with some degree of capsular exposure.[32] However, capsular exposure does not seem to correlate directly with recurrence. Separating the tumor directly off the facial nerve and thus potentially having positive margins is something that every parotid surgeon has experienced. Surprisingly, this has a very low correlation to recurrence of tumor. Microscopic positive margins show only a slight increase in recurrence compared with negative margins.[45] Recurrence therefore seems to be a statistical risk, and as the number of microscopic tumor cells (pseudopodia) left behind increases, the odds of recurrence also increase; having a few tumor cells left behind does not equate to certainty of recurrence. Advocates of ECD believe this to be true, which is why they also take a narrow margin of unaffected parotid tissue along with their specimens,[50] and also advise gentle handling of the tumor so as to not rupture the capsule and cause spillage, all to enhance the odds against recurrence.

The morbidity data for ECD are favorable. They show similar recurrence and permanent facial paralysis rates, with a much lower incidence of facial nerve paresis, salivary fistulas, and Frey's syndrome. The lower facial nerve weakness is likely caused by less manipulation, exposure, and stretching of the facial nerve branches because they are

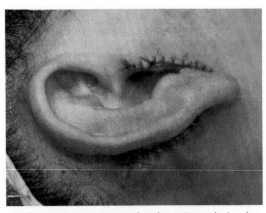

Fig. 7. Incision closed after reconstruction and Jackson-Pratt drain placement.

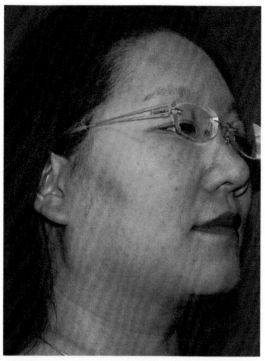

Fig. 8. Right parotid tumor.

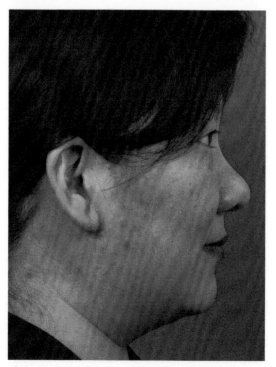

Fig. 9. Six months after microparotidectomy and reconstruction.

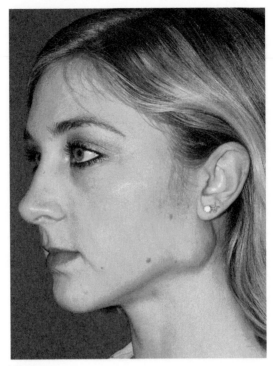

Fig. 10. Left parotid tumor.

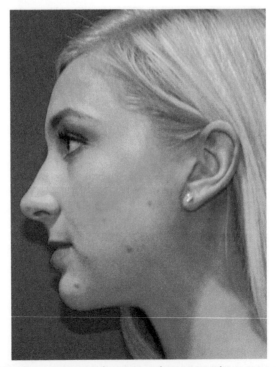

Fig. 11. Two weeks after microparotidectomy and reconstruction.

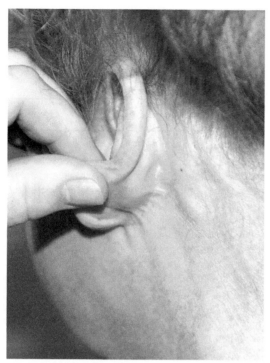

Fig. 12. Postauricular scar 6 weeks after surgery.

not identified. The lowered fistula and Frey's syndrome rate is clearly caused by a lesser degree of salivary tissue transection and exposure. The similarity in recurrence, as discussed earlier, is understandable as well. However, a point of interest is similarities in permanent facial paralysis rates. It is common to find PAs intimately involved with the facial nerve, with branches of the facial nerve being embedded in the tumor capsule. Under these circumstances, not entirely identifying and dissecting the facial nerve and it's heavy arborization would seem to lead to a much higher rate of facial nerve paralysis, especially if the tumor is anteriorly or superiorly positioned in areas where parotid tissue is thin and contact with the nerve unavoidable; the risk in these areas are probably minimized by nerve stimulation and meticulous branch dissection and offset by the fact that the facial nerve has redundancy of innervation of the facial muscles in the mid-face. The ECD studies advocate making an intraoperative decision as to what type of parotidectomy to perform, making it inherently biased toward less complex tumors. In addition, all the studies come from high-volume tertiary referral centers where the surgical experience and expertise is high, especially as it relates to facial nerve anatomy. Despite the challenges discussed here there is a role for minimally invasive parotid surgery; we advocate a systematic approach that includes all types of parotid surgery except enucleation procedures.

The decision as to what type of surgical approach, incision and extent is based on five factors: histology, size, mobility, location of tumor, as well as expertise of surgeon. Clearly malignant histology necessitates a more extensive procedure. Size less then 4 cm and mobility of the tumor are associated with lower morbidity.[50,51] Location is of utmost importance when considering approach, incision and extent (**Table 2**).

Table 2					
Anatomic divisions of the parotid gland					
Superficial			**Deep**		
Anterior (Anterior to the posterior border of mandibular ramus)	Posterior Upper Posterior Lower	Upper Lower	Superior-Inferior Dividing line is at the mid-point between upper and lower border of the parotid.		
Tail (Anatomically lower then Marginal Mandibular Nerve)		—			

The parotid can be subdivided into six different divisions: deep upper, deep lower, posterior superficial upper, Posterior superficial lower, tail, and anterior division. These divisions are made based on anatomical landmarks which include a plane created by the facial nerve subdividing the deep and superficial lobes; a coronal plane from the posterior edge of medial pterygoid muscle (also the mandible) going superficially to the skin and subdividing the superficial lobe into anterior and posterior divisions; a plane halfway between the upper and lower border of the parotid gland subdividing the posterior superficial lobe and the deep lobe into upper and lower divisions; and finally the marginal mandibular nerve separating the posterior lower superficial lobe from the lower division (essentially the tail).[24]

The areas of the parotid gland that have the most amount of salivary tissue or substance also have the lowest risk of facial nerve injury. This includes the tail, the posterior superficial lower division and the deep lower lobe. Historically, even followers of extensive parotidectomy have been performing extracapsular dissection in the deep lower parotid through a trans-cervical approach with great success and low morbidity. It only makes sense to extend the same methodology to tumors of the tail and with caution in the posterior superficial lower division as there is greater possibility of injury to the marginal mandibular nerve here. In the case of the superficial tumors a micro-parotidectomy incision can be used to minimize tissue trauma, as well as any of the traditional incisions.

The posterior superficial upper division, anterior division, and deep upper lobe carry a much higher risk of facial nerve injury for different reasons. As the frontal branch of the facial nerve in the posterior superficial upper parotid division quickly become superficial to go over the zygomatic arch multiple dedicated terminal branches can occur, along with paucity of salivary tissue overlying the mandible in this area the possibility of intimate contact between tumor and nerve increases thus creating the highest risk of injury to the facial nerve. The anterior parotid has a small amount of salivary substance (which lessens distally), and the most amount of branching (with the caveat of increased cross connectivity), which causes this area to have the second highest rate of facial nerve dysfunction; facial nerve redundancy here allows the midface some margin of safety in the hands of surgeons with great facial nerve expertise. These two areas can be accessed easily through all 3 types of incision, and require either anterograde facial nerve dissection or retrograde, mostly determined by the surgeons experience with the incision type and direction of facial nerve dissection. As experience is gained in operating in these areas and dealing with the facial nerve and it's variations more minimal surgery (ECD) can be done successfully.

The deep upper lobe carries the third highest incidence of facial nerve dysfunction because of the need to extensively dissect and transpose the nerve branches, especially the lower division of the facial nerve.[24] Access to this area often requires more extensive incisions, but the surgery can commence with a more minimal incision and, if access is then found to be inadequate, extending the incision to a TPTCA.[64]

The ECD technique relies heavily on technology; the facial nerve monitor and stimulator are necessities, because the facial nerve branches surrounding the nerve must be identified via stimulation and then exposed and separated from the tumor.[3] Any fault in these devices can have severe and permanent consequences. This equipment must be checked and rechecked throughout the procedure to ensure continuous function. However, the traditional main trunk facial nerve dissection techniques rely more on anatomic knowledge, patience, skill, and experience than on technology. The expertise gained in performing traditional parotidectomy leads to better appreciation of the limitations to appropriately selected patients and the performance of ECD in a safe and sound fashion.

Parotidectomy for recurrent benign disease is a complex issue, especially as it relates to RPA. Even when the number of RPA nodules seems limited on clinical and imaging assessment, microscopically there are numerous seedings. Facial nerve involvement is common, especially if the primary surgery involved dissection of the facial nerve. The more limited the facial nerve dissection at primary surgery, the less likely and less widespread is its involvement at reoperation. The incidence of TFND is 90% or more, and permanent loss is reported as many as 40%.[36,40,67] Intraoperative facial nerve monitoring and stimulation are necessary to help identify the nerve branches and help preserve them. It is recommended that dissection of previously exposed nerves be limited to prevent further trauma and devascularization, which can be done in areas away from the site of recurrence; however, the areas where the nerve is most manipulated at the original surgery is usually the site of the primary tumor and recurrence.

The treatment of RPA is extremely challenging without a clear standard. Each case is thus considered individually. Observation is suggested in elderly patients and those who are in poor health.[46] The likelihood of success mostly depends on what was done at the initial operation; if the tumor was enucleated and the facial nerve was fully exposed, the chances of cure are remote. However, if a partial parotidectomy was performed with limited nerve exposure then the odds of success are greater. However, a total parotidectomy and facial nerve sacrifice may reduce the rate of recurrence but does not prevent it.[68]

Whatever the type of primary surgery, reoperative parotidectomy needs to be more extensive because the microscopic extent of RPA is unclear. This procedure can be anything from a partial parotidectomy and facial nerve dissection, as in the case of a patient who had a simple open biopsy in the tail of the parotid without facial nerve exposure; superficial parotidectomy and facial nerve dissection for a recurrence in the superficial lobe from previous superficial posterior PA; to a total parotidectomy and facial nerve dissection for a deep lobe recurrence with multiple nodules. Again, each case must be considered based on its individual circumstances, taking into account age, location of the original tumor, original tumor–facial nerve interface, facial nerve risk, feasibility of removal, and the patient's desires and risk aversion. The patient must be fully aware that the chance of recurrence after reoperation is significant (43%–45%).[36,40] Although the risk of recurrence is lower for deep lobe PAs, potentially because of a thicker capsule,[35] once a recurrence occurs here the chance of cure is lower and the risk of subsequent recurrences much higher.[69]

Adjuvant radiation therapy (RT) is an option when complete removal of recurrent PA is not possible because of either multinodularity or facial nerve involvement.[43] Although there are no prospective studies comparing radiation alone with surgery or surgery combined with RT, improved local control has been reported in patients with multinodular disease or multiple recurrences; the incidence of second recurrence has been shown to decrease from 30% to 40% down to 4% to 10%, especially in multinodular RPA.[13,70]

For successful parotid surgery, a graded approach to parotidectomy must be taken. A high degree of experience is gained in training and afterward by doing parotid cancer surgery, which requires extensive resections and a high degree of facial nerve dissection, thus gaining expertise in superficial and total parotidectomy. In time, more minimally invasive approaches can be exercised when a better understanding of the anatomy is gained and a respect for the facial nerve has become ingrained. In experienced hands, ECD is an important option that should be part of the armamentarium of parotid surgeons. The graded nature of parotid surgeons' development is intended to diminish the chances of complications and recurrence. Recurrent PAs are especially challenging because they are commonly incurable and have a high degree of malignant transformation. Individualized treatment of RPA and consideration for adjuvant RT are more effective.

REFERENCES

1. Benedict EB, Meigs JV. Tumors of the parotid gland: a study of two hundred and twenty-five cases with complete end-results in eighty cases. Surg Gynecol Obstet 1930;51:626–47.
2. Rawson AJ, Howard JM, Royster HP, et al. Tumors of the salivary glands: a clinicopathological study of 160 cases. Cancer 1950;3:445–58.
3. Klintworth N, Zenk J, Koch M, et al. Postoperative complications after extracapsular dissection of benign parotid lesions with particular reference to facial nerve function. Laryngoscope 2010;120:484–90.
4. McFarland J. Mysterious mixed tumors of salivary glands. Surg Gynecol Obstet 1943;76:23–34.
5. Johnson JT, Ferlito A, Fagan JJ, et al. Role of limited parotidectomy in management of pleomorphic adenoma. J Laryngol Otol 2007;121:1126–8.
6. McFarland J. Three hundred mixed tumors of the salivary glands of which 69 recurred. Surg Gynecol Obstet 1936;63:457–68.
7. Patey D, Thackray A. The treatment of parotid tumours in the light of a pathological study of parotidectomy material. Br J Surg 1958;45:477–87.
8. Mantsopoulos K, Koch M, Klintworth N, et al. Trends in surgery for benign parotid tumors. Laryngoscope 2015;125:122–7.
9. Albergotti WG, Nguyen SA, Zenk J, et al. Extracapsular dissection for benign parotid tumors: a meta-analysis. Laryngoscope 2012;122:1954–60.
10. Iro H, Zenk J, Koch M, et al. Follow-up of parotid pleomorphic adenomas treated by extracapsular dissection. Head Neck 2013;35:788–93.
11. Rehberg E, Schroeder H, Kleinsasser O. Surgery in benign parotid tumors: individually adapted or standardized radical interventions? Laryngorhinootologie 1998;77:283–8 [in German].
12. Roh J, Kim H, Park C. Randomized clinical trial comparing partial parotidectomy versus superficial or total parotidectomy. Br J Surg 2007;94:1081–7.
13. Renehan A, Gleave EN, McGurk M. An analysis of the treatment of 114 patients with recurrent pleomorphic adenomas of the parotid gland. Am J Surg 1996;172:710–4.
14. George KS, McGurk M. Extracapsular dissection—minimal resection for benign parotid tumours. Br J Oral Maxillofac Surg 2011;49:451–4.
15. McGurk M, Combes J. Controversies in the management of salivary gland disease. Oxford (United Kingdom): Oxford University Press; 2012.
16. Que Hee CG, Perry CF. Fine-needle aspiration cytology of parotid tumours: is it useful? ANZ J Surg 2001;71:345–8.

17. Zbären P, Schär C, Hotz MA, et al. Value of fine-needle aspiration cytology of parotid gland masses. Laryngoscope 2001;111:1989–92.
18. Laccourreye H, Laccourreye O, Cauchois R, et al. Total conservative parotidectomy for primary benign pleomorphic adenoma of the parotid gland: a 25-year experience with 229 patients. Laryngoscope 1994;104:1487–94.
19. Dulguerov P, Marchal F, Lehmann W. Postparotidectomy facial nerve paralysis: possible etiologic factors and results with routine facial nerve monitoring. Laryngoscope 1999;109:754–62.
20. Gaillard C, Périé S, Susini B, et al. Facial nerve dysfunction after parotidectomy: the role of local factors. Laryngoscope 2005;115:287–91.
21. Zernial O, Springer IN, Warnke P, et al. Long-term recurrence rate of pleomorphic adenoma and postoperative facial nerve paresis (in parotid surgery). J Craniomaxillofac Surg 2007;35:189–92.
22. Mehle ME, Kraus DH, Wood BG, et al. Facial nerve morbidity following parotid surgery for benign disease: the Cleveland Clinic Foundation experience. Laryngoscope 1993;103:386–8.
23. Mra Z, Komisar A, Blaugrund SM. Functional facial nerve weakness after surgery for benign parotid tumors: a multivariate statistical analysis. Head Neck 1993;15: 147–52.
24. Ikoma R, Ishitoya J, Sakuma Y, et al. Temporary facial nerve dysfunction after parotidectomy correlates with tumor location. Auris Nasus Larynx 2014;41: 479–84.
25. Cannon CR, Replogle WH, Schenk MP. Facial nerve in parotidectomy: a topographical analysis. Laryngoscope 2004;114:2034–7.
26. Yang H, Kim H, Hu K. Anatomic and histological study of great auricular nerve and its clinical implication. J Plast Reconstr Aesthet Surg 2015;68:230–6.
27. Ryan WR, Fee WE Jr. Long-term great auricular nerve morbidity after sacrifice during parotidectomy. Laryngoscope 2009;119:1140–6.
28. Leverstein H, van der Wal JE, Tiwari RM, et al. Surgical management of 246 previously untreated pleomorphic adenomas of the parotid gland. Br J Surg 1997;84: 399–403.
29. Norman JED. Recurrent mixed tumours of the major and minor salivary glands. In: Norman JED, McGurk M, editors. Salivary glands. St Louis (MO): Mosby; 1995. p. 229–42.
30. Yamashita T, Tomoda K, Kumazawa T. The usefulness of partial parotidectomy for benign parotid gland tumors. Acta Otolaryngol Suppl 1993;500:113–6.
31. Spiro RH. Salivary neoplasms: overview of a 35-year experience with 2,807 patients. Head Neck Surg 1986;8:177–84.
32. Witt R. The significance of the margin in parotid surgery for pleomorphic adenoma. Laryngoscope 2002;112:2141–54.
33. Zbären P, Schüpbach J, Nuyens M, et al. Carcinoma of the parotid gland. Am J Surg 2003;186:57–62.
34. Zbären P, Vander Poorten V, Witt RL, et al. Pleomorphic adenoma of the parotid: formal parotidectomy or limited surgery? Am J Surg 2013;205:109–18.
35. Fliss DM, Rival R, Gullane P, et al. Pleomorphic adenoma: a preliminary histopathologic comparison between tumors occurring in the deep and superficial lobes of the parotid gland. Ear Nose Throat J 1992;71:254–7.
36. Zbären P, Tschumi I, Nuyens M, et al. Recurrent pleomorphic adenoma of the parotid gland. Am J Surg 2005;189:2003–7.
37. Krolls SO, Boyers RC. Mixed tumors of salivary glands. Long-term follow-up. Cancer 1972;30:276–81.

38. Batsakis JG. Quality assurance. Sisyphean or sibylline? Arch Pathol Lab Med 1990;114:1173–4.
39. Hamada T, Matsukita S, Goto M, et al. Mucin expression in pleomorphic adenoma of salivary gland: a potential role for MUC1 as a marker to predict recurrence. J Clin Pathol 2004;57:813–21.
40. Philips PP, Olsen KD. Recurrent pleomorphic adenoma of the parotid gland: report of 126 cases and a review of the literature. Ann Otol Rhinol Laryngol 1995;104:100–4.
41. Niparko JK, Beauchamp ML, Krause CJ, et al. Surgical treatment of recurrent pleomorphic adenoma of the parotid gland. Arch Otolaryngol Head Neck Surg 1986;112:1180–4.
42. Stennert E, Wittekindt C, Klussmann JP, et al. Recurrent pleomorphic adenoma of the parotid gland: a prospective histopathological and immunohistochemical study. Laryngoscope 2004;114:158–63.
43. Gleave EN, Whittaker JS, Nicholson A. Salivary tumours—experience over thirty years. Clin Otolaryngol 1979;4:247–57.
44. Beahrs OH, Woolner LB, Kirklin JW, et al. Carcinomatous transformation of mixed tumors of the parotid gland. AMA Arch Surg 1957;75:605–13.
45. Thackray AC, Lucas RB. Tumors of the major salivary glands. In: Atlas of tumor pathology, 2nd series, Fascicle 10. Washington, DC: Armed forces Institute of Pathology; 1983. p. 107–17.
46. Witt RL, Eisele DW, Morton RP, et al. Etiology and management of recurrent parotid pleomorphic adenoma. Laryngoscope 2015;125:888–93.
47. Natvig K, Søberg R. Relationship of intraoperative rupture of pleomorphic adenomas to recurrence: an 11–25 year follow-up study. Head Neck 1994;16:213–7.
48. Manstopoulos K, Koch M, Klintworth N, et al. Evolution and changing trends in surgery for benign parotid tumors. Laryngoscope 2015;125:122–7.
49. Barzan L, Pin M. Extra-capsular dissection in benign parotid tumors. Oral Oncol 2012;48:977–9.
50. McGurk M, Thomas BL, Renehan AG. Extracapsular dissection for clinically benign parotid lumps: reduced morbidity without oncological compromise. Br J Cancer 2003;89:1610–3.
51. Piekarski J, Nejc D, Szymczak W, et al. Results of extracapsular dissection of pleomorphic adenoma of parotid gland. J Oral Maxillofac Surg 2004;62:1198–202.
52. Donovan DT, Conley JJ. Capsular significance in parotid tumor surgery: reality and myths of lateral lobectomy. Laryngoscope 1984;94:324–9.
53. O'Brien CJ. Current management of benign parotid tumors – the role of limited superficial parotidectomy. Head Neck 2003;25:946–52.
54. Mehta V, Nathan CA. Extracapsular dissection versus superficial parotidectomy for benign parotid tumors. Laryngoscope 2015;125:1039–40.
55. Blair VP. Surgery and diseases of the mouth and jaws. 3rd edition. St Louis (MO): CV Mosby; 1918. p. 492–523.
56. Bailey H. The treatment of tumors of the parotid glands. Br J Surg 1941;111:337–46.
57. Foustanos A, Zavrides H. Face-lift approach combined with a superficial musculoaponeurotic system advancement flap in parotidectomy. Br J Oral Maxillofac Surg 2007;45:652–5.
58. Wasson J, Karim H, Yeo J, et al. Cervicomastoidfacial versus modified facelift incision for parotid surgery: a patient feedback comparison. Ann R Coll Surg Engl 2010;92:40–3.

59. Lin TC, Chen PR, Wen YH, et al. Intra-auricular modification of facelift incision with sternocleidomastoid flap—a cosmetic approach for parotidectomy: how we do it. Clin Otolaryngol 2011;36:375–9.
60. Bianchi B, Ferri A, Ferrari S, et al. Improving aesthetic results in benign parotid surgery: statistical evaluation of facelift approach, sternocleidomastoid flap, and superficial musculoaponeurotic system flap application. J Oral Maxillofac Surg 2011;69:1235–41.
61. Appiani E. Plastic incisions for facial and neck tumors. Ann Plast Surg 1984;13: 335–52.
62. Lee SY, Koh WY, Kim BG, et al. The extended indication of parotidectomy using the modified facelift incision in benign lesions: retrospective analysis of a single institution. World J Surg 2011;35:2228–37.
63. Martí-Pagès C, García-Díez E, García-Arana L, et al. Minimal incision in parotidectomy. Int J Oral Maxillofac Surg 2007;36(1):72–6.
64. Casani AP, Cerchiai N, Dallan I, et al. Benign tumours affecting the deep lobe of the parotid gland: how to select the optimal surgical approach. Acta Otorhinolaryngol Ital 2015;35:80–7.
65. Presutti L, Molteni G, Malve L. Parapharyngeal space tumors without mandibulotomy: our experience. Eur Arch Otorhinolaryngol 2012;269:265–73.
66. Yang TL, Hsiao TY, Wang CP, et al. Extracapsular dissection for minimal resection of benign parapharyngeal tumor. Eur Arch Otorhinolaryngol 2012;269:2097–102.
67. Wittekindt C, Streubel K, Arnold G, et al. Recurrent pleomorphic adenoma of the parotid gland: analysis of 108 consecutive patients. Head Neck 2007;29:822–8.
68. Piorkowski RJ, Guillamondegui OM. Is aggressive surgical treatment indicated for recurrent benign mixed tumors of the parotid gland? Am J Surg 1981;142: 434–6.
69. Maran AG, Mackenzie IJ, Stanley RE. Recurrent pleomorphic adenoma of the parotid gland. Arch Otolaryngol 1984;110:167–71.
70. Dawson AK. Radiation therapy in recurrent pleomorphic adenoma of the parotid. Int J Radiat Oncol Biol Phys 1989;16:819–21.

Parotidectomy for Parotid Cancer

Jennifer R. Cracchiolo, MD*, Ashok R. Shaha, MD

KEYWORDS

- Parotid cancer • Parotidectomy • Facial nerve • Accessory parotid gland carcinoma

KEY POINTS

- Adequate excision of a parotid cancer should be based on the extent of the primary tumor.
- Every attempt should be made to remove all gross tumor. Radiation therapy does not compensate for inadequate surgery.
- The extent of parotidectomy depends more on the extent and location of the tumor than the histology of the tumor.
- The anatomic relationship of the tumor to the nerve dictates the extent of surgery, not the histologic classification of the neoplasm.

INTRODUCTION

Malignancy of the parotid gland requiring surgical management can be considered in 3 groups. First include primary parotid salivary malignancies. Although this group represents a small minority of head and neck tumors overall, parotid cancers represent a high percentage of salivary malignancies. Next, when working up a parotid malignancy, metastatic disease must be considered. This second group most commonly includes cutaneous malignancies (melanoma and nonmelanoma), however, may rarely involve metastatic disease from a distant site. A third less common but encountered situation that requires surgical management is direct extension of tumor into the parotid gland. This extension can be seen in cutaneous malignances, such as in neglected basal cell carcinoma or extension from an advanced oral cavity tumor. For all 3 categories, local control goals and the anatomy encountered may be similar. However, long-term outcomes may vary greatly; therefore, overall goals of surgery should be considered when deciding the extent of surgery, degree of radicality, and preservation/sacrifice of structure and function. The histology of primary salivary malignancies is vast and outcomes vary. For metastatic disease to the parotid gland, this often represents a biologically aggressive tumor, which may harbor features of

Disclosure: This research was funded in part through NIH/NCI Cancer Center Support Grants P30 CA008748 and T32 CA009685-23.
Head and Neck Service, Department of Surgery, Memorial Sloan Kettering Cancer Center, 1275 York Avenue, New York, NY 10065, USA
* Corresponding author.
E-mail address: cracchij@mskcc.org

0030-6665/16/$ – see front matter © 2016 Elsevier Inc. All rights reserved.

perineural invasion and a propensity for distant spread. In the current article, the authors discuss parotidectomy for parotid cancer: preoperative evaluation, technique, adjunct tools, and the controversies.

PREOPERATIVE EVALUATION

The preoperative approach to malignant disease in parotid tumors focuses on having adequate knowledge to plan the surgery as well as counsel patients and manage expectations. As discussed, most parotid tumors are benign; other than a detailed history and physical examination, additional diagnostic testing rarely alters surgical planning in most cases with well-circumscribed, mobile, slowly growing masses. However, when the history is atypical, the mass is ill defined, facial nerve (FN) involvement is present, or there is skin involvement, additional testing may offer information that defines anatomic boundaries when planning the extent of surgery as well as be useful with patient consulting. Additionally, if preoperative evaluation suggests FN sacrifice is likely, acquiring a team that can address facial reanimation at the time of surgery is beneficial. The authors discuss the history and physical examination with emphasis on findings associated with malignancy, radiographic assessment, and tissue diagnosis.

History and Physical Examination

Stigmata of parotid malignancy
- Rapid growth-fixed mass
- Pain
- FN paralysis
- Skin involvement
- Nodal metastasis

Rapid growth, pain, and FN paralysis represent the stigmata of parotid malignancy; however, in three-quarters of cases,[1] patients will present with an asymptomatic preauricular mass. While pain can sometimes point to infection or inflammatory disease is present in 44% of patients with carcinoma.[2] Facial palsy should always raise suspicion for malignancy and is present in 12% to 19% of patients with a malignant parotid mass independent of tumor size.[1–3] Importantly, in patients diagnosed with Bell palsy that does not improve or worsens, parotid carcinoma should remain high on the differential. In these patients the deep lobe parotid gland can harbor an occult cancer; therefore, attention should be given to the oral cavity as patients can present with swelling of the lateral oropharyngeal wall or soft palate in these cases. Other findings consistent with malignancy include skin involvement and cervical lymph node metastasis. Although skin involvement is a late and alarming sign of parotid malignancy, cervical metastasis is more dictated by the biology of the tumor. For example, in salivary ductal carcinoma and high-grade mucoepidermoid carcinoma, metastatic lymph nodes at presentation are quite high.

Tissue Diagnosis

Indications for preoperative biopsy of parotid lesions
- Is it something other than a salivary gland tumor?
- Will a histologic diagnosis change the management?
- Is the FN dissection likely to be tedious or is FN sacrifice likely?

Options for preoperative tissue diagnosis
- Fine-needle aspiration (FNA)
- Ultrasound-guided core biopsy
- Open biopsy

There is much debate surrounding the need for tissue diagnosis before proceeding to the operating room for parotidectomy. Those that disagree with tissue diagnosis before surgery suggest surgery remains the primary treatment independent of tissue diagnosis. Alternatively, others note tissue diagnosis offers the surgeon the ability to risk-stratify patients, to counsel them appropriately, and to avoid surgery in those cases whereby it is not appropriate or unnecessary. The authors consider FNA beneficial in evaluating poorly defined salivary gland masses and to confirm clinical suspicion of malignant disease. FNA can be particularly useful if FN paralysis/paresis is present in order to counsel patients before surgery. FNA is also useful in the scenario of metastatic disease in order to restage and direct adjuvant therapy. Finally, if patients are poor surgical patients, a benign FNA can justify an observation protocol. Alternatively, if the FNA shows lymphoma, surgery is generally not indicated and, therefore, can be avoided. In general, FNA has a relatively low sensitivity in malignant disease, however, is fairly specific. The reported numbers are broad. It could be hypothesized this is secondary to the technique used (image guided vs without imaging), the experience of the person taking the sample (surgeon vs pathologist), the broad range of pathologies associated with salivary malignancies, as well as the expertise of the cytopathologist. Mallon and colleagues[4] reported, for malignant disease, FNA has a sensitivity and specificity of 52% and 92%, respectively. In the authors' practice whereby FNA is used selectively, the authors have reported that FNA in the diagnosis of a malignant or suspicious lesion had positive and negative predictive values of 84% and 77%, respectively.[5] Many of the authors' false-negative FNAs (10 out of 20) were identified as low-grade lymphoma on final histology; therefore, cytologic findings of a lymphocyte-predominant lesion should prompt further work-up to rule out lymphoma. This work-up may involve a core biopsy. Ultrasound-guided core needle biopsy has been reported to be safe with a higher sensitivity and specificity than FNA in management of parotid lesions.[6–8] If FNA is nondiagnostic and a more definitive diagnosis is required or findings are concentrated with lymphocytes, ultrasound core biopsy should be considered to further clarify before proceeding to parotidectomy. Importantly, the predictive value of a negative FNA finding is low and should not take the place of clinical suspicion of malignancy. Additionally, FNA diagnosis is not used to make a critical intraoperative decisions regarding FN management or if the nerve is to be sacrificed. The management of FN in the operating room depends on the intraoperative findings.

Open biopsy of a discrete parotid lesion as a preoperative assessment before definitive surgery is rarely indicated secondary to the risk of FN palsy when the nerve is not defined intraoperatively, such as in a formal parotidectomy. Additionally, biopsy of a discrete lesion may result in tumor spillage and may predispose to tumor dissemination into surrounding skin and soft tissues. Open biopsy may be warranted in a very select group, including patients with a high suspicion of malignancy with likely FN sacrifice or in patients with suspected lymphoma and diagnosis cannot be made on FNA or core needle biopsy.

Imaging in Parotid Gland Malignancy

Indications for imaging in parotid malignancy
- Uncertain extent of disease
- Fixation to surrounding structures
- Parapharyngeal location
- Recurrent tumor
- Facial paresis or paralysis
- Cervical nodal involvement
- Patient under observation to document change in growth

Although imaging of parotid lesions can accurately predict malignant histology (MRI alone sensitivity 88% and specificity 77%),[9] the role of imaging in parotid gland malignancy is often to define the extent of disease. This definition includes local invasion into surrounding structures, perineural invasion, regional involvement such as in cervical metastasis, and evaluation of distant dissemination in the case of metastatic disease to the parotid or advanced primary salivary malignancies. A detailed discussion of parotid gland imaging is presented in another article of this publication. Briefly, for preoperative evaluation of parotid gland malignancies computed tomography (CT) is used for tumors extending into bony structures, for instance, into the mandible or temporal bone such as when an extended lateral temporal bone resection is planned to resect a locally invasive cutaneous malignancy or primary/metastatic lesion of the gland. MRI is useful in evaluating deep lobe versus parapharyngeal space tumors, base of skull extension, and cranial nerve involvement. Neurotrophic tumors, such as adenoid cystic carcinoma or cutaneous squamous cell carcinoma (cSSC), can often spread to via cranial nerves centrally. Identifying these characteristics may change the surgical approach and in some cases classifies patients as unresectable. Often both MRI and CT are complementary and contributory studies in advanced malignant tumors of the parotid gland.

EXTENT OF SURGERY FOR PAROTID MALIGNANCY

Variations in the extent of parotidectomy for malignancy
- Partial parotidectomy: limited, wide excision
- Superficial parotidectomy
- Total parotidectomy
- Radical parotidectomy
- Extended radical parotidectomy

Certainly parotidectomy using the technique of FN identification and parotid tissue resected is reasonably well standardized; however, the extent of parotid tissue needed to be excised to adequately address a malignant parotid neoplasm is a point of debate. Historically, surgical enucleation of parotid tumors resulted in high rates of FN palsy and tumor recurrence. Evolution of a less than superficial parotidectomy has been reported. This discussion mostly pertains to benign lesions.[10,11] For primary parotid cancers, if a partial parotidectomy is oncologically equivalent to a more extensive operation is difficult to assess given the rarity of the tumors, the vast number of histologies and the long time interval for recurrence. There is little evidence that more extensive operations result in better outcomes. Retrospectively, conservative parotidectomy, defined as any procedure that is less than a superficial parotidectomy whereby less than a full FN is dissected, has been reported in a small series[12] with comparable results with superficial parotidectomy. Importantly, about one-quarter of the patients in this series received adjuvant radiation; there was a median follow-up of less than 5 years, and only 43 patients were reported. Partial FN paralysis or paresis was 12%, comparable with Bron and O'Brien's[13] reported rates of 34% facial weakness for malignant tumors treated with complete superficial parotidectomy compared with 13% of those treated with a conservative parotidectomy.[13] It seems reasonable that, for small tumors whereby an adequate margin can be achieved while limiting FN dissection, a more conservative approach may result in improved postoperative FN function without compromising oncologic outcomes.

Total parotidectomy involves removal of all parotid tissue superficial to the FN as well as tissue deep to the FN. A discussion of indications for a deep lobe parotidectomy must first begin with an understanding of the concept that the division between the superficial and deep portions of the parotid is iatrogenic, not embryologic. Removal of the parotid tissue deep to the FN, representing 20% of the parotid glandular tissue, can be considered as 2 entities. The first group includes primary malignant parotid tumors originating from the deep lobe. In this case removal of the primary tumor with a cuff of margin will require a total parotidectomy, including a superficial parotidectomy for nerve identification and access and deep lobe of the parotid gland to excise the tumor. It should be noted that some deep lobe parotid tumors, located mostly in the parapharyngeal space, may be amenable to an isolated cervical approach; therefore, a superficial parotidectomy may not be required. These tumors represent a small minority of tumors and are often benign pleomorphic adenomas. These tumors can generally be easily removed through a stylohyoid window.

The second scenario is considered in metastatic disease and requires an understanding of the parotid gland as a lymphatic basin. The parotid gland is the first draining site for cutaneous malignancies on the cheek, pinna, forehead, and temple.[14] Anatomic studies have reported 7 lymph nodes in the superficial lobe (range, 3–19) and 2 in the deep lobe (range, 0–9).[15–17] Although there are fewer lymph nodes that reside within the tissue deep to the FN, this is consistent with less volume of glandular tissue in the deep lobe. Sites including the conjunctiva, oropharynx, and middle ear can also involve parotid lymph nodes.[16,18,19] Deep lobe lymph node metastasis can also arise from primary salivary gland malignances arising from the superficial gland. Controversy exists if total parotidectomy (extending the operation to clear tissue deep to the FN) is required when managing metastatic lesions to the parotid gland. Certainly, there is prognostic value to the identification of involved lymph nodes in the deep lobe tissue. Work by Thom and colleagues[20] showed that deep lobe metastasis from cSCC was a significant risk factor of distant metastatic disease, disease recurrence, death from disease, and overall survival. However, does extending radicality to involve the tissue deep to the FN alter outcomes? Although this question has not been answered in a randomized prospective fashion, analysis of retrospective studies indicates there may be a benefit to total parotidectomy in some select cases. When considering increasing radicality locally, local recurrence rates without this maneuver should be recognized. In a large series from Australia of 87 patients with clinical metastasis to the parotid gland, 82% had a superficial parotidectomy and 86% had adjuvant radiation.[21] Of the series, there was a local recurrence rate of 20%, with two-thirds observed in the deep bed of the parotid lobe. It is unclear if the recurrences were isolated to the group that underwent radical parotidectomy that were more likely to have a positive margin or if leaving tissue deep to the FN was a source of recurrence. Others have reported parotid bed recurrences ranging from 11% to 44%.[22–25] The Mayo Clinic has published on their experience with the use of total parotidectomy for primary salivary and metastatic disease involving the parotid gland.[20,26] Local parotid control rates of 93% (median follow-up 36.4 months) with metastatic cSCC and melanoma of 100% (median follow-up 30.6 months) was reported with the routine use of total parotidectomy for metastatic cutaneous malignancies.[20] Although local control in the parotid bed was superior to other series, overall survival remained poor. With the goal of improving local control, deep lobe parotidectomy can be considered when metastasis to the deep lymph nodes is likely. These cases include patients with metastasis to any intraparotid lymph nodes, high-grade primary parotid cancers, and primary parotid cancer with metastasis to lymph nodes of the parotid gland or neck nodes.

Radical parotidectomy involves removal of all parotid tissue as well as sacrifice of the FN. This procedure is done in cases whereby the FN has been invaded by tumor or if preoperative FN function was impaired in the presence of malignant disease.

Further discussion of indications and outcomes are included in the management of FN section.

Extended radical parotidectomy is carried out when the parotid tumor (primary salivary, metastatic disease, or through direct extension from a cutaneous malignancy) invades adjacent structures, such as the temporal bone, the mandibular bone, or the skin. These cases may require the performance of an extended total parotidectomy, which can include adjunct procedures, such as mandibulectomy, skin resection, infratemporal fossa dissection, and skull base or temporal bone resection. Prognosis for these patients is poor. Mehra and colleagues[27] reported on 12 patients that underwent lateral temporal bone resection (LTBR) as part of an extended parotidectomy as part of management of primary parotid malignancies. In addition to LTBR, 58% had partial mandibulectomy and 83% had FN sacrifice. Aggressive management of the primary site resulted in locoregional control of 75%. However, the 5-year survival was 22%. These data would support that the inclusion of LTBR as an adjunctive procedure in extended radical parotidectomy achieves reasonable rates of locoregional control and palliates local symptoms; however, overall survival remains poor secondary to distant failure. Of note, extending the parotidectomy may be needed in order to provide an FN segment with negative margins in order to graft. Overall, temporal bone surgery is an important adjunct to the management of advanced, recurrent, and metastatic parotid malignancies.

Extent of Surgery for Accessory Parotid Gland Carcinoma

Sometimes, primary salivary malignancies can arise in the accessory salivary tissue. This tissue follows the Stensen duct and, therefore, can present as a cheek mass. In general, surgery for accessory parotid tumor involves the identification of the FN by first completing a superficial parotidectomy and then tracing out the branches distally. However, in some cases, if the tumor is discrete and separate from the parotid gland, superficial parotidectomy can be avoided, as there is no oncologic justification for removal of the superficial parotid tissue in this scenario if total excision with negative margins can be achieved. This surgical technique involves identification of the buccal and zygomatic branches distally at the anterior edge after elevation of the anterior skin flap. The branches are then meticulously dissected and preserved.

INTRAOPERATIVE CONSIDERATIONS

Role of frozen sections in parotidectomy for malignancy
- Jugulodigastric node
- Periparotid node
- Confirm benign versus malignant or carcinoma versus lymphoma in primary salivary tumor
- Before sacrificing functioning nerve
- Tissue surrounding FN

As discussed, preoperative FNA is limited by its high false-negative rate; the extent of the operation can often depend on histology. Frozen section may provide an opportunity to refine the presurgical diagnosis intraoperatively among patients who are undergoing parotidectomy for presumed malignancy. Frozen section may be useful in 3 scenarios: confirmation/clarification of preoperative diagnosis, assessment of surgical margins, and determine whether nerve or neck involvement is present. Intraoperative frozen section has been shown to be useful in distinguishing benign from malignant tumors[28,29]; however, this may not add much when deciding how to manage FN involvement, extending the operation to address the deep lobe or cervical lymph nodes or terminating surgery in the case of lymphoma. Olson and colleagues[26] reported on the use of intraoperative frozen section in stratifying lymphoma or carcinoma, low-grade or high-grade malignant tumor, and the status of the intraparotid nodes in a high-volume setting. Although this group found frozen section useful as an intraoperative discussion tool, it must be considered that the variation in sensitivity and specificity will exist depending on the experience of the institution with salivary malignancies. Margin assessment is a tool unique to frozen section, which can be especially useful in the management of a resected FN. First it can be used to ensure proximal and distal control of the perineural spread before primary neural reconstruction. Additionally, for tumors that are located adjacent to the stylomastoid foramen and involve the FN, frozen section may be helpful in determining if an extended radical parotidectomy or dissection into the facial canal is required to control the proximal FN margin.

Frozen section assessment of the jugulodigastric lymph node (important for cutaneous malignancy) or periparotid lymph nodes may eliminate the need for a staged neck dissection if confirmed positive for metastatic disease during the primary surgery. This assessment may avoid, in some cases, the need to stage the neck dissection for high-grade lesions with high likelihood of regional cervical lymph node involvement.

FACIAL NERVE MANAGEMENT

> *In seventh nerve paralysis, joy, happiness, sorrow, shock, surprise, all the emotions have for their common expression the same blank stare.*
> —*Sterling Bunnell, 1827*[30]

A discussion of parotidectomy does not come without significant attention to FN management. This topic has been the subject of many sections of this publication. FN sacrifice is sometimes inevitable; however, protecting the nerve in cases whereby FN sacrifice does not add to an oncologic resection, when to take the FN versus when to peel the tumor off the nerve, and what tools are useful in helping make these intraoperative decisions are subjects of debate and represent an area for which a significant body of literature exists, sometimes with conflicting findings. In general, many would approach FN sacrifice with the philosophy of if the FN is functioning normally preoperatively, and not invading the nerve intraoperatively, then effort should be made to preserve it. This approach is based on the feeling that sacrifice of the nerve may add little to the surgical margin, however, results in significant morbidity to patients. Additionally, sacrifice of the FN does not avoid the need for adjuvant therapy in most cases. These statements, however, should not undervalue that every attempt should be made to achieve a clear surgical margin.

In patients with confirmed carcinoma and a nonfunctioning FN at the time of surgery, management of FN is more straightforward, including excision of involved portion, conformation of proximal and distal margin, and FN repair/reanimation procedure when appropriate. However, this scenario represents a small portion of patients presenting with parotid malignancy. Therefore, emphasis should be on patients presenting with carcinoma and a functioning FN. Tumor location as it relates to proximity of the FN and extent of tumor infiltration should be considered before sacrifice of a preoperatively functioning FN. If direct infiltration is seen at the time of the operation, FN sacrifice would be indicated. Larger tumors that are aggressive and infiltrative will often necessitate FN sacrifice.

FN involvement is a poor prognostic indicator[31–33]; however, it is unclear if increasing radically with FN sacrifice improves outcomes. In a comparison of patients treated with radical surgery versus conservative surgery, O'Brien and colleagues,[21] in a cohort of patients with metastatic cSCC, did not report a survival benefit (62% vs 54% at 5 years). Although Renehan and colleagues[34] reported a 10-year survival for patients having nerve sacrifice of 45% compared with 74% among those cases in which the nerve was spared. It is difficult to compare these 2 studies, as most cases in the later study were primary salivary malignancies. Additionally, more aggressive, infiltrative tumors with FN involvement requiring sacrifice are more likely to have poor survival outcomes. Although positive margins predict for local recurrence and poor outcomes,[21] FN sacrifice did not reduce the positive margin rate (FN sacrifice vs preservation O'Brien and colleagues[21] 53% vs 12%; Renehan and colleagues[34] 57% vs 53%) and local recurrences were equivalent for preservation versus sacrifice of the FN (FN sacrifice vs preservation O'Brien and colleagues 40% vs 24%) for cSCC. In the Renehan and colleagues'[34] cohort whereby primary parotid histology dominated, FN sacrifice versus preservation resulted in local recurrence rates of 21% versus 12%; however, as mentioned previously, 10-year survival was not significantly different.

SUMMARY

Parotidectomy for parotid cancer represents 3 entities, including management for primary salivary cancer, metastatic cancer to lymph nodes, and direct extension from surrounding structures or cutaneous malignancies. Preoperative evaluation should provide the surgeon with enough information to plan an oncologically sound operation, reconstruction when needed, and adequately counsel patients. FN sacrifice is sometimes required; but in preoperative functioning nerves, effort should be taken to preserve function. Although nerve involvement predicts poor outcome, with a sound oncologic procedure and adjuvant therapy, survival of around 50% has been reported for primary parotid malignancy. Metastatic cSSC is often a high-grade aggressive histology whereby local control for palliation with an extended parotidectomy can be achieved; however, overall survival remains poor, most often secondary to distant metastasis.

REFERENCES

1. Spiro RH, Huvos AG, Strong EW. Cancer of the parotid gland. A clinicopathologic study of 288 primary cases. Am J Surg 1975;130(4):452–9.
2. Poorten VV, Hart A, Vauterin T, et al. Prognostic index for patients with parotid carcinoma: international external validation in a Belgian-German database. Cancer 2009;115(3):540–50.
3. Johns ME. Parotid cancer: a rational basis for treatment. Head Neck Surg 1980; 3(2):132–41.
4. Mallon DH, Kostalas M, MacPherson FJ, et al. The diagnostic value of fine needle aspiration in parotid lumps. Ann R Coll Surg Engl 2013;95(4):258–62.
5. Cohen EG, Patel SG, Lin O, et al. Fine-needle aspiration biopsy of salivary gland lesions in a selected patient population. Arch Otolaryngol Head Neck Surg 2004; 130(6):773–8.
6. Haldar S, Mandalia U, Skelton E, et al. Diagnostic investigation of parotid neoplasms: a 16-year experience of freehand fine needle aspiration cytology and ultrasound-guided core needle biopsy. Int J Oral Maxillofac Surg 2015;44(2): 151–7.
7. Howlett DC, Skelton E, Moody AB. Establishing an accurate diagnosis of a parotid lump: evaluation of the current biopsy methods - fine needle aspiration

cytology, ultrasound-guided core biopsy, and intraoperative frozen section. Br J Oral Maxillofac Surg 2015;53(7):580–3.

8. Huang YC, Wu CT, Lin G, et al. Comparison of ultrasonographically guided fine-needle aspiration and core needle biopsy in the diagnosis of parotid masses. J Clin Ultrasound 2012;40(4):189–94.

9. Bartels S, Talbot JM, DiTomasso J, et al. The relative value of fine-needle aspiration and imaging in the preoperative evaluation of parotid masses. Head Neck 2000;22(8):781–6.

10. Huang G, Yan G, Wei X, et al. Superficial parotidectomy versus partial superficial parotidectomy in treating benign parotid tumors. Oncol Lett 2015;9(2):887–90.

11. Roh JL, Kim HS, Park CI. Randomized clinical trial comparing partial parotidectomy versus superficial or total parotidectomy. Br J Surg 2007;94(9):1081–7.

12. Lim YC, Lee SY, Kim K, et al. Conservative parotidectomy for the treatment of parotid cancers. Oral Oncol 2005;41(10):1021–7.

13. Bron LP, O'Brien CJ. Facial nerve function after parotidectomy. Arch Otolaryngol Head Neck Surg 1997;123(10):1091–6.

14. Vauterin TJ, Veness MJ, Morgan GJ, et al. Patterns of lymph node spread of cutaneous squamous cell carcinoma of the head and neck. Head Neck 2006;28(9):785–91.

15. McKean ME, Lee K, McGregor IA. The distribution of lymph nodes in and around the parotid gland: an anatomical study. Br J Plast Surg 1985;38(1):1–5.

16. Pisani P, Ramponi A, Pia F. The deep parotid lymph nodes: an anatomical and oncological study. J Laryngol Otol 1996;110(2):148–50.

17. Garatea-Crelgo J, Gay-Escoda C, Bermejo B, et al. Morphological study of the parotid lymph nodes. J Craniomaxillofac Surg 1993;21(5):207–9.

18. Nuyens M, Schüpbach J, Stauffer E, et al. Metastatic disease to the parotid gland. Otolaryngol Head Neck Surg 2006;135(6):844–8.

19. Mehlum DL, Parker GS, Strom CG, et al. Conjunctival squamous cell carcinoma with parotid gland metastasis. Otolaryngol Head Neck Surg 1986;94(2):246–9.

20. Thom JJ, Moore EJ, Price DL, et al. The role of total parotidectomy for metastatic cutaneous squamous cell carcinoma and malignant melanoma. JAMA Otolaryngol Head Neck Surg 2014;140(6):548–54.

21. O'Brien CJ, McNeil EB, McMahon JD, et al. Significance of clinical stage, extent of surgery, and pathologic findings in metastatic cutaneous squamous carcinoma of the parotid gland. Head Neck 2002;24(5):417–22.

22. Andruchow JL, Veness MJ, Morgan GJ, et al. Implications for clinical staging of metastatic cutaneous squamous carcinoma of the head and neck based on a multicenter study of treatment outcomes. Cancer 2006;106(5):1078–83.

23. Hinerman RW, Indelicato DJ, Amdur RJ, et al. Cutaneous squamous cell carcinoma metastatic to parotid-area lymph nodes. Laryngoscope 2008;118(11):1989–96.

24. Palme CE, O'Brien CJ, Veness MJ, et al. Extent of parotid disease influences outcome in patients with metastatic cutaneous squamous cell carcinoma. Arch Otolaryngol Head Neck Surg 2003;129(7):750–3.

25. Ch'ng S, Maitra A, Lea R, et al. Parotid metastasis–an independent prognostic factor for head and neck cutaneous squamous cell carcinoma. J Plast Reconstr Aesthet Surg 2006;59(12):1288–93.

26. Olsen KD, Moore EJ. Deep lobe parotidectomy: clinical rationale in the management of primary and metastatic cancer. Eur Arch Otorhinolaryngol 2014;271(5):1181–5.

27. Mehra S, Morris LG, Shah J, et al. Outcomes of temporal bone resection for locally advanced parotid cancer. Skull Base 2011;21(6):389–96.

28. Arabi Mianroodi AA, Sigston EA, Vallance NA. Frozen section for parotid surgery: should it become routine? ANZ J Surg 2006;76(8):736–9.

29. Olsen KD, Moore EJ, Lewis JE. Frozen section pathology for decision making in parotid surgery. JAMA Otolaryngol Head Neck Surg 2013;139(12):1275–8.

30. Bunnell S. Suture of the facial nerve within the temporal bone, with a report of the first successful case. Surg Gynecol Obstet 1827;45:7–12.

31. Terakedis BE, Hunt JP, Buchmann LO, et al. The prognostic significance of facial nerve involvement in carcinomas of the parotid gland. Am J Clin Oncol 2014. [Epub ahead of print].

32. Gallo O, Franchi A, Bottai GV, et al. Risk factors for distant metastases from carcinoma of the parotid gland. Cancer 1997;80(5):844–51.

33. Pedersen DE, Overgaard J, Søgaard H, et al. Malignant parotid tumors. Therapeutic results and prognosis in 110 consecutive patients. Ugeskr Laeger 1993; 155(29):2255–9 [in Danish].

34. Renehan AG, Gleave EN, Slevin NJ, et al. Clinico-pathological and treatment-related factors influencing survival in parotid cancer. Br J Cancer 1999;80(8): 1296–300.

Parotid Gland Tumors and the Facial Nerve

Michele M. Gandolfi, MD, William Slattery III, MD*

KEYWORDS

- Parotid tumor • Facial nerve • Paralysis • Paresis • Facial nerve weakness

KEY POINTS

- The different types of parotid gland tumors, nonneoplastic and both benign and malignant neoplasms, are discussed.
- In general, benign tumors do not affect facial nerve function. However, there are some rare cases of benign tumors invading the stylomastoid foramen, and through compression, presenting with facial nerve paresis/paralysis.
- Facial nerve paresis/paralysis is a poor prognostic indication and is associated with size and aggressiveness of parotid tumor.

INTRODUCTION

Approximately 25% of parotid masses are nonneoplastic; the remaining 75% are neoplastic.[1] Salivary gland tumors are relatively rare and constitute only 3% to 4% of all head and neck neoplasms. Approximately 70% of salivary gland tumors arise in the parotid gland.[2] Although most minor salivary gland tumors are malignant, three-fourths of parotid tumors are benign.[1] The most common malignant types of tumor in the parotid gland are mucoepidermoid carcinoma (30%), adenoid cystic carcinoma, and malignant mixed tumors.[1] Traditionally, facial nerve paralysis or paresis is an ominous sign that a parotid mass is most likely malignant and has invaded the facial nerve. However, this is not always the case because there have been case reports indicating that some benign tumors of the parotid gland can invade the stylomastoid foramen, and through compression, can cause paresis or paralysis.

At least 2 theories of tumorigenesis have been proposed for salivary gland neoplasms. In the first, the multicellular theory, each type of neoplasm is thought to originate from a distinctive cell type within the salivary gland unit. Therefore, Warthin and oncocytic tumors are thought to arise from striated ductal cells, acinic cell tumors from acinar cells, and mixed tumors from intercalated duct and myoepithelial cells.[1,2] This theory is supported by the observation that all differentiated salivary cell types retain

House Clinic, 2100 West 3rd Street, Los Angeles, CA 90057, USA
* Corresponding author.
E-mail address: Wslattery@hei.org

Otolaryngol Clin N Am 49 (2016) 425–434
http://dx.doi.org/10.1016/j.otc.2015.12.001
0030-6665/16/$ – see front matter © 2016 Elsevier Inc. All rights reserved.

the ability to undergo mitosis and regenerate.[1] The second theory, the bicellular reserve cell theory, assumes that the origin of the various types of salivary neoplasms can be traced to the basal cells of either the excretory or the intercalated duct. According to this theory, either of these 2 cells can act as a reserve cell with the potential for differentiation into a variety of epithelial cells.[1,2] So despite the seeming heterogeneity of salivary tumors, all of them are thought to arise from 1 of 2 pluripotent stem cell populations. In this theory, adenomatoid tumors, including pleomorphic adenoma, and oncocytic tumors are derived from the reserve cell of the intercalated duct, whereas epidermoid tumors, such as squamous cell and mucoepidermoid carcinomas, are derived from the reserve cells of the excretory duct.[1,2] Some reports provide molecular evidence to support the reserve cell theory of salivary gland tumorigenesis.

FACIAL NERVE

The main trunk of the facial nerve exits the skull base via the stylomastoid foramen, immediately producing 3 small branches: the posterior auricular, posterior digastric, and stylohyoid nerves.[1] The facial nerve then courses laterally around the styloid process and is immediately superficial to the posterior belly of the digastric muscle. As the nerve continues caudally, it pierces the posterior capsule of the parotid gland. The main trunk typically bifurcates in to the zygomaticotemporal branch and the cervicofacial branch at the pes anserinus, also known as the goose's foot, and thereafter into the temporal, zygomatic, buccal, marginal, and cervical branches.[1] The pes anserinus is about 1.3 cm from the stylomastoid foramen. The nerve continues within the gland, going lateral to the posterior facial vein or retromandibular vein and the more medially situated external carotid artery. The nerve then divides via variable anatomic patterns into the temporal, zygomatic, buccal, mandibular, and cervical branches (**Fig. 1**). There is an important nerve that connects the facial nerve and the mandibular nerve (V3): the auriculotemporal nerve. Tumor from a parotid malignancy can extend along this nerve and then spread in a retrograde manner along the trigeminal nerve. Thus, transection of this nerve in appropriate cases is an important surgical consideration when dealing with parotid malignancies.[1]

Regardless of whether they are benign or malignant, tumors of the parotid gland usually present as a painless swelling. There are some nonneoplastic parotid tumors that should be also be considered, such as lymphoepithelial lesions caused by lymphomas or human immunodeficiency virus, and granulomatous masses caused by sarcoidosis and Sjorgren syndrome. These masses tend to present as diffuse swelling or multiple swellings and less so as a discrete parotid tumor.[1,2] They do not typically cause any deficit in the function of the facial nerve. Neoplastic benign tumors are usually present for a long duration and have a slow growth rate. However, patients may indicate that they incidentally noticed the appearance of a lump. Rapid increase in the size of a long-standing mass should raise the suspicion of malignant transformation of a pre-existing benign tumor but may be due to inflammation or cystic degeneration, most commonly associated with Warthin tumor.[1] Patients who come to medical attention with a mass in the parotid gland should be asked about a history of cancer of the scalp or facial skin. Metastasis to the parotid gland from skin cancer, including melanoma, may be diagnosed by a careful examination of these areas for evidence of a skin cancer or a scar from a previous excision.[1]

On examination, benign tumors of the parotid gland are usually well defined, nontender, and freely mobile. They are commonly located in the "tail" of the parotid gland but may be present anywhere in the superficial or deep lobe. Tumors may originate entirely from the deep lobe or they may extend from the superficial to the deep lobe

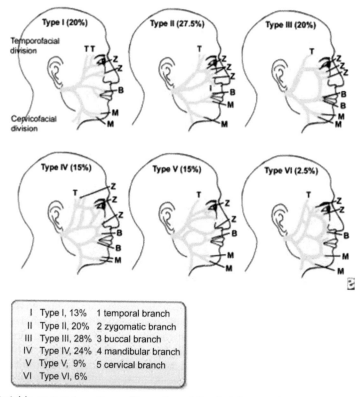

I	Type I, 13%	1 temporal branch
II	Type II, 20%	2 zygomatic branch
III	Type III, 28%	3 buccal branch
IV	Type IV, 24%	4 mandibular branch
V	Type V, 9%	5 cervical branch
VI	Type VI, 6%	

Fig. 1. Variable anatomic pattern of branches of the facial nerve. (*From* Standring S. Gray's anatomy. 40th edition. Philadelphia, PA: Elsevier; 2008; with permission.)

through the relatively narrow stylomandibular tunnel, which gives the appearance of a dumbbell tumor. In either case, the tumor may extend to the parapharyngeal space and may displace the oropharyngeal wall medially. The presence of pain, facial nerve paresis or paralysis, fixation of the mass to the overlying skin or underlying structures, and associated cervical adenopathy usually indicates the presence of malignancy.[1] It should be noted, however, that these findings usually indicate local or regional extension of the tumor, and the diagnosis of parotid malignancy should not await the development of these signs and symptoms. The possibility of malignancy should be ruled out in patients with any mass in the parotid gland. A mass in the parotid gland will usually require cytologic or histologic evaluation with fine-needle aspiration (FNA) biopsy or parotidectomy.

Facial nerve paralysis is most commonly associated with parotid undifferentiated carcinoma (24%), squamous cell carcinoma (19%), adenoid cystic carcinoma (17%), adenocarcinoma (11%), mucoepidermoid carcinoma (9%), carcinoma ex pleomorphic adenoma (7%), and acinic cell carcinoma (1%).[1,2] Overall, if the facial nerve is paralyzed at clinical presentation, the 5-year survival rate is only between 9% and 14%.[1] Pain on presentation of a parotid mass most likely indicates perineural invasion, which greatly increases the likelihood of malignancy in a patient with a parotid mass. Of patients with malignant parotid tumors, 7% to 20% present with facial nerve weakness or paralysis, which rarely accompanies benign lesions and indicates a poor prognosis. Facial nerve tumor invasion and therefore functional paresis or paralysis often correlate directly with an increased rate of nodal metastasis of up to 66% to 77%.[1] These patients have an average survival of 2.7 years and a 10-year survival of 14% to 26%.[1]

The House-Brackmann Facial Nerve Grading System is widely used to characterize the degree of facial paralysis.[1] Having common nomenclature in order to communicate the severity of the facial nerve paresis is important to standardize. In this scale, grade I is assigned to normal function, and grade VI represents complete paralysis. Intermediate grades vary according to function at rest and with effort (**Tables 1** and **2**).

PREOPERATIVE IMAGING OF PAROTID MASSES

In terms of evaluation of a parotid mass, plain film radiography and sialography have more recently been replaced with computed tomography (CT) and MRI, due to improvement in sensitivity and resolution.[2] CT is very useful for evaluating salivary gland masses, providing thin-section (3–5 mm) slices and on multislice CT as thin as 0.6- to 0.725-mm slices.[2] CT allows detection of location, size, and relationship with other large anatomic structures, especially bony landmarks, which are achieved with ease.

MRI appears to be complementary and may be superior to CT in portrayal of tissue characterization and extent of disease.[2] MRI may be better than CT in segregating parotid from extraparotid space masses, such as paraganglioma, schwannoma, or minor salivary gland masses. MRI also appears to have greater sensitivity and higher resolution than CT.[2] On T1-weighted images, all parotid masses are isointense to muscle in signal intensity and can be separated from the normal hyperintense signal intensity of the rest of the parotid gland. Along with fat-saturated T1-weighted postcontrast images for the delineation of the tumor borders as well as illustration of perinerual spread, these 2 sequences may be used to determine boundary and extent of lesion.[2] T2-weighted images are in general not specific in separating tumor types because

Table 1 House-Brackmann facial nerve paresis description				
Grade	Description	Gross Function	Resting Appearance	Dynamic Appearance
1	Normal	Normal	Normal	Normal
2	Mild dysfunction	Slight weakness with effort, may have mild synkinesis	Normal	Mild oral and forehead asymmetry; complete eye closure with minimal effort
3	Moderate dysfunction	Obvious asymmetry with movement, noticeable synkinesis, or contracture	Normal	Mild oral asymmetry, complete eye closure with effort, slight forehead movement
4	Moderately severe dysfunction	Obvious asymmetry, disfiguring asymmetry	Normal	Asymmetrical mouth, incomplete eye closure, no forehead movement
5	Severe dysfunction	Barely perceptible movement	Asymmetric	Slight oral/nasal movement with effort, incomplete eye closure
6	Total paralysis	None	Asymmetric	No movement

From House JW, Brackmann DE. Facial nerve grading system. Otolaryngol Head Neck Surg 1985;93(2):146; with permission.

Table 2
House-Brackmann facial nerve paresis estimated function

Grade	Description	Measurement	Function, %	Estimated Function, %
I	Normal	8/8	100	100
II	Slight	7/8	76–99	80
III	Moderate	5/8–6/8	51–75	60
IV	Moderately severe	3/8–4/8	26–50	40
V	Severe	1/8–2/8	1–25	20
VI	Total	0/8	0	0

From House JW, Brackmann DE. Facial nerve grading system. Otolaryngol Head Neck Surg 1985;93(2):147; with permission.

most tumors are hyperintense in signal intensity. One should keep in mind that those lesions that demonstrate isointense to hypointense signal intensity relative to muscle may be indicative of malignancy. MRI is less useful in demonstrating calcification, which is better with CT. MRI is contraindicated for patients with severe claustro-phobia, pacemakers, intracranial ferromagnetic aneurysm clips, and most cochlear implants and brainstem implants.[2] Although the use of gadolinium does not add very much additional useful information and usually is not given, it may aid in depiction of perineural spread in such cases of adenoid cystic carcinoma. Extraglandular tumor infiltration may be better defined with gadolinium also.[1,2]

In most instances, a CT with and without contrast is ordered when a parotid mass is encountered. If there is any suspicion based on history, symptoms, or FNA that tumor could be malignant, then an MRI with and without gadolinium is ordered if possible perinueral spread or extraglandular infiltration is suspected.

NONNEOPLASTIC PAROTID TUMORS AND THE FACIAL NERVE

Causes of nonneoplastic tumors of the parotid include granulomatous, lymphoepithe-lial, and certain inflammatory diseases. Most of these manifest by an asymptomatic, gradual diffuse enlargement of a lymph node or lymphatic cells within the gland. In sarcoidosis, salivary gland involvement may cause duct obstruction, pain associated with the duct, xerostomia, or enlargement of the gland. Unlike neoplasms, these can cause pain in their early stages. They are also distinguished from neoplasms because they begin with diffuse enlargement of one or more salivary glands.[3] This category of tumors usually does not cause involvement of the facial nerve. However, there have been a few rare case reports of Heerfordt syndrome characterized by fever uveitis, pa-rotid gland enlargement, and facial nerve palsy.[4–7] In addition, there have also been case reports of lymphoepithelial cysts causing facial paralysis.[8] These cases resolved with systemic treatment with high-dose steroids and medical treatment.

BENIGN PAROTID TUMORS AND THE FACIAL NERVE

Pleomorphic adenomas are by far the most common of the benign tumors of the parotid gland. Warthin tumor, or papillary cystadenoma lymphomatosum, is the sec-ond most common, accounting for 6% to 10%. Pleomorphic adenomas, also known as benign mixed tumors, are the most common neoplasms of the salivary gland. The term pleomorphic was chosen to describe these tumors, because they possess morphologic diversity with both epithelial and mesenchymal components in various proportions.[1,2] Pleomorphic adenoma constitutes approximately 75% of all benign tumors of the major salivary glands.

In the parotid gland, approximately 90% of pleomorphic adenomas originate superficial to the facial nerve.[3] Occasionally, tumors of the superficial lobe extend to the deep lobe medial of the facial nerve. If they extend to the parapharyngeal space through the stylomandibular "tunnel" bounded by the stylomandibular ligament, they may have a narrow isthmus that connects the superficial and deep components, which can give the tumor a dumbbell appearance.[3] Approximately 10% of pleomorphic adenomas originate entirely from the deep lobe and are usually located deep to the stylomandibular ligament; therefore, they have a more rounded appearance on high-resolution imaging.

Clinically, pleomorphic adenoma is characterized as a painless, slow-growing mass. Multiple primary pleomorphic adenomas are extremely rare, although they have been reported.[3,9] Pathologically, pleomorphic adenomas are solitary, firm, round tumors. The cut surface is characteristically solid and may be hard, rubbery, or soft in consistency with a whitish gray to pale yellow color. Pleomorphic adenoma of the parotid typically has a capsule, although it varies in thickness and completeness, whereas pleomorphic adenoma of the minor salivary glands is usually unencapsulated.[9] On histologic examination, pleomorphic adenoma consists of an epithelial component that may take the form of ducts, nests, cords, or solid sheets of cells and myoepithelial cells that appear plasmacytoid or spindled in a fibrocollagenous, myxochondroid, or chondroid background. Myoepithelium in pleomorphic adenoma is considered to be responsible for the development of the characteristic myxoid or chondroid stroma. Variations in the histologic appearance of this tumor type are common and may include squamous metaplasia, calcification, cartilaginous tissue, oxyphilic cells, tyrosine-calcium oxalate crystals, and a palisading appearance of the underlying stroma. Lipomatous and osseous changes have been occasionally reported in pleomorphic adenoma.[3,9]

Malignant transformation of pleomorphic adenoma is rare and occurs most frequently in patients with long-standing tumors. The risk of malignant transformation in pleomorphic adenoma is 1.5% within the first 5 years of diagnosis, but this increases to 10% if observed for more than 15 years.[9] Cases of benign pleomorphic adenoma metastasizing to cervical lymph nodes have been reported.

Although most benign neoplasms such as pleomorphic adenomas do not commonly cause facial nerve paralysis on presentation, there have been a few case reports of invasion of pleomorphic adenomas into the stylomastoid foramen causing compressing and paresis of the facial nerve.[10,11] These cases were initially thought to be Bell palsy; however, once it did not resolve and imaging was done, the mass was discovered in the stylomastoid foramen.

Warthin tumor most commonly occurs in the parotid gland and typically presents in older men, and it has a correlation with smoking history.[1,2] This tumor usually presents as a slow-growing mass in the tail of the parotid. Tumors can be multicentric in up to 21% of cases and approximately 10% are bilateral.[2] The gross appearance of the tumor is smooth with a well-defined capsule. Cut sections contain multiple cystic spaces of different sizes filled with thick, mucinous material. There also have been rare reports of Warthin tumors of the parotid causing facial nerve paresis.[12] However, this was also superinfected, and the inflammatory process most likely contributed to the paresis. Return to function on antibiotic treatment and superficial parotidectomy was the outcome with no residual sequel.

Oncocytoma occurs almost exclusively within in the parotid gland and accounts for less than 1% of all parotid neoplasms.[13] The tumor occurs in the sixth or seventh decade of life with equal predilection for men and women. They are noncystic, firm, and rubbery. Microscopically, they contain plump granular eosinophilic cells and a mitochondria-filled cytoplasm. Like the other benign neoplasms, there are rare case reports of oncocytoma causing facial nerve paralysis,[14] usually caused by a superinfection, and medical treatment and surgical intervention does lead to resolution.[14] Other benign neoplasms, such as monomorphic adenomas, and intraductal papilloma are rare and usually epithelial in origin and do not affect the function of the facial nerve.[2,3] Benign nonepithelial tumors such as hemangioma and lymphangiomas are commonly found in children and also do not commonly affect facial nerve function.[3]

MALIGNANT PAROTID TUMORS AND THE FACIAL NERVE

Mucoepidermoid carcinoma is the most common malignant tumor of the parotid gland, roughly one-third of all parotid cancers, and it is classified into low and high grade based on histologic amount of mucinous versus epidermoid cells. Low-grade tumors usually contain more mucoid cells. High-grade tumors require selective neck dissection, and postoperative radiation is often necessary. Such tumors still have a 5-year survival rate of 52%.[9]

Adenoid cystic carcinoma is an aggressive tumor with a predilection for perineural spread with skip metastasis along the facial nerve and its branches; the incidence of such increases with higher tumor stages.[9] The incidence of local recurrence is also very high, and postoperative radiation therapy is often necessary for those with perineural invasion or positive margins.[3,9] Cervical lymph node metastasis is relatively low; however, distant metastasis to the lung and liver has been reported to be as high as 38%.[3,9]

Adenocarcinoma is a malignant parotid neoplasm that has decreased in incidence due to reclassification into variants of other subtypes and histopathologies.[3,9] They are aggressive tumors with high rates of facial nerve involvement, regional disease, and distant metastasis. It should be managed as a high-grade parotid tumor, and radiation postoperatively is necessary.

Acinic cell carcinoma is a low-grade tumor with a female predominance of about 60%, bilateral presentation 3% of the time, and a 20-year overall survival rate of 90%.[9] These tumors are well circumscribed, but a small percentage of them do have cervical metastasis. They can be managed with surgery alone, but some histopathological findings that suggest aggressiveness warrant radiation therapy. A recent study found that patients with undifferentiated or poorly differentiated histologic grades of acinic cell carcinoma had dramatically lower 10- and 20-year survival rates.[15]

Primary squamous cell carcinoma of the parotid gland is rare, and most are due to skin cancer that has metastasized to the periparotid lymph nodes. Primary lymphoma is also uncommon with only 5% of parotid masses having this diagnosis. Sarcomas and neuroendocrine tumors (small cell and Merkel cell carcinomas) are rare and require surgical along with adjunctive radiation and chemotherapy.[3,9]

NERVE SHEATH TUMORS OF THE PAROTID GLAND

Neurogenic intraparotid benign tumors may be either schwannoma or neurofibroma. Schwannoma are an encapsulated tumor. Microscopically, the typical palisading nuclei of Schwann cell Antoni type A or type B pattern will be evident. Neurofibromas are nonencapsulated tumors and composed of an admixture of all elements of a peripheral nerve. The histologic difference between schwannomas and neurofibromas of the facial nerve may dictate the type of surgical resection.[16] Theoretically, schwannomas can be stripped free of the nerve without sacrificing the nerve. In contrast, fibers from the facial nerve pass directly through a neurofibroma, and separation of the nerve fibers from the tumor is rarely possible.[16]

Schwannomas of the facial nerve arise from either the extratemporal or the intratemporal course of this nerve.[17] Most of these tumors are intratemporal, whereas 9% are located extracranially and usually appear as an asymptomatic parotid mass.[18] Intraparotid facial nerve schwannomas account for only 2 types of 142 parotid tumors.[17] Hence, it is difficult to establish a correct preoperative diagnosis for facial nerve schwannoma.[17] Some investigators, however, point toward a trend of facial nerve schwannomas having a predilection toward growth along the facial canal more so than other more common tumors such as pleomorphic adenomas.[19]

The typical presentation of an intraparotid facial nerve schwannoma is a slow-growing, painless parotid mass mimicking the most common benign parotid tumor, pleomorphic adenoma. In addition, intraparotid facial nerve schwannoma intraparotid may present with pain or facial palsy and may raise suspicion of a malignant parotid tumor. The incidence of facial nerve palsy in intraparotid facial nerve schwannoma is about 20% to 27%.[17] Although most patients with intraparotid schwannomas do not present with facial nerve palsy, it is important to suggest this diagnosis preoperatively because postoperative facial nerve paresis or palsy is common, and these patients can be better informed of this complication before surgery.

Malignant peripheral nerve sheath tumor (MPNST) refers to spindle cell sarcomas arising from or separating in the direction of cells of the peripheral nerve sheath[20]; this is most commonly Schwann cells, but multiple cell origins have been speculated. The MPNST of the parotid gland is an extremely rare tumor, usually having a poor prognosis, and only a few cases been described in the literature.[20]

METASTASIS TO THE PAROTID GLAND

Metastasis to the parotid does commonly occur with skin squamous cell carcinoma as previously mentioned. Melanoma additionally can present this way. Cutaneous squamous cell and melanoma are exceedingly the most common metastatic parotid malignancies, and unfortunately, despite proper treatment, 25% to 50% will have local or distant failure.[21–23] Other cancers that have been reported to metastasize to the parotid include basal cell, Merkel cell, and small cell carcinomas.[9] All of these have the potential to infiltrate the facial nerve and affect its function.

DISCUSSION

Overwhelmingly, malignant tumors of the parotid gland have a higher incidence of facial nerve involvement and functional deficits. In a recent study on how parotid tumor size predicts proximity to facial nerve, they found malignant tumors were most likely to have positive facial nerve margin (63% vs 53% of pleomorphic adenomas and 37% of Warthin tumors).[24] For all type tumors 5 cm or larger, 82.3% had a positive facial nerve margin. Tumors less than 2 cm were least likely to have a positive facial nerve margin. Logistic regression showed that diameter was correlated with risk of facial nerve margin positivity as predicted. These results demonstrate that parotid tumor diameter is both a convenient and a functional means of predicting proximity of a tumor to the facial nerve and for preoperative risk stratification. These observations have important clinical implications for surgical planning.[24]

In some malignant parotid tumors, preoperative imaging (ultrasonography, CT, and magnetic resonance) does not have the resolution for nerve structure visualization.[25] Therefore, intraoperative nerve assessment is crucial in the decision-making process as to whether the nerve should be resected. A study by Wierzbicka and colleagues[25] aimed to assess the frequency of facial paralysis and undiagnosed nerve infiltration in patients with parotid malignancies and evaluate the duration of symptoms before presentation. In addition, they wanted to define risk factors for nerve impairment and the impact of facial nerve involvement in treatment methods, outcomes, and survival.

In this study, facial nerve palsy appeared in 33% (32/103), and this included 28 patients with total paralysis and 4 with partial paralysis.[25] Facial nerve palsy was the clinical symptom in 60% of patients with adenoid cystic carcinoma and in 66% with squamous cell cancer. Paralysis (33.3%) was less frequent in cancers developing from mixed tumors. They also showed that tumor size played a significant role in facial palsy because it occurred more in tumors greater than 4 cm. Also, the duration of symptoms in patients with facial nerve palsy was nearly 3 months longer than in patients whose only symptoms was a tumor.[25] Terhaard and colleagues[26] also presented similar findings. They demonstrated that facial nerve palsy correlated with a significantly lower percentage of survival and tumor size correlated with severity of symptoms.

SUMMARY

Although there are rare cases of nonneoplastic and benign neoplasms of the parotid gland causing facial nerve paralysis or paresis, malignant tumors have a much higher rate of paresis. One should be highly suspicious of any diagnosis of Bell palsy that does not resolve with time, and imaging should be done to evaluate for a tumor causing facial nerve paresis. Tumors such as adenoid cystic and squamous cell carcinoma have higher rates of facial nerve involvement than other malignant parotid tumors.

REFERENCES

1. Haughey BH, Thomas JR, Niparko JK, et al. Cummings otolaryngology. In: Flint PW, Haughey BH, Lund VJ, et al, editors. Head and neck surgery, 3 Volume Set, 6th edition. Philadelphia, PA: Elsevier; 2012. p. 1133–78.
2. Johnson JT, Rosen CA, Bailey BJ. Baileys head and neck surgery. In: Otolaryngology. 5th edition. Philadelphia, PA: Wolters Kluwer Health/Lippincott Williams & Wilkins; 2014. p. 689–814.
3. Shaha AR. ACS surgery: principles and practice. Chapter 2 parotid mass. Head and Neck. 2006. Available at: http://www.med.unc.edu/surgery/education/files/articles/Parotid%20Mass.pdf.
4. Petropoulos IK, Zuber JP, Guex-Crosier Y. Heerfordt syndrome with unilateral facial nerve palsy: a rare presentation of sarcoidosis. Klin Monbl Augenheilkd 2008;224(5):453–6.
5. Tamme T, Leibur E, Kulla A. Sarcoidosis (Heerfordt syndrome): a case report. Stomatologija 2007;9(2):61–4.
6. Fieb A, Frisch I, Wicht S, et al. A rare manifestation of sarcoidosis. Ophthalmologe 2012;109(8):794–7.
7. Kato K, Kato Y, Tanaka Y, et al. Case of Heerfordt's syndrome presenting polyneuropathy. Nippon Ganka Gakkai Zaashi 2011;115(5):460–4.
8. Watts SJ, Turner NO, San Juan J, et al. Facial paralysis caused by a lymphoepithelial cyst located in the parotid gland. J Laryngol Otol 1996;110(8):799–801.
9. Lin HW, Bhattacharyya N. Chapter: parotid mass head and neck. Scientific American Surgery; Decker Intelletual Properties Inc; 2014.
10. Blevins NH, Jackler RK, Kaplan MJ. Facial paralysis due to benign parotid tumors. Arch Otolaryngol Head Neck Surg 1992;118:427–30.

11. Nader M, Bell D, Sturgis EM, et al. Facial nerve paralysis due to a pleomorphic adenoma with the imaging characteristics of a facial nerve schwannoma. J Neurol Surg Rep 2014;75:e84–8.

12. Grosheva M, Ortmann M, Beutner D. Facial nerve palsy due to a benign parotid gland tumor. HNO 2010;58(12):1197–8.

13. Stavrianos SD, McLean NR, Soames JV. Synchronous unilateral parotid neoplasms of different histological types. Eur J Surg Oncol 1999;25:331–2.

14. Roden DM, Levy FE. Oncocytoma of the parotid gland presenting with nerve paralysis. Otolaryngol Head Neck Surg 1994;110(6):587–90.

15. Patel NR, Sanghvi S, Khan MN, et al. Demographic trends and disease-specific survival in salivary acinic cell carcinoma: an analysis of 1129 cases. Laryngoscope 2014;124:172–8.

16. Verma KR, Prasad RK, Bharti S, et al. Intraparotid facial nerve schannoma involving the deep lobe: a case report. Egyptian J of ENT and Allied Sciences 2011;12:163–6.

17. Balle VH, Greisen O. Neurilemomas of the facial nerve presenting as parotid tumors. Ann Otol Rhinol Laryngol 1984;93:70–2.

18. Forton GE, Moeneclaey LL, Offeciers FE. Facial nerve neuroma: report of two cases including histological and radiological imaging studies. Eur Arch Otorhinolaryngol 1994;251:17–22.

19. Shimizu K, Iwai H, Ikeda K, et al. Intraparotid facial nerve schannoma: a report of five cases and an analysis of MR imaging results. AJNR Am J Neuroradiol 2005; 26:1328–30.

20. Chris O, Albu S. Malignant peripheral nerve sheath tumor of the parotid gland. J Craniofac Surg 2014;25(5):e424–6.

21. Bron LP, Traynor SJ, McNeil EB, et al. Primary and metastatic cancer of the parotid: comparison of clinical behavior in 232 cases. Laryngoscope 2003;113: 1070–5.

22. O'Brian CJ, McNeil EB, McMahon JD, et al. Significance of clinical stage, extent of surgery, and pathologic findings in metastatic cutaneous squamous carcinoma of the parotid gland. Head Neck 2002;24:417–22.

23. Andruchow JL, Veness MJ, Morgan GJ, et al. Implication for clinical staging of metastatic cutaneous squamous carcinoma of the head and neck on a multicenter study of treatment outcomes. Cancer 2006;106:1078–83.

24. Domenick NA, Johnson JT. Parotid tumor size predicts proximity to the facial nerve. Laryngoscope 2011;121:2366–70.

25. Wierzbicka M, Kopec T, Szyfter W. The presence of facial nerve weakness on diagnosis of a parotid gland malignant process. Eur Arch Otorhinolaryngol 2012;269:1177–82.

26. Terhaard CH, Lubsen H, Va der Tweel I, et al. Salivary gland carcinoma: independent prognostic factors for locoregional control, distant metastases, and overall survival: results of the Dutch head and neck oncology cooperative group. Head Neck 2004;26(8):681–92.

Locoregional Parotid Reconstruction

 CrossMark

Leslie E. Irvine, MD[a], Babak Larian, MD[b], Babak Azizzadeh, MD[b],*

KEYWORDS

- Parotidectomy • Parotidectomy reconstruction • Sternocleidomastoid muscle flap
- Supraclavicular artery island flap • Acellular dermis

KEY POINTS

- Reconstruction after parotidectomy is customized to patients' needs.
- Exposure of both sides of the face during parotidectomy allows accurate reconstruction based on the contralateral side.
- Local and regional flaps can be used for most benign and malignant tumors and the sternocleidomastoid muscle flap is a useful first choice in most cases.
- Reconstruction after radical parotidectomy involves volume restoration, commonly with the supraclavicular artery island flap or free tissue transfer, as well as facial nerve reconstruction.

INTRODUCTION

Most salivary gland tumors are located in the parotid gland, and 70% to 80% of these neoplasms are benign.[1,2] Tumor resection may involve partial, superficial, total, or radical parotidectomy, depending on pathology findings and location.[3] Regardless of the extent of resection, patients are often left with a cosmetic deformity in the preauricular, infra-auricular, and retromandibular regions. This cosmetic deformity can cause disfigurement and decrease patients' quality of life.[4,5]

The principal goals of reconstruction after parotidectomy include correcting any facial nerve abnormality, preventing gustatory sweating (Frey syndrome), and restoring facial symmetry and contour. A cosmetically pleasing reconstruction is especially important given the preponderance of benign tumors among a fairly young

Disclosure: The authors have nothing to disclose.
[a] Caruso Department of Head and Neck Surgery, Keck School of Medicine, University of Southern California, 1540 Alcazar Street, Los Angeles, CA 90033, USA; [b] Department of Head and Neck Surgery, Center for Advanced Facial Plastic Surgery, David Geffen School of Medicine, University of California, 9401 Wilshire Boulevard, Los Angeles, Beverly Hills, CA 90212, USA
* Corresponding author. Center for Advanced Facial Plastic Surgery, 9401 Wilshire Boulevard #650, Beverly Hills, CA 90212.
E-mail address: drazizzadeh@gmail.com

population.[6] Single-stage surgery improves patient satisfaction, prevents the need for revision surgeries, and has not been shown to interfere with postoperative tumor surveillance.[7] Most parotidectomy reconstructions can be completed with local or regional flaps. This article provides an algorithm for reconstruction of parotidectomy defects using predominantly locoregional flaps and allografts.

SURGICAL MANAGEMENT

The parotid gland is the largest salivary gland. Its deep and superficial lobes are artificially divided by the facial nerve, which courses though it. The superficial lobe contains 80% of the substance of the gland, and approximately 90% of parotid tumors arise here.[8] Most tumors can be removed with a partial parotidectomy.[2] Radical parotidectomy, including resection of the facial nerve, is reserved for malignant tumors with aggressive features and/or perineural invasion.

Preoperative Planning

Preoperative planning for parotidectomy includes fine-needle aspiration and at times MRI or computed tomography, along with appropriate patient counseling. In addition, the senior authors (B.A., B.L.) take preoperative frontal, oblique, and lateral three-dimensional photographs of all patients undergoing parotidectomy (**Fig. 1**).

In the operating room, both sides of the face are exposed and prepped. When a local flap such as the sternocleidomastoid (SCM) muscle flap will be used, the incision is carefully planned to allow for adequate exposure. The senior authors prefer a short-scar facelift incision (microparotidectomy incision) in most benign tumors. This incision extends from the superior portion of the tragus, around the earlobe, and onto the posterior surface of the concha. They have successfully used this technique in tumors as large as 5 cm. In larger tumors, when access becomes difficult, the incision can be extended along the temporal and/or occipital hairlines. The classic modified Blair incision is rarely used in benign disorders, with the exception of very large tumors.

Reconstruction

After tumor resection, the defect is analyzed and compared with the contralateral side. Most benign tumors can be reconstructed with an SCM muscle flap with or without freeze-dried acellular human dermis. Local fascia flaps including the superficial muscular aponeurotic system (SMAS) and the temporoparietal fascia (TPF) flap are reserved for small contour abnormalities or anterior or superior defects that cannot be reached with the SCM muscle flap. Larger defects requiring significant tissue bulk, such as those from radical parotidectomy, are best reconstructed with axial flaps, such as the supraclavicular artery island (SAI) flap. The anterolateral thigh (ALT) free flap is the most commonly used free tissue flap and is generally reserved for radical defects involving mandibulectomy.

Acellular dermis

Freeze-dried acellular human dermis has gained popularity in parotid reconstruction.[9] After tumor resection, it can be sutured to the remaining parotid tissue to add bulk and fill contour defects (**Fig. 2**). By acting as a mechanical barrier to aberrant auriculotemporal nerve regeneration, acellular human dermis is associated with a reduced incidence of Frey syndrome.[10–14] The material is incorporated into surrounding fibrous tissue and minimally resorbed over the first 6 months, after which time its volume remains stable.[15] An increased incidence of seroma has been noted with acellular human dermis; however, the use of prolonged suction drainage reduces seroma formation significantly.[10–12]

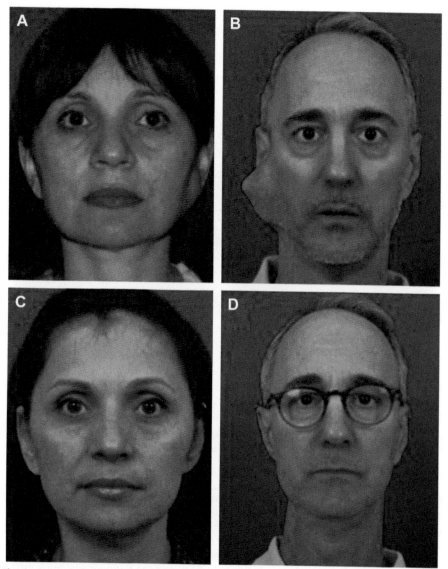

Fig. 1. Preoperative (*A, B*) and postoperative (*C, D*) views of 2 patients with pleomorphic adenoma who underwent parotidectomy with superiorly based sternocleidomastoid muscle flaps and thick AlloDerm.

In the senior authors' practice, acellular dermis is primarily used in conjunction with locoregional reconstruction such as the SCM muscle flap. A thick sheet, folded into no more than 2 layers, is placed superiorly or inferiorly to the flap if extra volume or length is needed. For small defects located anteriorly or superiorly, outside of the range of the SCM flap, acellular dermis is used as a stand-alone reconstruction.

Sternocleidomastoid muscle flap

The SCM muscle flap is the most commonly used flap for parotidectomy reconstruction and is sufficient for correction of most defects (**Fig. 3**). Like acellular dermis, the SCM

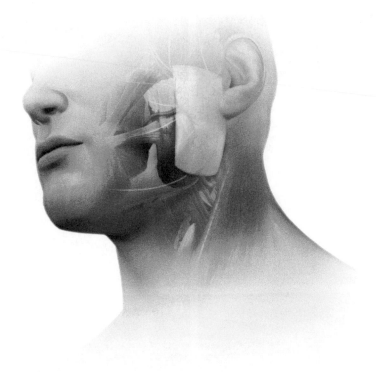

Fig. 2. Parotid reconstruction with AlloDerm. AlloDerm can be sutured to the parotid bed, SCM muscle, tragus, and mastoid fascia. (Used with permission from LifeCell Corporation.)

muscle flap has been shown to reduce the incidence of Frey syndrome.[16–21] A significant amount of bulk can be obtained by transposing part of the muscle to fill depressions in the preauricular and infra-auricular areas.[22,23] Compared with the SMAS flap (discussed later), the SCM muscle flap shows improved correction of contour abnormalities.[24,25]

Blood supply to the SCM muscle is derived from the occipital artery in the superior third, the superior thyroid artery in the middle third, and the thyrocervical trunk inferiorly.[26] The flap can be superiorly or inferiorly based, or the central portion can be advanced anteriorly. The superiorly based SCM muscle flap is the most commonly used (**Fig. 4**). The senior authors' technique involves skeletonizing the SCM muscle and making a vertical incision along the midline portion of the muscle. Care is taken to identify and preserve the greater auricular and spinal accessory nerves (see **Fig. 4**). The distance from the pivot point at the superior portion of the muscle to the edge of the defect is measured, and a horizontal cut is made using electrocautery. The SCM muscle is then rotated into the defect to cover the entire parotid bed and sutured using horizontal mattress sutures. If the posterior pull from the SCM muscle flap causes the SMAS to advance slightly, the skin is undermined anteriorly to prevent dimpling. If the defect is larger or more superior, then a wider and/or longer section of the SCM muscle is transposed. A suction drain is placed, and a small amount of

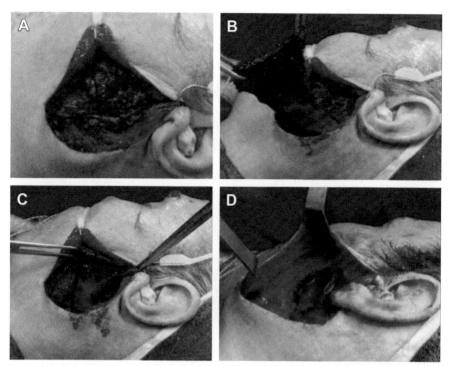

Fig. 3. Intraoperative views of a patient undergoing superficial parotidectomy with reconstruction using the SCM muscle flap. (*A*) The tumor and superficial lobe of the parotid gland are removed with the facial nerve visible in the parotid bed. The superiorly based SCM muscle flap is mobilized (*B*) and rotated anteriorly (*C*). (*D*) The SCM muscle is inset and sutured to the remaining parotid gland.

skin is excised if necessary. Atrophy of the SCM muscle may occur with time, so slight overcorrection can be advantageous. In addition, a posterior defect over the region of the muscle harvest can be corrected by advancing the lateral aspect of the posterior belly of the SCM muscle.[27]

Superficial muscular aponeurotic system flap
The SMAS flap is an easily accessible local flap that can be used for small defects (**Fig. 5**). It also provides a physical barrier for prevention of Frey syndrome, and it is useful for anterior defects that cannot be reached with the SCM muscle flap alone. At the beginning of the parotidectomy, the SMAS can be dissected out between the subcutaneous flap and the parotidomasseteric fascia. After resection, the SMAS can be folded, laid over the parotid bed, and sutured to the remaining parotid tissue and zygomatic fascia.[28–33] This flap cannot be used in cases in which the tumor involves the SMAS, and it does not provide sufficient soft tissue bulk to fill moderate to large defects. In the senior author's practice, this flap is rarely used as a stand-alone procedure and is more commonly used to complement acellular dermis and SCM muscle flap.

Temporoparietal fascia flap
A flap based on the superficial temporal artery can also be used as an interposition flap. In this case, the parotidectomy incision is extended into the temporal hair line and a double-layered fascia graft, consisting of the TPF and the deep temporal fascia,

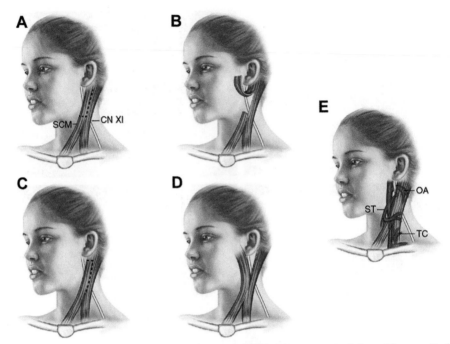

Fig. 4. Superiorly and inferiorly based SCM muscle flaps. For a superiorly based flap, vertical and horizontal incisions are made (*A*), and the freed muscle is rotated into the defect (*B*). For an inferiorly based flap, incisions are made superiorly and laterally (*C*) and rotated to fill the defect (*D*). (*E*) The usual blood supply to the SCM muscle. Key elements are the 2 muscle bellies of the SCM (*brown*) and the spinal accessory nerve (*in orange*). OA, occipital artery; ST, superior thyroid artery; TC, transverse cervical artery.

is harvested.[34] This graft is pedicled inferiorly, folded over the zygomatic arch, and sutured to the edges of the parotid bed. It has been used to fill gaps larger than 3 cm and may reduce the incidence of Frey syndrome.[35] However, this flap is rarely used in our practice because of the likelihood of injury to the superficial temporal artery during parotidectomy surgery. Furthermore, there is potential for alopecia, damage to the frontal nerve, and hematoma formation.

Fat grafting
Fat can be harvested from the abdomen or thighs and placed in the parotid bed to fill contour defects.[7] It may also be combined with the SMAS flap.[36,37] The SMAS flap plus fat grafting for reconstruction after malignant parotid tumor resection has been reported with successful take of the fat even after radiation therapy.[29] Disadvantages of fat grafting include donor site morbidity, increased blood loss and operative time, and unpredictable loss of fat.

Cervicofacial advancement flaps
In patients with tumor involving the overlying skin but without large volume deficits, local tissue advancement flaps are used to provide skin coverage and modest bulk. The cervicofacial advancement flap can be used to rotate skin, subcutaneous tissue, and platysma muscle from the neck to the face. This flap is inferiorly based and is designed based on the extent of the defect. For patients undergoing neck dissection, the inferior neck incision can be planned to allow for flap advancement. The posterior

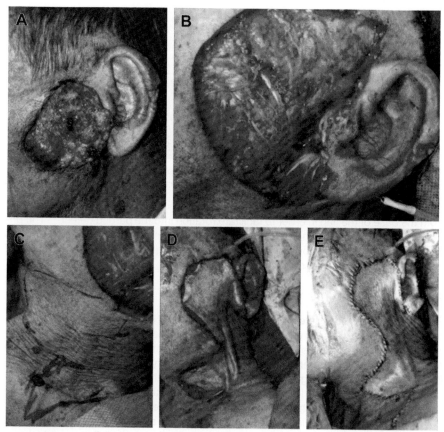

Fig. 5. Bilobed cervicofacial advancement flap for reconstruction of skin and parotid tissue defect. (*A*) Malignant tumor involving skin. (*B*) Defect after removal of mass and superficial parotid gland. (*C*) Skin markings for bilobed cervicofacial advancement flap. (*D*) Skin is rotated into the defect. (*E*) Final skin closure.

inferior limb of the incision extends inferiorly as far as necessary, even onto the chest wall, to provide adequate arc of rotation and tissue coverage.[38] The plane of dissection is supra-SMAS in the face, subplatysmal in the neck, and subcutaneous (supra-deltopectoral fascia) if it extends into the chest. The blood supply to the facial portion of the flap is in a random pattern from the subdermal plexus. The platysmal portion of the flap derives its blood supply primarily from submental artery perforators anteriorly.[39] Defects as large as 7 × 6 cm and extending as far superiorly as the supra-orbital rim have been reconstructed with this flap.[40]

The cervicofacial flap can be modified to a bilobed configuration. The bilobed flap technique is well known for its use on many areas of the face and neck, and a large bilobed flap has been used for postburn scar contractures in the neck.[41] The senior authors have found a modification of this flap useful for parotidectomy defects involving the overlying skin (**Fig. 6**). It is based posteriorly in the neck and uses the principles described by Zitelli[42] for the bilobed flap in nasal reconstruction. The primary lobe of the flap is measured to be the same diameter as the defect, and the secondary lobe is approximately half the size of the primary lobe (see **Fig. 6**C). The posterior limb of the secondary lobe can be extended and curved slightly away

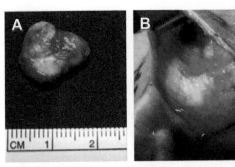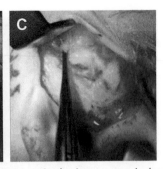

Fig. 6. An 8-year old boy with a pilomatricoma. (*A*) Tumor was excised using a preauricular incision and skin flap elevation. (*B*) The defect after resection. (*C*) Reconstruction with a superficial musculoaponeurotic system flap.

from the base of the flap in order to facilitate rotation into the parotid defect.[41] The primary lobe is rotated into the defect and the secondary lobe is closed primarily. This flap provides excellent color and texture match, although it necessitates an extended incision and relies on a random blood supply.

POST–RADICAL PAROTIDECTOMY RECONSTRUCTION

Radical parotidectomy defects may include skin, muscle, mandible, maxilla, or temporal bone. This extensive resection combined with facial nerve sacrifice and possible radiation therapy lead to significant deformity and disfigurement.[43] If possible, the facial nerve is reconstructed at the time of initial surgery. Facial nerve reconstruction is possible if negative margins are obtained distally in the peripheral branches of the facial nerve and proximally in the temporal bone. Sural nerve graft is usually harvested using a single-incision technique with a tendon stripper (Azizzadeh, prepublication, 2015). Regardless, immediate static reconstruction is almost always chosen, using facial static sling with acellular dermis or tensor fascia lata.[44,45] Some centers use orthodromic temporalis tendon transfer (OTTT) in the ablative setting.[46] At our institution, we usually reserve OTTT for secondary facial reanimation. Most patients with primary or metastatic malignancies in the parotid gland are not good candidates for more advanced reanimation techniques, such as gracilis free flap innervated by masseteric or cross-facial nerve graft. If skin is involved, the SAI flap, cervicofacial, or cervicofacial bilobed flap can be used to provide the best color match with short operating time.[47] Free tissue transfer is generally used for large volume deficits in cases in which mandibulectomy is necessary.

Supraclavicular Artery Island Flap

The SAI flap is a pedicled fasciocutaneous flap that can be used to cover a broad range of defects. Originally described in 1949 by Drs. Kazanjian and Converse,[48] the SAI flap was repopularized in the 1990s as a local flap to treat postburn contractures in the head and neck.[49,50] This flap is based on the supraclavicular artery, a branch of the transverse cervical artery. It can be used for reconstruction of combined parotid, skin, lateral skull base, and auriculectomy defects.[51] The flap's significant length allows access to the superior limit of parotidectomy dissection. The soft tissue bulk can fill a deep facial defect and support an auricular remnant. It provides good skin color match and excellent pliability, and can be sensate if the cervical plexus nerves are preserved.[52,53] If skin coverage is not needed, the flap is deepithelialized and placed in the defect to fill contour abnormalities.[54]

Although significant length can be obtained, a flap longer than 22 cm may increase the risk of necrosis. The width should be no more than 6 to 7 cm to allow primary donor site closure, although up to 12 cm has been described. Smoking increases the risk of flap dehiscence.[55] Disadvantages of the SAI flap include a long scar along the ipsilateral shoulder and arm and a dog ear deformity at the site of the pedicle. Secondary procedures are occasionally required for debulking or scar revision.

Free tissue transfer

In general, the senior authors reserve free tissue transfer for complex parotid defects, including resection of skin, muscle, parotid tissue, and mandibulectomy. The ALT free fasciocutaneous flap is the most commonly used free tissue flap in parotidectomy reconstruction. A portion of the vastus lateralis muscle can be harvested for additional bulk when necessary.[56] Adjunctive procedures, including nerve grafting, oral commissuroplasty with fascia lata, or dynamic reanimation with the OTTT, can be performed simultaneously.[46] The lateral femoral cutaneous nerve or the nerve to the vastus lateralis muscle can be used for neural coaptation.

SUMMARY

After parotidectomy, patients are often left with facial contour abnormalities. Given the increasing emphasis on cosmesis, reconstruction after partial or total parotidectomy can significantly improve patient satisfaction. Local and regional flaps can be used to reconstruct most of these defects and it is important to tailor reconstruction to the extent of the defect. To this end, the contemporary management of soft tissue defects after parotidectomy has been described.

REFERENCES

1. Skolnik EM, Friedman M, Becker S, et al. Tumors of the major salivary glands. Laryngoscope 1977;87(6):843–61.
2. Spiro RH. Salivary neoplasms: overview of a 35-year experience with 2,807 patients. Head Neck Surg 1986;8(3):177–84.
3. Mantsopoulos K, Koch M, Klintworth N, et al. Evolution and changing trends in surgery for benign parotid tumors. Laryngoscope 2015;125(1):122–7.
4. Nitzan D, Kronenberg J, Horowitz Z, et al. Quality of life following parotidectomy for malignant and benign disease. Plast Reconstr Surg 2004;114(5):1060–7.
5. Marshall AH, Quraishi SM, Bradley PJ. Patients' perspectives on the short- and long-term outcomes following surgery for benign parotid neoplasms. J Laryngol Otol 2003;117(8):624–9.
6. Shah SA, Riaz U, Zubair M, et al. Surgical presentation and outcome of parotid gland tumours. J Coll Physicians Surg Pak 2013;23(9):625–8.
7. Conger BT, Gourin CG. Free abdominal fat transfer for reconstruction of the total parotidectomy defect. Laryngoscope 2008;118(7):1186–90.
8. Debets JM, Munting JD. Parotidectomy for parotid tumours: 19-year experience from The Netherlands. Br J Surg 1992;79(11):1159–61.
9. Shridharani SM, Tufaro AP. A systematic review of acelluar dermal matrices in head and neck reconstruction. Plast Reconstr Surg 2012;130(5 Suppl 2):35s–43s.
10. Sachsman SM, Rice DH. Use of AlloDerm implant to improve cosmesis after parotidectomy. Ear Nose Throat J 2007;86(8):512–3.
11. Sinha UK, Saadat D, Doherty CM, et al. Use of AlloDerm implant to prevent Frey syndrome after parotidectomy. Arch Facial Plast Surg 2003;5(1):109–12.

12. Govindaraj S, Cohen M, Genden EM, et al. The use of acellular dermis in the prevention of Frey's syndrome. Laryngoscope 2001;111(11 Pt 1):1993–8.
13. Athavale SM, Rangarajan S, Dharamsi L, et al. AlloDerm and DermaMatrix implants for parotidectomy reconstruction: a histologic study in the rat model. Head Neck 2013;35(2):242–9.
14. Li C, Yang X, Pan J, et al. Graft for prevention of Frey syndrome after parotidectomy: a systematic review and meta-analysis of randomized controlled trials. J Oral Maxillofac Surg 2013;71(2):419–27.
15. Sclafani AP, Romo T 3rd, Jacono AA, et al. Evaluation of acellular dermal graft (AlloDerm) sheet for soft tissue augmentation: a 1-year follow-up of clinical observations and histological findings. Arch Facial Plast Surg 2001;3(2):101–3.
16. Asal K, Köybaşioğlu A, Inal E, et al. Sternocleidomastoid muscle flap reconstruction during parotidectomy to prevent Frey's syndrome and facial contour deformity. Ear Nose Throat J 2005;84(3):173–6.
17. Casler JD, Conley J. Sternocleidomastoid muscle transfer and superficial musculoaponeurotic system plication in the prevention of Frey's syndrome. Laryngoscope 1991;101(1 Pt 1):95–100.
18. Dai XM, Liu H, He J, et al. Treatment of postparotidectomy Frey syndrome with the interposition of temporalis fascia and sternocleidomastoid flaps. Oral Surg Oral Med Oral Pathol Oral Radiol 2015;119(5):514–21.
19. Liu H, Li Y, Dai X. Modified face-lift approach combined with a superficially anterior and superior-based sternocleidomastoid muscle flap in total parotidectomy. Oral Surg Oral Med Oral Pathol Oral Radiol 2012;113(5):593–9.
20. Liu DY, Tian XJ, Li C, et al. The sternocleidomastoid muscle flap for the prevention of Frey syndrome and cosmetic deformity following parotidectomy: a systematic review and meta-analysis. Oncol Lett 2013;5(4):1335–42.
21. Demirci U, Basut O, Noyan B, et al. The efficiacy of sternocleidomastoid muscle flap on Frey's syndrome via a novel test: galvanic skin response. Indian J Otolaryngol Head Neck Surg 2014;66(Suppl 1):291–8.
22. Bianchi B, Ferri A, Ferrari S, et al. Improving esthetic results in benign parotid surgery: statistical evaluation of facelift approach, sternocleidomastoid flap, and superficial musculoaponeurotic system flap application. J Oral Maxillofac Surg 2011;69(4):1235–41.
23. Chow TL, Lam CY, Chiu PW, et al. Sternomastoid-muscle transposition improves the cosmetic outcome of superficial parotidectomy. Br J Plast Surg 2001;54(5):409–11.
24. Zhao HW, Li LJ, Han B, et al. Preventing post-surgical complications by modification of parotidectomy. Int J Oral Maxillofac Surg 2008;37(4):345–9.
25. Sanabria A, Kowalski LP, Bradley PJ, et al. Sternocleidomastoid muscle flap in preventing Frey's syndrome after parotidectomy: a systematic review. Head Neck 2012;34(4):589–98.
26. Ariyan S. One-stage reconstruction for defects of the mouth using a sternomastoid myocutaneous flap. Plast Reconstr Surg 1979;63(5):618–25.
27. Alvarez GE, Escamilla JT, Carranza A. The split sternocleidomastoid myocutaneous flap. Br J Plast Surg 1983;36(2):183–6.
28. Cesteleyn L, Helman J, King S, et al. Temporoparietal fascia flaps and superficial musculoaponeurotic system plication in parotid surgery reduces Frey's syndrome. J Oral Maxillofac Surg 2002;60(11):1284–97 [discussion: 1297–8].
29. Ambro BT, Goodstein LA, Morales RE, et al. Evaluation of superficial musculoaponeurotic system flap and fat graft outcomes for benign and malignant parotid disease. Otolaryngol Head Neck Surg 2013;148(6):949–54.

30. Barberá R, Castillo F, D'Oleo C, et al. Superficial musculoaponeurotic system flap in partial parotidectomy and clinical and subclinical Frey's syndrome. Cosmesis and quality of life. Head Neck 2014;36(1):130–6.
31. Foustanos A, Zavrides H. Face-lift approach combined with a superficial musculoaponeurotic system advancement flap in parotidectomy. Br J Oral Maxillofac Surg 2007;45(8):652–5.
32. Meningaud JP, Bertolus C, Bertrand JC. Parotidectomy: assessment of a surgical technique including facelift incision and SMAS advancement. J Craniomaxillofac Surg 2006;34(1):34–7.
33. Arden RL, Miguel GS. Aesthetic parotid surgery: evolution of a technique. Laryngoscope 2011;121(12):2581–5.
34. Ahmed OA, Kolhe PS. Prevention of Frey's syndrome and volume deficit after parotidectomy using the superficial temporal artery fascial flap. Br J Plast Surg 1999;52(4):256–60.
35. Dell'aversana Orabona G, Salzano G, Petrocelli M, et al. Reconstructive techniques of the parotid region. J Craniofac Surg 2014;25(3):998–1002.
36. Harada T, Inoue T, Harashina T, et al. Dermis-fat graft after parotidectomy to prevent Frey's syndrome and the concave deformity. Ann Plast Surg 1993;31(5): 450–2.
37. Nosan DK, Ochi JW, Davidson TM. Preservation of facial contour during parotidectomy. Otolaryngol Head Neck Surg 1991;104(3):293–8.
38. Moore BA, Wine T, Netterville JL. Cervicofacial and cervicothoracic rotation flaps in head and neck reconstruction. Head Neck 2005;27(12):1092–101.
39. Hurwitz DJ, Rabson JA, Futrell JW. The anatomic basis for the platysma skin flap. Plast Reconstr Surg 1983;72(3):302–14.
40. Liu FY, Xu ZF, Li P, et al. The versatile application of cervicofacial and cervicothoracic rotation flaps in head and neck surgery. World J Surg Oncol 2011;9:135.
41. Aranmolate S, Attah AA. Bilobed flap in the release of postburn mentosternal contracture. Plast Reconstr Surg 1989;83(2):356–61.
42. Zitelli JA. The bilobed flap for nasal reconstruction. Arch Dermatol 1989;125(7): 957–9.
43. Ia-Kotola T, Goldstein DP, Hofer SO, et al. Facial nerve reconstruction and facial disfigurement after radical parotidectomy. J Reconstr Microsurg 2015;31(4): 313–8.
44. Fisher E, Frodel JL. Facial suspension with acellular human dermal allograft. Arch Facial Plast Surg 1999;1(3):195–9.
45. Leckenby JI, Harrison DH, Grobbelaar AO. Static support in the facial palsy patient: a case series of 51 patients using tensor fascia lata slings as the sole treatment for correcting the position of the mouth. J Plast Reconstr Aesthet Surg 2014; 67(3):350–7.
46. Revenaugh PC, Knott PD, Scharpf J, et al. Simultaneous anterolateral thigh flap and temporalis tendon transfer to optimize facial form and function after radical parotidectomy. Arch Facial Plast Surg 2012;14(2):104–9.
47. Ch'ng S, Ashford BG, Gao K, et al. Reconstruction of post-radical parotidectomy defects. Plast Reconstr Surg 2012;129(2):275e–87e.
48. Kazanjian VH, Converse JM. The Surgical Treatment of Facial Injuries. Baltimore: Williams & Wilkins; 1949.
49. Pallua N, Machens HG, Rennekampff O, et al. The fasciocutaneous supraclavicular artery island flap for releasing postburn mentosternal contractures. Plast Reconstr Surg 1997;99(7):1878–84 [discussion: 1885–6].

50. Vinh VQ, Van Anh T, Ogawa R, et al. Anatomical and clinical studies of the supraclavicular flap: analysis of 103 flaps used to reconstruct neck scar contractures. Plast Reconstr Surg 2009;123(5):1471–80.
51. Emerick KS, Herr MW, Lin DT, et al. Supraclavicular artery island flap for reconstruction of complex parotidectomy, lateral skull base, and total auriculectomy defects. JAMA Otolaryngol Head Neck Surg 2014;140(9):861–6.
52. Granzow JW, Suliman A, Roostaeian J, et al. The supraclavicular artery island flap (SCAIF) for head and neck reconstruction: surgical technique and refinements. Otolaryngol Head Neck Surg 2013;148(6):933–40.
53. Kokot N, Mazhar K, Reder LS, et al. Use of the supraclavicular artery island flap for reconstruction of cervicofacial defects. Otolaryngol Head Neck Surg 2014; 150(2):222–8.
54. Epps MT, Cannon CL, Wright MJ, et al. Aesthetic restoration of parotidectomy contour deformity using the supraclavicular artery island flap. Plast Reconstr Surg 2011;127(5):1925–31.
55. Kokot N, Mazhar K, Reder LS, et al. The supraclavicular artery island flap in head and neck reconstruction: applications and limitations. JAMA Otolaryngol Head Neck Surg 2013;139(11):1247–55.
56. Elliott RM, Weinstein GS, Low DW, et al. Reconstruction of complex total parotidectomy defects using the free anterolateral thigh flap: a classification system and algorithm. Ann Plast Surg 2011;66(5):429–37.

Microvascular Reconstruction of the Parotidectomy Defect

Michael A. Fritz, MD[a],*, Bryan Nicholas Rolfes, MD[b]

KEYWORDS

- Total parotidectomy • Anterolateral thigh (ALT) free flap • Facial paralysis
- Temporalis tendon transfer • Contour defect

KEY POINTS

- The contour deformity created when volume is not replaced after parotidectomy can be disfiguring and can significantly affect quality of life.
- Large-volume deficits are best corrected with vascularized adipose tissue because it is accurate acute contour restoration and provides a stable result over time.
- The preferred donor graft is the anterolateral thigh (ALT) free flap, because the donor site morbidity is minimal, it provides an ample tissue source that does not include denervated muscle, it can be harvested with a skin paddle if needed, and it allows access to neural and fascial graft tissue if needed.
- In the setting of facial paralysis, concurrent orthodromic temporalis tendon transfer is safe, adds minimal morbidity, and makes a significant contribution to facial symmetry.

Parotidectomy is commonly performed to address benign and malignant processes involving the parotid gland itself, aggressive cutaneous facial tumors, and adjacent head and neck malignancies. The surgical spectrum includes partial and superficial gland resection, total gland resection, and more radical procedures that include sacrifice of the facial nerve and adjacent structures. Complications also cover a broad spectrum and include facial nerve weakness to complete paralysis, sialocele, Frey syndrome, infection, hematoma, and contour deformities.[1,2] Due to its location at the lateral cheek and angle of the mandible, a volume deficit in the parotid bed can lead to an obvious and unappealing deformity that is easily visible on both direct and lateral facial views. As a result, resection of substantial soft tissue in the process

[a] Cleveland Clinic Head and Neck Institute, Cleveland Clinic Main Campus, Mail Code A71, 9500 Euclid Avenue, Cleveland, OH 44195, USA; [b] Department of Facial Plastic and Reconstructive Surgery, Boston University, 830 Harrison Avenue, Moakley Building Ground Floor, Boston, MA 02118, USA
* Corresponding author.
E-mail address: fritzm1@ccf.org

Otolaryngol Clin N Am 49 (2016) 447–457
http://dx.doi.org/10.1016/j.otc.2015.10.008
0030-6665/16/$ – see front matter © 2016 Elsevier Inc. All rights reserved.

of parotidectomy, irrespective of facial nerve status, can result in dramatic and obvious disfigurement.

Facial symmetry is widely accepted as one of the key measurements of human beauty and, even more importantly, facial asymmetry and deformity have been shown to impart a social penalty beyond self-image.[3] More than 50% of patients report being affected by facial contour abnormalities after parotidectomy.[4] In the setting of radical parotidectomy, the effects of volume loss are arguably as profound and debilitating as the facial paralysis, because they compound the deformities imparted by loss of facial tone and movement.[5,6]

There are several methods that have been described to fill the surgical defect created by parotidectomy, including sternocleidomastoid rotation flaps, superficial musculoaponeurotic system (SMAS) interposition flaps, temporoparietal biparietal fascia (TPF) flaps, autologous free fat or dermal/fat grafts, and processed alloplastic dermal implants. These may provide benefit for limited or superficial gland resection, but none of these methods provides enough bulk to restore facial symmetry after total gland resection. Additionally, many patients who require total and especially radical parotidectomy are subjected to postoperative radiation therapy. This assault can diminish volume achieved by tissue with a tenuous vascular supply. Furthermore, the use of acellular dermal implants has been associated with higher complication rates in the setting of previous or postoperative radiation.[7] Critically, denervated muscle flaps provide short-term contour improvement, but long-term volume restoration is unreliable, because denervated muscle flaps lose bulk over time due to atrophy.

As the use of vascularized free tissue grafts has become commonplace in the reconstruction of complex head and neck defects, microvascular technique has become safe, reliable, and efficient. This has led to an expansion of indications to optimize facial form and function, including reconstruction of the isolated facial contour defects.[5,6,8,9] The benefits provided by this method include accurate, lasting, and radiation-resistant volume correction (**Fig. 1**); access to additional tissue at donor sites for nerve grafting and facial reanimation; and potential protection from radiation-induced complications. As a result, free tissue transfer is becoming the criterion standard for management of large-volume parotidectomy defects.

Past critiques of aggressive volume correction have argued that addition of tissue for the sake of contour can interfere with a surgeon's surveillance of the surgical site for recurrence and that free tissue transfer adds additional morbidity at the donor and anastomosis sites. With current imaging techniques, any neoplastic tissue is

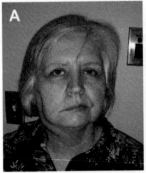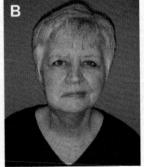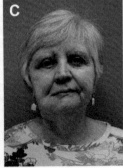

Fig. 1. (*A*) Contour correction 6 weeks after ALT free flap and nerve grafting after radical parotidectomy and neck dissection. (*B*) Result at 1 year after radiation therapy. (*C*) Result at 5 years after contour flap and 6 months after temporalis tendon transfer for recurrent paralysis.

readily distinguished from reconstructive tissue, mitigating the potential compromise of oncologic surveillance. Many total parotidectomies in the setting of malignancy are performed with concurrent neck dissection, eliminating the need for additional surgery required to locate donor vessels for microvascular anastomosis. When no concurrent neck dissection is planned, suitable vessels for anastomosis can generally be accessed through the existing parotidectomy defect. In cases of these vessels found insufficient, the pedicle can be tunneled under the skin to a minimal access incision.[10] Furthermore, with newer flap harvest sites and techniques, donor site morbidity is minimal, not significantly more than the harvest of a nerve graft.[11]

Many different free flaps, including radial forearm,[12] lateral arm,[13] gastrocnemius,[14] groin,[15] inferior epigastric perforator,[16] and parascapular,[17] have been described in the reconstruction of the parotidectomy defect. For several reasons, the authors find that an ALT flap is the preferred option in almost every instance.[18] The most compelling argument for its use is a lack of donor site morbidity. The only long-term evidence left at the harvest site is a scar less obvious than that left by procuring a skin graft.[11] Careful design and closure of the incision, for instance, with the application of a distal m-plasty, allows a surgeon to harvest a flap with a large skin paddle and achieve primary closure with the incision terminating above the hem of a pair of shorts. The donor site also allows access for the concurrent harvest of a tensor fascia lata graft if facial reanimation is to be performed as well as the motor nerve to the vastus lateralis (MNVL) when needed as a graft for facial reinnervation. The area and bulk of the ALT flap can be adjusted over a wide range depending on body habitus and volume needs, incorporating fascia, subcutaneous fat, and/or dermis. Thin flaps may be folded and thick flaps may be primarily thinned to create an ideal fit for the defect.[19] Finally, the ALT flap is easily concurrently harvested by a second surgical team, minimizing added operative time for reconstruction.

PRIMARY VOLUME RESTORATION

Given ready access to both the surgical defect and vessels for microvascular anastomoses, total parotidectomy soft tissue defects are optimally managed at the same operative setting as the ablative procedure. Furthermore, in the setting of malignancy and anticipated postoperative radiation therapy, immediate reconstruction with vascularized tissue may convey an additional radioprotective effect. This concept is supported by well-established evidence of revascularization of surrounding structures after transplantation of an adjacent vascular pedicle.[20]

If immediate reconstruction is planned, flap harvest is optimally begun and completed concomitantly with the ablative procedure. Given the distance of the thigh from the head and neck region and the lack of requirement of a tourniquet, the ALT harvest site is optimally suited for this method. Furthermore, presence of ample skin and soft tissue in the typical thigh allows for harvest of a flap that accommodates an extended defect yet is still amenable to complete advancement flap closure. This volume can then be adjusted for size and contour once full margin clearance has been attained.

In the setting of radical parotidectomy, ALT free flap harvest is performed in a manner that allows for concomitant facial nerve reinnervation and reanimation if this is also required. In this instance, a vascularized contour flap is performed along with spanning grafts from the MNVL and orthodromic temporalis tendon transfer combined with a fascia lata extension for lower lip suspension. Aside from the temporalis tendon, all these elements are readily available in a single harvest site.

ALT flap harvest is begun with Doppler probe identification and marking of perforators to the overlying skin near the midpoint between the anterosuperior iliac spine and the superolateral patella. A cutaneous paddle amenable to primary advancement closure is always included in the flap harvest regardless of whether a skin defect is anticipated. This facilitates closure without significant contour defect in the thigh, allows for flap manipulation with less trauma to underlying structures, and provides an external monitor paddle when this is desired. Furthermore, this technique provides a vascularized dermal graft if additional bulk is required in patients with thin thighs.

Harvest is first begun with a single vertical incision at the medial aspect of the skin paddle, dissection to and then through the fascia overlying rectus femoris muscle, and identification of septocutaneous or, far more commonly, musculocutaneous perforators. In cases of the musculocutaneous perforators, these are followed through the vastus lateralis muscle until the vascular pedicle is reached. Once the location and vascular origin of the perforators are confirmed, full cutaneous flap design is completed, and the incisions are created. Commonly, an area of vascularized fascia lata of significantly greater dimensions than the skin paddle is harvested. This allows for further versatility with regard to volume replacement without additional harvest site morbidity. At this point, perforators are followed circumferentially through the vastus lateralis muscle with complete sparing of the surrounding musculature (perforator flap technique) (**Fig. 2**). This method is critical to maximize the length of the vascular pedicle and, most importantly, to minimize the importation of denervated muscle into the volume correction because it is subject to tissue atrophy over time.

During pedicle dissection, MNVLs are encountered and dissected away from the vessels. These nerves, with their long branching pattern and redundant nature, provide an ideal substrate for reinnervation if this is required (**Fig. 3**).[5,6] Because of their redundancy proximally, nerve harvest or sacrifice is not associated with functional impairment.[11] Harvest concomitantly with the ALT flap avoids an additional donor site morbidity and provides a potential advantage of motor nerve grafts for motor nerve replacement.[21,22] Additionally, in instances of radical parotidectomy and anticipated temporalis tendon transfer, a nonvascularized 2-cm by 10-cm slip of remaining fascia lata is removed separately from the lateral thigh.

After the ALT free flap is revascularized, it is draped in the parotid bed and any existing neck dissection defect and then circumferentially suspended to SMAS and deep soft tissues. The flap is then modified to establish symmetric facial contour and skin and subcutaneous tissue is removed as required to accomplish this goal. Facial contour is slightly overcorrected to compensate for flap edema during harvest and reperfusion; however, gross overcorrection is not performed, because the soft tissue volume remains stable over time.[18] This ability to reliably maintain established contour differentiates this reconstruction from the inevitable atrophy of both free and pedicled

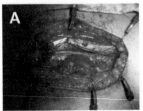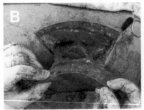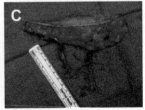

Fig. 2. (*A*) ALT musculocutaneous perforators identified and followed through vastus lateralis. (*B*) Perforators dissected circumferentially to vascular pedicle. (*C*) Harvested flap with complete muscle sparing.

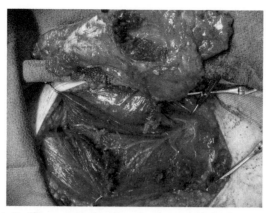

Fig. 3. ALT harvest site (flap superior) with redundant and branching MNVL.

denervated muscle flaps. If pedicle geometry and soft tissue orientation permit, a cutaneous monitoring segment is created during flap modification and secured between the native skin flaps prior to closure (**Fig. 4**).

Although external skin defect reconstruction with color-mismatched ALT skin is not optimal, restoration of large areas of skin with locoregional flaps often requires extensive dissection and skin tension that can obscure precise volume correction and accuracy of facial suspension. As a result, these defects are often addressed by an ALT skin paddle, which can be reduced in size by locoregional advancement. At a later point after completion of treatment, and often in the office setting under local anesthesia, color-mismatched skin can often be removed or minimized with serial excisions and local advancement flaps.

Management of the Radical Parotidectomy Defect

The setting of radical parotidectomy with facial nerve sacrifice presents issues and challenges beyond the scope of facial contour correction. Simultaneous management of facial nerve and reanimation issues allows for the best potential for recovery and provides the most rapid return to functional status. Immediate facial nerve grafting provides the best potential for long-term recovery of tone and function; however, grafting alone is not an ideal option in this patient population for several reasons. The potential for a good clinical outcome with nerve grafting alone is significantly decreased in typically elderly patients with parotid cancer based on age alone.[23,24]

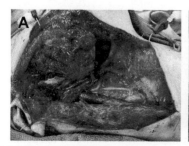
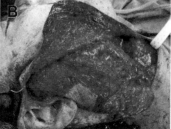

Fig. 4. (*A*) Radical parotidectomy and neck defect. (*B*) Vascularized ALT flap in position with volume correction and monitor paddle.

In addition, the high potential for tumor recurrence and greater functional compromise of paralysis in this group make the lag time of up to 12 months for experiencing clinical effects of reinnervation less tolerable or acceptable.[25] As a result, the authors typically use a combined approach with both nerve grafting and facial reanimation performed at the same setting as contour correction (**Fig. 5**).[5,6]

Both static facial suspensions and dynamic muscle transfer have been endorsed to provide immediate rehabilitation at the time of radical parotidectomy. Orthodromic temporalis tendon transfer, a well-established and increasingly popular reanimation technique, can impart both facial symmetry at rest and voluntary facial movement without creation of a secondary harvest site defect. Also favoring this option in the setting of parotidectomy, access to the insertion of the temporalis tendon on the coronoid is easily obtained through the same incision. Furthermore, this procedure can be performed without compromising the potential for reinnervation. Although the degree of voluntary facial movement generated through this procedure is variable and

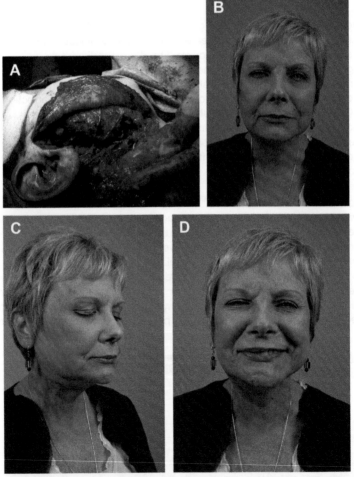

Fig. 5. (*A*) Radical parotidectomy defect with flap retracted inferiorly, temporalis tendon transfer sutures passed into nasolabial fold, and MNVL grafts in place. (*B, C*) Symmetry and contour maintained at 13 months after radiation therapy. (*D*) Dynamic smile at 13 months.

possibly affected by radiation therapy, surgical outcomes that establish immediate facial symmetry and support are nearly universal.[5,6,26,27] These latter benefits are the most critical to attain in this oncologic patient population.

Although free muscle transfer is often cited as the ideal reanimation method to provide the greatest potential for restoration of dynamic facial function, this method is not considered a component of primary rehabilitation in the oncologic setting. Functional recovery using this technique is delayed as it may take months for reinnervation to occur, and radiation therapy compounds the unpredictable effects of long-term function of transferred free muscle. In select patients, such as those who are young and have a favorable oncologic prognosis, rehabilitation with free muscle flaps may be considered in delayed fashion.

Reanimation Technique

In the setting of both contour correction and reanimation, the ALT flap is typically revascularized and then carefully oriented inferiorly and monitored while nerve grafting and temporalis tendon transfer are under way (see **Fig. 5B**). Attention is then focused on accessing the tendon of the temporalis muscle on the coronoid process. The masseter muscle, if unresected, is elevated off the lateral mandible and retracted medially to expose the coronoid process. The motor nerve to the masseter muscle is carefully preserved and in some instances identified and isolated for grafting purposes. The lateral coronoid is fully exposed and the tendon on the medial aspect is carefully elevated with superiostial dissection and protected by a right angle hemostat before coronoidectomy is performed with a sagittal saw (**Fig. 6A**). The underlying temporalis tendon is now fully exposed and the full length is preserved. The portion of the tendon attached on the medial coronoid base and to the posterior-medial aspect of the mandibular angle that provide optimal length and avoid the need for fascia lata extension grafts (except to the midline lower lip). It is the authors' opinion that minimizing use of extension grafts is critical to ensuring reliable movement and position after postoperative radiation therapy.

Prior to suture placement, the remnant coronoid bone is elevated off the tendon and discarded (**Fig. 6B**). Four to 5 sutures (4.0 Prolene) are then placed in horizontal mattress fashion in the tendon. Keys to optimizing outcomes are to avoid use of the short proximal tendon slips and to ensure that the temporalis muscle is fully detached from the mandible and moves freely. The sutures are then passed medial to the masseter through an incision created along the full length of the nasolabial fold (**Fig. 6C**). The passage between the nasolabial fold and temporalis dissection is created with sharp and blunt dissection, identifying and sparing neurovascular structures. After the sutures are passed through the incision, the tendon slips are secured to the orbicularis oris/SMAS along the length of the nasolabial fold.

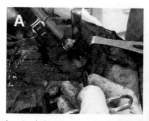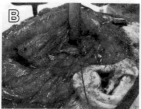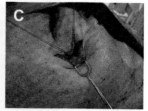

Fig. 6. (*A*) Coronoid process exposed and removed. (*B*) Sutures in distal temporalis tendon. (*C*) Sutures and tendon passed into nasolabial fold incision.

The addition of a fascia lata lower lip suspension improves oral competence and adds volume to compensate for orbicularis atrophy over time. The medial aspect of the fascia lata (previously obtained from the ALT harvest site) is secured to the central orbicularis in the midline lower lip through a small mucosal incision. The fascia is then passed through a tunnel created in the lower lip orbicularis marginalis muscle to the inferior aspect of the nasolabial fold incision and then secured to the lowest slip of the temporalis tendon (**Fig. 7**). The fascia is trimmed for the inset to the tendon so that the lower lip is well supported without external distortion. This lower lip suspension technique has significantly improved long-term function and appearance and has eliminated the need for lower lip wedge resections previously performed due to lip lengthening and atrophy over time.

In the surgical setting where temporalis muscle has been resected, static facial suspension with fascia lata is performed; vascularized fascia as a component of the free flap is used if this can be achieved without compromise of flap geometry or contour correction. Nonvascularized fascia lata suspension may also be performed. In this setting of high likelihood of adjuvant radiation therapy, suspension with nonautogenous tissue is typically avoided.

Reinnervation Technique

Using the previously harvested MNVL graft, facial nerve grafting is performed after the orthodromic temporalis tendon transfer is completed. In this patient population, in which modest outcomes of House-Brackmann Scale 3 to 4 are anticipated, all available major nerves are grafted. Again, the long and multiple branches of the harvested MNVL typically allow for this to be performed easily. If proximal facial nerve is not available for motor input, the masseteric nerve is isolated and used for this purpose. In younger patients in whom a more robust outcome is anticipated, nerve grafting alone may be performed, deferring free or regional muscle transfer until the full potential of reinnervation is attained.

SECONDARY VOLUME RESTORATION

Secondary contour deformities are often more difficult to correct due to irradiated and/or scarred operative beds and potential proximity of remaining facial nerve branches to the elevated skin flaps. To allow optimal tissue recovery, contour restoration is typically deferred for at least 12 months after completion of surgery and adjunctive

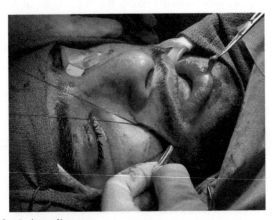

Fig. 7. Lower lip fascia lata sling.

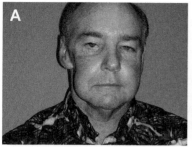
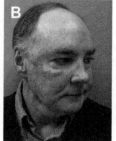
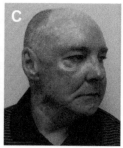

Fig. 8. (*A*) Radical parotidectomy defect after temporalis tendon transfer alone without contour flap. (*B*) ALT flap contour correction 1 year postoperatively. (*C*) Stable volume correction at 5 years postoperatively.

therapy. Given the commonly compromised vascularity of the recipient bed, avascular free grafts are prone to resorption and are rarely considered in this setting.

To attain volume correction and re-establish symmetry, skin flaps are typically elevated through existing parotidecomy scars to include the skin envelope 2 cm to 3 cm beyond the circumferential limits of the contour defect. Vessels for microvascular anastomosis are either accessed through the same incision or via a minimal access approaches.[10] After revascularization, the flap is sculpted for optimal contour replacement without overcorrection and then suspended in position with percutaneous bolster sutures, which are left in place for at least 1 week. The posterior aspect of the flap is then secured to preauricular soft tissues prior to wound closure.

Using free vascularized tissue without denervated muscle, accurate and lasting volume correction can be attained (**Fig. 8**). Surgical morbidity is minimized by subcutaneous dissection, minimal access vessel approaches, and ALT perforator flap harvest. As a result, postoperative hospital stays can often be abbreviated (typically <3 days).

SUMMARY

As facility and reliability of free tissue transfer increase, reconstructive indications continue to expand. Vascularized soft tissue flaps yield stable volume correction, which is resistant to the effects of radiation, and are becoming the criterion standard for managing contour defects after large volume parotidectomy. Low harvest site morbidity, ample soft tissue volume, and readily available nerve and fascia grafts make the ALT flap the ideal harvest site in this setting. Should facial nerve grafting and reanimation be required, a tripartite approach, including reinnervation, orthodromic temporalis tendon transfer, and vascularized ALT flap contour replacement, provides optimal postoperative form and function.

REFERENCES

1. Casler JD, Conley J. Sternocleidomastoid muscle transfer and superficial musculoaponeurotic system plication in the prevention of Frey's syndrome. Laryngoscope 1991;101:95–100.
2. Upton DC, McNamar JP, Connor NP, et al. Parotidectomy: ten-year review of 237 cases at a single institution. Otolaryngol Head Neck 2007;136:788–92.
3. Dey JK, Ishii LE, Byrne PJ, et al. The social penalty of facial lesions: new evidence supporting high-quality reconstruction. JAMA Facial Plast Surg 2015;17(2):90–6.

4. Nitzan D, Kronenberg J, Horowitz Z, et al. Quality of life following parotidectomy for malignant and benign disease. Plast Reconstr Surg 2004;114:1060–7.

5. Revenaugh PC, Knott D, McBride JM, et al. Motor nerve to the vastus lateralis. Arch Facial Plast Surg 2012;14(5):365–8.

6. Revenaugh PC, Knott PD, Scharpf J, et al. Simultaneous anterolateral thigh flap and temporalis tendo transfer to optimize facial form and function after parotidectomy. Arch Facial Plast Surg 2012;14(2):104–9.

7. Shridharani SM, Tufaro AP. A systemic review of acellular dermal matices in head and neck reconstuction. Plast Reconstr Surg 2012;130:35S–43S.

8. Hanasono MM, Skoracki RJ, Silva AK, et al. Adipofascial perforator flaps for "Aesthetic" head and neck reconstruction. Head Neck 2011;33(10):1513–9.

9. Wolff KD, Kesting M, Löffelbein D, et al. Perforator based anterolateral thigh adipofacial or dermal fat flaps for facial contour augmentation. J Reconstr Microsurg 2007;23:497–503.

10. Revenaugh PC, Fritz MA, Haffey TM, et al. Minimizing morbidity in microvascular surgery: small-caliber anastomotic vessels and minimal access approaches. JAMA Facial Plast Surg 2015;17(1):44–8.

11. Hanasono MM, Skoracki RJ, Yu P. A prospective study of donor-site morbidity after anterolateral thigh fasciocutaneous and myocutaneous free flap harvest in 220 patients. Plast Reconstr Surg 2010;125:209–14.

12. Urken ML, Weinberg H, Vickery C, et al. The neurofasciocutaneous radial forearm flap in head and neck reconstruction: a preliminary report. Laryngoscope 1990; 100(2):161–73.

13. Teknos TN, Nussenbaum B, Bradford CR, et al. Reconstruction of complex parotidectomy defects using the lateral arm free tissue transfer. Otolaryngol Head Neck Surg 2003;129:183–91.

14. Hyodo I, Ozawa T, Hasegawa Y, et al. Management fo the total parotidecotmy defect with a gastrocnemius muscle transfer and vascularized sural nerve grafting. Ann Plast Surg 2007;58:677–82.

15. Baker DC, Shaw WW, Conley J. Reconstruction of radial parotidectomy defects. Am J Surg 1979;138:550–4.

16. Allen RJ, Kaplan J. Reconstruction of a parotidectomy defect using a paraumbilical perforator flap without deep inferior epigastric vessels. J Reconstr Microsurg 2000;16(4):255–7.

17. Biglioli F, Autelitano L. Reconstruction after total parotidectomy using de-epithelialized free flap. J Craniomaxillofac Surg 2007;35:364–8.

18. Cannady SB, Seth R, Fritz MA, et al. Total parotidectomy defect reconstruction using burried free flap. Otolaryngol Head Neck Surg 2010;143:637–43.

19. Seth R, Nabili V, Fritz MA, et al. Volume-directed facial soft tissue reconstruction. Facial Plast Surg 2010;26:494–503.

20. Pribaz JJ, Weiss DD, Mulliken JB, et al. Prelaminated free flap reconstruction of complex central facial defects. Plast Reconstr Surg 1999;104(2):357–65.

21. Lloyd BE, Luginbuhl RD, Brenner MJ, et al. Use of motor nerve material in peripheral nerve repair with conduits. Microsurgery 2007;27:38–45.

22. Brooks DN, Weber RV, Chao JD, et al. Processed nerve allografts for peripheral nerve reconstruction: a multicenter study of untilization and outcomes in sensory, mixed, and motor nerve reconstructions. Microsurgery 2012;32: 1–14.

23. Brown PD, Eshleman JS, Foote RL, et al. An analysis of facial nerve function in irradiated and unirradiated facial nerve grafts. Int J Radiat Oncol Biol Phys 2000;48(3):737–43.

24. Reddy PG, Arden RL, Mathog RH. Facial nerve rehabilitation after radical paroti-dectomy. Laryngoscope 1999;109(6):894–9.
25. Kopec T, Mikaszewski B, Jackowska J, et al. Treatment of parotid malignancies - 10 year of experience. J Oral Maxillofac Surg 2015;73:1397–402.
26. Byrne PJ, Kim M, Boahene K, et al. Temporalis tendon transfer as part of a comprehensive approach to facial reanimation. Arch Facial Plast Surg 2007; 9(4):234–41.
27. Sidle DM, Fishman AJ. Modification of the orthodromic temporalis tendon transfer technique for reanimation of the paralyzed face. Otolaryngol Head Neck Surg 2011;145(1):18–23.

Facial Paralysis Reconstruction

Ali Razfar, MD[a], Matthew K. Lee, MD[b], Guy G. Massry, MD[c],
Babak Azizzadeh, MD[d],*

KEYWORDS

- Facial nerve • Facial nerve paralysis • Static facial reconstruction
- Dynamic facial reconstruction

KEY POINTS

- Optimal facial rehabilitation must address each affected zone of the face: lower lip, oral commissure, midface, ocular region, and brow.
- Since its introduction, the gracilis free muscle flap has revolutionized facial reanimation by achieving the critical goals of restoring spontaneous facial motion and functionality to the paralyzed face.
- Reconstruction after radical parotidectomy involves both facial nerve reconstruction and volume restoration of the surgical defect commonly with free tissue transfer.

INTRODUCTION

Facial nerve paralysis is a debilitating condition that affects an estimated 20 to 30 per 100,000 people per year.[1] The facial nerve is responsible for the innervation and control of the muscles of facial expression, or the facial mimetic muscles. With loss of this function, there is a pathologic relaxation and droop of the eyebrow, eyelid, cheek, and corner of the mouth.[2] Speech, oral competence, vision, and expression of emotion may be compromised, with significant effects on the overall quality of life of affected patients.[3,4] The psychological and social implications of this disorder cannot be understated, because facial expressions play a pivotal role in interpersonal communications. Facial paralysis can encumber this critical function, giving rise to feelings of social isolation and depression in affected individuals.[3,5]

The authors have nothing to disclose.
[a] Division of Facial Plastic and Reconstructive Surgery, Center for Facial Cosmetic Surgery, University of Michigan School of Medicine, 19900 Haggerty Hwy, Livonia, MI 48152, USA;
[b] Division of Facial Plastic and Reconstructive Surgery, Stanford University School of Medicine, 801 Welch Rd, Palo Alto, CA, 94305 USA; [c] Ophthalmic Plastic and Reconstructive Surgery, Keck School of Medicine, University of Southern California, 9401 Wilshire Blvd., Suite 650, Beverly Hills, CA 90212, USA; [d] Department of Head and Neck Surgery, Center for Advanced Facial Plastic Surgery, David Geffen School of Medicine, University of California, Los Angeles, 9401 Wilshire Blvd., Suite 650, Beverly Hills, CA 90212, USA
* Corresponding author.
E-mail address: drazizzadeh@gmail.com

Otolaryngol Clin N Am 49 (2016) 459–473
http://dx.doi.org/10.1016/j.otc.2015.12.002
0030-6665/16/$ – see front matter © 2016 Elsevier Inc. All rights reserved.

A facial paralysis is referred to as acute paralysis within the first year of onset and chronic paralysis thereafter. Pathologic conditions that target structures along the course of the facial nerve such as brainstem masses, temporal bone trauma, parotid neoplasms, or traumatic injury to the face may impair the function the facial nerve, resulting in facial paralysis.[6] Given its divergent origins, the variety of settings on which it may first be diagnosed, and its wide-ranging effects on the affected individual, facial nerve paralysis is best managed through a multispecialty, team-oriented approach. The goal of the current review is to provide a contemporary summary of the surgical management of facial nerve paralysis, procedures that are collectively referred to as facial reanimation.

SURGICAL MANAGEMENT

The facial nerve has a long, circuitous course, traveling from the brainstem through the temporal bone to eventually emerge via the stylomastoid foramen. The nerve then enters into the parotid gland and divides into 5 major branches: temporal, zygomatic, buccal, marginal mandibular, and cervical. Facial nerve paralysis may affect some or all branches of the facial nerve. The facial nerve innervates the facial musculature in a zonal pattern, and as such, the specific disabilities suffered are contingent on the affected facial subunits. Historically, the goals of facial reanimation were simply to provide eye closure for corneal protection and oral competence to prevent drooling. However, advances in facial reanimation techniques have made it possible to achieve these basic goals as well as to attain facial symmetry both at rest and with movement. To this end, attempts at optimal facial reanimation must address each affected zone of the face: lower lip, oral commissure, midface, ocular region, and brow. Furthermore, defects following radical parotidectomy offer unique challenges for the reconstructive surgeon.

Lower Face and Midface

The facial musculature acts to provide oral competence, express emotion through smiling, and augment nasal breathing by flaring of the nostrils. With loss of this function, patients may suffer from drooling, nasal airway obstruction, esthetic deformity, and emotional distress.[2,3,6] Surgical interventions are therefore targeted at restoring or replicating the native function of the facial musculature.

Static reconstruction

Generally, facial paralysis reconstructive techniques may be classified as static or dynamic. Static reconstruction techniques have historically acted as the workhorse of facial reanimation by repositioning the pathologically relaxed soft tissues of the face to counteract the effects of gravity (ie, facial droop) and provide symmetry at rest.[2] In addition, static reconstruction can restore oral competence as well as improve external nasal valve collapse.[5] Static reconstruction of the lower face can be accomplished with the use of "sling" suspension techniques. Using a facelift approach, a skin flap is elevated in the subcutaneous plane medial to the oral commissure and nasolabial fold, exposing the muscle fibers of the orbicularis oris if present. A "static sling" is then sutured medially to the oral commissure, lower lip, and nasolabial fold. The lateral aspect of the sling is then secured to the temporalis fascia or the zygomatic arch, to provide appropriate elevation of the soft tissue and symmetry at rest (**Fig. 1**).

Expanded polytetrafluoroethylene (ePTFE; Gore-Tex, W.L. Gore & Associates, Flagstaff, AZ) is a common synthetic material that has been used for static facial reanimation of the lower face.[7,8] However, concerns have been raised regarding the high rate of complications, including loss of tensile strength with time, graft infection, and need for revision surgery.[2] Alternatively, freeze-dried acellular human dermis

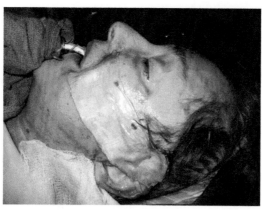

Fig. 1. Tensor fascia lata static sling position.

(AlloDerm, Lifecell Corporation, The Woodlands, TX) and porcine dermis (Surgisis, Cook Surgical, Cook Biotech, Inc, West Lafayette, IN) are other commercially available options that may be used.[9,10] Like ePTFE, use of acellular dermis spares the patient donor site morbidity; however, acellular dermis slings give less oral commissure support compared with ePTFE or autologous tensor fascia lata.[11] Tensor fascia lata is the most common autologous material used for static suspension. Autogenous tissue carries the advantage of providing superb tensile strength while having no immunologic response but does have increased morbidity from a second surgical site.[12]

Dynamic reanimation

Although static reanimation as a stand-alone procedure can improve facial symmetry at rest, it does fall short of the key goals of restoring voluntary facial movement and symmetric facial expressions. To this end, dynamic reanimation techniques have been developed with the goal of re-establishing voluntary facial movements. Dynamic reanimation techniques may be further divided into those that produce either volitional or spontaneous facial movement. With volitional movement, patients must be actively conscious of their attempts to move their face, as the patterns of innervation of facial musculature are different than that of the native face. As such, significant muscular retraining must take place for the patient to obtain optimal results. By contrast, with techniques that restore spontaneous facial movement, the patient needs only to attempt facial expressions as he or she normally would before onset of their facial paralysis.

Volitional reanimation

Dynamic facial reanimation techniques that reproduce volitional movement include cranial nerve substitution techniques and local muscle transfer. Importantly, cranial nerve substitution techniques may only be performed when the distal portion of the facial nerve is intact and facial musculature has not atrophied, thereby having the ability to reinnervate. This situation may arise when there is proximal injury to the facial nerve, as in the case of intracranial facial nerve injury during the extirpation of cerebellopontine tumors, or intratemporal facial nerve injury as a result of trauma or mastoid surgery.[13]

The most well-described cranial nerve substitution technique is the hypoglossal-facial nerve transfer (XII-VII transfer). The XII-VII transfer (**Fig. 2**A–D) involves using the hypoglossal nerve, which controls the movement of the tongue, to reinnervate the distal facial nerve. The hypoglossal nerve may be split in half in a linear fashion, and the superior nerve bundle is then coapted to the recipient distal facial nerve stump (**Fig. 2**B). A split

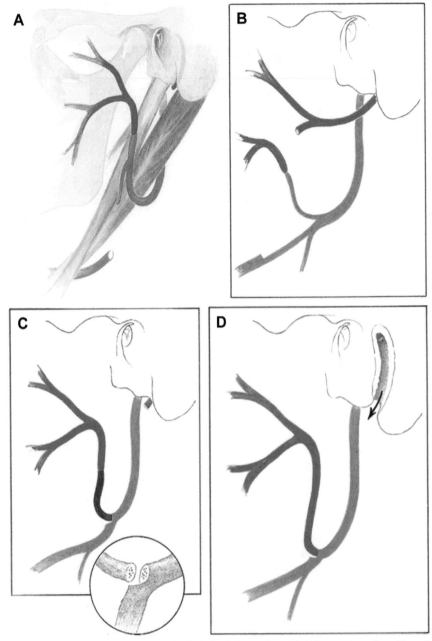

Fig. 2. Hypoglossal facial nerve transfer. (*A*) Classic hypoglossal facial nerve transfer with entire hypoglossal nerve transected. (*B*) Hypoglossal facial nerve modification with partial segment of nerve secured to lower division. (*C*) Hypoglossal facial nerve jump graft (*purple*) uses interposition graft harvested from great auricular or sural nerve to connect a partially transected hypoglossal nerve to the facial nerve. (*D*) In the facial translocation modification of hypoglossal facial nerve transfer, the facial nerve is identified in the mastoid bone and reflected into the neck and sutured to a partially transected hypoglossal nerve. This allows only one suture line. *Arrow* indicates the facial nerve being translocated from the temporal bone prior to anastamosis to the hypoglossal nerve. (*From* Hadlock TA, Cheney ML, McKenna MJ. Facial reanimation surgery. In: Nadol JB Jr, McKenna MJ, editors. Surgery of the ear and temporal bone. 2nd edition. Netherlands: Wolters Kluwer; 2004. p. 458; with permission.)

hypoglossal graft is preferred to sacrificing the entire hypoglossal nerve, because the latter may produce significant hemitongue atrophy and difficulty with speech articulation and swallowing.[14,15] Alternatively, a "jump" graft may be performed in which the hypoglossal nerve is partially incised, and a donor nerve (typically the sural or greater auricular nerve) is interpositioned between the hypoglossal and the facial nerve (**Fig. 2**C).[16]

Alternative donor nerves have also been suggested as candidates for nerve substitution procedures, with the masseteric branch of the trigeminal nerve showing particular promise (**Fig. 3**A, B). Use of masseteric-facial transfer for reanimation is particularly advantageous because it provides robust neurotization of the facial nerve with minimal donor site morbidity.[17,18] Most importantly, the masseteric nerve has demonstrated the ability to produce the most natural excursion of the oral commissure with smiling, providing an indispensible alternative to the hypoglossal-facial transfer (**Fig. 3**C, D).[19]

Regardless of which technique is used, the nerve substitution procedures all aim to facilitate neurotization of the distal facial nerve. Grafting to the facial nerve, however, may be impossible in a variety of scenarios. These scenarios include situations in which sufficient time has passed since onset of the facial nerve injury that the facial muscle motor end plates have undergone fibrosis, or when a distal segment of the facial nerve was sacrificed for oncologic purposes.[4] For these patients, muscle transfer (either local muscle flaps or microvascular free muscle flaps) provides an additional option for reanimation.

The temporalis muscle transfer is one technique that can restore volitional facial movement (**Fig. 4**A). In this procedure, the central one-third of the temporalis muscle is elevated off the temporal fossa, transposed over the zygomatic arch, and sutured to the orbicular oris at the oral commissure. This procedure elevates the lower lip and provides volitional lateral and superior excursion of the corner of the mouth. Thus, by biting down and activating the temporalis muscle, the patient is able to mimic the action of the muscles normally used to produce smiling.[20] Although efficacious, the temporalis muscle transfer is accompanied by significant donor site morbidity, including esthetic deformity secondary to depression of the temple and fullness over the zygomatic arch[4,20]; this has been addressed by development of the temporalis tendon transfer. In this procedure, the temporalis tendon is detached from its insertion at the coronoid process and transferred in an orthodromic fashion to the oral commissure (**Fig. 4**B),[4] providing similar volitional movement of the face without the temporal donor site (**Fig. 5**).

Spontaneous reanimation

All of the procedures described thus far rehabilitate facial nerve paralysis with varying degrees of success. Static reanimation corrects soft tissue laxity and allows for restoration of oral competence. Volitional dynamic reanimation allows for the reproduction of the smile mechanism and facial expression, albeit with conscious effort and neuromuscular retraining. However, the loftiest goal of facial reanimation is the restoration of spontaneous motion, in which facial movement on the paralyzed side can be reproduced without conscious effort. These goals have been realized with the advent of spontaneous dynamic reanimation procedures.

The first technique described that attempted to restore spontaneous reanimation of the face was the cross-facial nerve graft (CFNG). This procedure takes advantage of the contralateral, unaffected facial nerve (and for this reason, can only be used in patients with a unilateral facial nerve paralysis). Motor axons from the contralateral facial nerve are delivered via interpositional nerve grafts to the paralyzed side and then

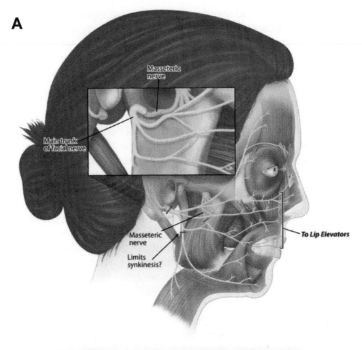

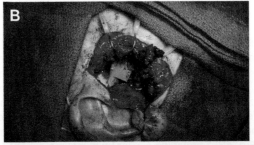

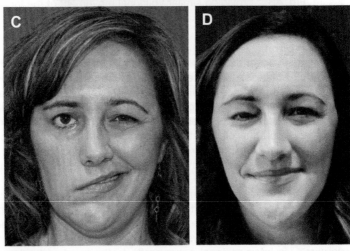

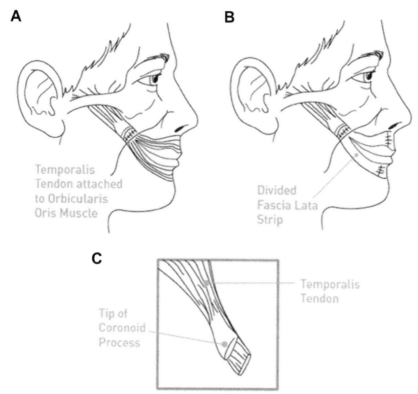

Fig. 4. Orthodromic temporalis tendon transfer: through a direct nasolabial fold incision, the temporalis tendon can be attached to the orbicularis oris either (*A*) primarily or (*B*) via a tensor fascia lata extension graft. (*C*) Attachment of temporalis tendon to the coronoid process. (*Courtesy of* Babak Azizzadeh, MD, Beverly Hills, CA.)

coapted to distal stump of the facial nerve (**Fig. 6**).[21] Long-term studies evaluating the efficacy of this technique have tempered much of the enthusiasm surrounding this procedure, because results have been shown to be less than ideal.[22] Contributing to these poor outcomes is the prolonged recovery time required for axonal regrowth through the CFNG, which may take in excess of 9 months. During this time period, the facial musculature remains in a state of denervation during which muscular atrophy and motor endplate fibrosis may ensue. To prevent muscular atrophy, the CFNG may be combined along with a split hypoglossal-facial transfer, a technique known as the "babysitter" procedure. In this 2-stage procedure, a portion of the ipsilateral hypoglossal nerve is first coapted to the main trunk of the paralytic facial nerve, providing immediate reinnervation of the facial musculature and preventing muscular atrophy. During this same procedure, 3 or 4 CFNGs are connected to the unaffected

Fig. 3. (*A, B*) The senior author's approach to masseteric facial nerve transfer. The facial nerve is identified via a parotidectomy approach and is completely transected at the stylomastoid foramen. It is then anastomosed to the masseteric nerve. The lower division of the facial nerve is transected distally to limit synkinesis. (*C, D*) Preoperative and postoperative photographs of a patient who has undergone masseteric-facial nerve transfer for complete facial paralysis. ([*A*] *Courtesy of* Babak Azizzadeh, MD, Beverly Hills, CA.)

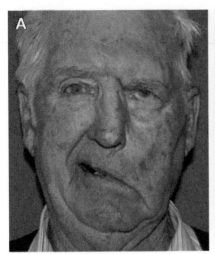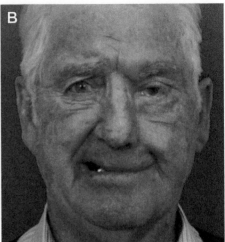

Fig. 5. (*A, B*) Preoperative and postoperative photographs of an individual who developed complete facial paralysis secondary to a parotid malignancy and underwent an orthodromic temporalis tendon transfer.

facial nerve and tunneled across the face to the paralytic side. In the second stage (performed approximately 9 months later), the distal ends of the CFNGs are coapted to the distal branches of the facial nerve, leaving the proximal hypoglossal-facial nerve anastomosis undisturbed.[23]

In addition to its utility as an independent procedure, the CFNG has played a critical role when combined with free muscle transfer, now considered the pinnacle of facial reanimation. Although several free muscle flaps have been described, the gracilis muscle is currently the most widely used. Since its introduction, the gracilis free muscle flap has revolutionized facial reanimation by achieving the critical goals of restoring spontaneous facial motion to the paralyzed face, re-establishing oral competence, correcting external nasal collapse, reintroducing a nasolabial fold, and providing voluntary facial expression.[23–26]

Typically, the reanimation using a gracilis free flap takes place as a 2-stage procedure. The first stage involves establishment of a CFNG. A large branch of the peripheral facial nerve on the unaffected side is identified via a facelift approach. A nerve graft (typically the sural nerve) is then harvested and primary neurorrhaphy is performed between the nerve graft donor facial nerve. The nerve graft is then tunneled across the upper lip to the contralateral gingivobuccal sulcus and tagged with a nonabsorbable suture and/or a vascular clip (see **Fig. 6**). After waiting approximately 9 months for axonal regrowth through the nerve graft, a gracilis free muscle transfer is then performed. A segment of gracilis muscle is harvested along with its neurovascular pedicle, including the obturator nerve and adductor artery and vein. A subcutaneous flap is then elevated on the paralytic side medially to the oral commissure and nasolabial fold. The gracilis muscle is then sutured to the oral commissure, and the donor vessels are anastomosed to the facial artery and vein under an operating microscope (**Fig. 7**). Finally, the obturator nerve is tunneled to the gingivobuccal sulcus, and a neurorrhaphy is performed with the CFNG.

Alternatively, the gracilis free muscle flap can also be performed as a single-stage reconstruction. In the single-stage procedure, the nerve to the donor muscle is kept long and tunneled across the upper lip to be connected to the contralateral intact facial

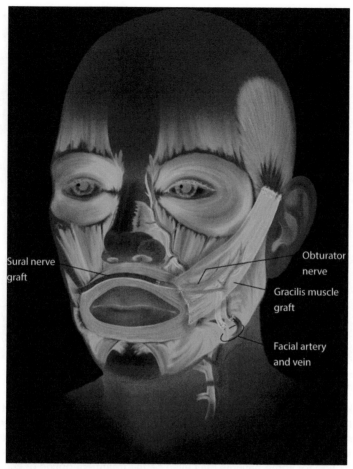

Sural nerve graft

Obturator nerve

Gracilis muscle graft

Facial artery and vein

Fig. 6. Gracilis free tissue transfer innervated by cross-facial sural nerve graft. (*Courtesy of* Babak Azizzadeh, MD, Beverly Hills, CA.)

nerve. Although both the 2-stage and single-stage gracilis flaps have grossly comparable results, the 2-stage procedure has been shown to achieve superior symmetry at rest, and for this reason, may generally be considered the more desirable technique.[27]

One unique circumstance in which the gracilis free muscle reanimation must be performed as a single-stage procedure is when a contralateral facial nerve is not available to serve as the source of reinnervation via a CFNG. This situation may arise in the case of bilateral facial paralysis, as can occur in Mobius syndrome wherein the patient suffers from congenital absence of bilateral facial nerves. For these patients, the nerve the masseter may be used as an alternative to the CFNG as source of muscle reinnervation.[26,28] Ostensibly, this would appear to be less ideal than cross-facial innervation because the masseteric nerve would be expected to produce a smile that is volitional rather than spontaneous. Interestingly, long-term studies have demonstrated that even with masseteric reinnervation of the gracilis muscle, most patients are eventually able to obtain a spontaneous smile (ie, smiling without thinking or having to consciously bite down to activate the masseteric nerve), possibly because of cerebral plasticity and cortical reorganization.[25] Furthermore, innervation by the masseteric

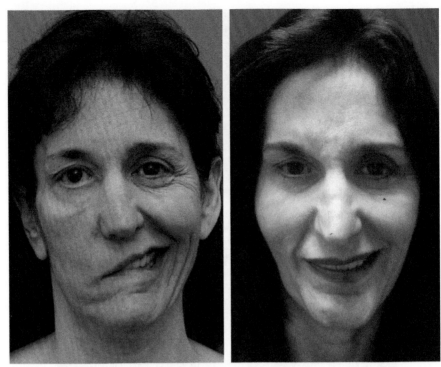

Fig. 7. Preoperative and postoperative outcome from staged CFNG, masseteric facial nerve transfer with secondary gracilis free flap.

nerve yields excursion of the oral commissure during smiling that is greater than that produced by cross-facial innervation and nearly equivalent to that produced by the native smile mechanism.[19] For these reasons, the single-stage gracilis flap with masseteric reinnervation is an invaluable alternative to the traditional 2-stage flap with CFNG, and for some patients may even be the treatment option of choice.

Upper Face

As with the lower face and midface, dysfunction from upper face paralysis is directly related to the loss of innervation to the facial musculature (specifically the orbicularis oculi and frontalis muscles) and resulting soft tissue laxity. For the upper face, this has been rectified with great success using static reanimation techniques. The loss of frontalis muscle tone leads to brow ptosis on the affected side, causing superior visual field impairment in addition to cosmetic deformity.[29] Furthermore, loss of function of the orbicularis oculi muscle results in an inability to close the eye and loss of the blink reflex. The subsequent absence of corneal protection may ultimately result in keratitis, corneal ulceration, and potentially, complete loss of vision on the affected side.[30] A successful reanimation of the upper face must therefore address both of these critical issues, correcting brow ptosis and allowing for complete closure of the eye.

Management of the brow

Paralysis of the frontal branch leads to loss of frontalis muscle tone and brow ptosis. Open brow-lifting techniques include the direct brow lift, the mid-forehead lift, and the coronal/pretrichial brow lift. The direct brow lift is performed via an incision just inside the superior brow hairline. An ellipse of soft tissue including skin and subcutaneous fat is then excised, and the height of the brow is adjusted to the desired level. A deep suture can be used to secure the brow at this height to the periosteum of the forehead. Alternatively, if the patient presents at a more advanced age and with deep forehead wrinkles, the incision can be placed within a mid-forehead skin crease.[29] Both of these variations of the open brow lift may place the patient at risk for a prominent scar. An alternative open option is the coronal brow lift, in which the incision is placed 4 to 6 cm posterior to the forehead hairline. This option does carry the potential of pulling the hairline further posteriorly, which may be unacceptable for patients with a high forehead or receding hairline. Alternatively, the pretrichial approach places the incision immediately posterior to the hairline. This approach allows the anteriorly excised skin to be non-hair-bearing, and thus preserving the location of the hairline.[29] Recently, endoscopic techniques have risen to favor because of their ability to achieve similar brow-lifting results with minimal incisions.[31] Typically, 3 to 5 small access incisions hidden posterior to the hairline are required. Once the depressor muscles of the brow (ie, corrugator and procerus muscles) are divided, the elevated brow can be secured with several fixation methods.[32]

Management of the eye
Upper eyelid With loss of innervation to the orbicular oculi, the patient suffers from an inability to attain complete closure of the eyelids, a debility known as lagophthalmos. Lid loading, in which a weight is placed in the upper eyelid and used to supply additional gravitational force to the upper eyelid, allows it to achieve full closure (**Fig. 8**).[33] This procedure is typically performed via an incision placed in an upper eyelid crease and deepened through the skin and orbicularis oculi muscle. A precise pocket for the lid weight is developed, and the lid weight is then secured to the superior tarsal plate with sutures.[34] Historically, lid loading has been accomplished with use of a gold weight. However, this has been marred by poor esthetic outcomes secondary to the thick profile of the gold weight and resulting contour deformity of the upper

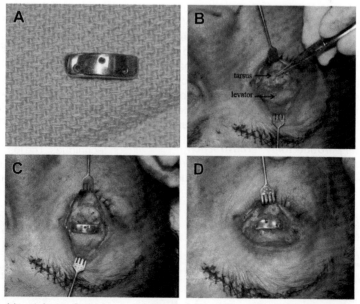

Fig. 8. Gold weight implantation surgical series. (*A*) Gold weight, 1.4 g. (*B*) Exposure of the tarsus and levator aponeurosis. (*C*) Gold weight placed in surgical site above tarsus and below recessed levator. (*D*) Gold weight sutured to tarsus below and levator above.

eyelid.[35] For these reasons, platinum weights have recently gained popularity, as the increased density of platinum allows for the weight to have a lower profile while maintaining the same degree of lid loading.[30,35,36] Regardless of which type of weight is used, lid loading has been demonstrated to be extremely efficacious, with complete eye closure and corneal protection achievable in nearly all cases.[33,34,36] Another method of aiding upper eyelid closure involves the placement of palpebral springs. This technique is not commonly used given high rates of extrusion and infection.[37]

Lower eyelid Paralysis of the lower half of the orbicularis oculi muscle results in significant laxity of the lower eyelid and subsequent disruption of the normal tear film mechanism, which results in corneal dessication that leads to exposure keratitis, corneal ulceration, and ultimately, loss of vision.[30] There are several techniques used for lower eyelid rehabilitation. Tarsorrhaphy is the classical method for providing corneal protection. Although effective, tarsorrhaphy is cosmetically unappealing and results in reduced peripheral vision and secondary complications, including trichiasis. Correction of lower lid laxity can be easily corrected through a lid-tightening procedure known as a "tarsal strip." After the lateral canthal tendon is transected, an inferior cantholysis is performed resulting in a "tarsal strip," which is then sutured to the periosteum of the lateral orbital rim.[34,38] This "tarsal strip" allows for the restoration of the normal tear film, improvement in ocular symptoms, and decreased exposure keratopathy.[39]

Lower lid laxity and severe paralytic ectropion can lead to chronic epiphora and cicatricial changes and to scarring down of the lower eyelid and an increase in the vertical palpebral fissure distance. One method to help elevate the retracted lower eyelid involves a "spacer" graft using septal and conchal cartilage, hard palate mucosa, fascia, or acellular dermal matrices.[40,41] Grafts are placed between the orbicularis oculi and the orbital septum for patients with anterior lamella deficiency.[42] In the case of posterior lamellar deficiency, the graft is placed between the tarsus and the retracted lid retractors.[42] Fascial slings use autogenous fascia such as tensor fascia lata to help suspend the lower eyelid.[43] Furthermore, the lower eyelid is thought of as an anatomic continuum with the soft tissue structures of the midface, particularly the suborbicularis oculi fat pad (SOOF). The SOOF lift is often used as an adjuvant to the lateral tarsal strip to give vertical support with improved ocular outcomes, reducing lagophthalmos and keratopathy.[44] The combination of hard palate spacer grafting, lateral canthoplasty, and midface suspension was effective in treating lower eyelid retraction with resolution of scleral show and improved cosmesis.[45] Given the multifactorial nature of lower eyelid laxity and ectropion, multiple procedures may be required to effectively improve functional and cosmetic outcomes (**Fig. 9**).

Postradical parotidectomy reconstruction
Parotid tumors that show aggressive features such as perineural invasion often require a radical parotidectomy. In addition to functional and cosmetic deficits from facial

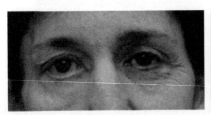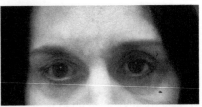

Fig. 9. Patient with right facial paralysis who underwent right gold weight and lower lid reconstruction.

nerve sacrifice, these defects result in severe contour defects secondary to resection of skin, muscle, mandible, and/or temporal bone. The reconstruction dilemma is 2-fold: facial nerve reconstruction as well as volume restoration of the surgical defect. After complete oncologic resection, if coaptable proximal and distal facial nerve stumps are available, a nerve graft using the greater auricular or sural nerve can be performed. An alloderm static sling procedure is performed at the same time as nerve grafting. Once radiation therapy is complete, a secondary orthodromic temporalis tendon transfer (OTTT) can be performed 6 to 12 months after the primary surgery. In a select group of younger patients who have nonirradiated skin and accessible facial vessels, secondary CFNG and gracilis flap is a reconstructive option. Given the predictable ocular symptoms, the eye is managed with an upper eyelid weight and lower eyelid tightening procedures as previously described.

Contour defects after radical parotidectomy require large volume reconstruction. Regional flaps such as pectoralis major, temporalis muscle, or sternocleidomastoid either lack volume or sculpting flexibility for adequate reconstruction. Free tissue transfer using the anterolateral thigh (ALT) flap has become the workhorse for single-stage reconstruction radical parotidectomy defects. The flap has minimal donor site morbidity, can be harvested with a 2-team approach, and has soft tissue versatility as both a cutaneous and a musculocutaneous flap. Furthermore, it has specific advantages for radical parotidectomy defects including access to motor nerves for grafting and fascia lata for static reanimation. The ALT flap combined with OTTT offers single-stage dynamic facial reanimation along with restoration of volume deficit.[46]

SUMMARY

Facial nerve paralysis is a debilitating condition with pervasive implications on patient quality of life. Given that facial nerve paralysis may be encountered by physicians in a wide range of specialties, including general surgeons, trauma surgeons, neurosurgeons, and emergency room physicians, a general understanding of facial reanimation is critical to ensure clear lines of communication in an increasingly collaborative medical environment. Accordingly, the contemporary surgical management of chronic, irreversible facial paralysis has been described.

REFERENCES

1. Lorch M, Teach SJ. Facial nerve palsy: etiology and approach to diagnosis and treatment. Pediatr Emerg Care 2010;26(10):763–9 [quiz: 770–63].
2. Constantinides M, Galli SK, Miller PJ. Complications of static facial suspensions with expanded polytetrafluoroethylene (ePTFE). Laryngoscope 2001;111(12): 2114–21.
3. Coulson SE, O'Dwyer NJ, Adams RD, et al. Expression of emotion and quality of life after facial nerve paralysis. Otol Neurotol 2004;25(6):1014–9.
4. Byrne PJ, Kim M, Boahene K, et al. Temporalis tendon transfer as part of a comprehensive approach to facial reanimation. Arch Facial Plast Surg 2007; 9(4):234–41.
5. Robey AB, Snyder MC. Reconstruction of the paralyzed face. Ear Nose Throat J 2011;90(6):267–75.
6. Hazin R, Azizzadeh B, Bhatti MT. Medical and surgical management of facial nerve palsy. Curr Opin Ophthalmol 2009;20(6):440–50.
7. Petroff MA, Goode RL, Levet Y. Gore-Tex implants: applications in facial paralysis rehabilitation and soft-tissue augmentation. Laryngoscope 1992;102(10):1185–9.

8. Konior RJ. Facial paralysis reconstruction with Gore-Tex Soft-Tissue Patch. Arch Otolaryngol Head Neck Surg 1992;118(11):1188–94.
9. Fisher E, Frodel JL. Facial suspension with acellular human dermal allograft. Arch Facial Plast Surg 1999;1(3):195–9.
10. Leventhal DD, Pribitkin EA. Static facial suspension with Surgisis ES (Enhanced Strength) sling. Laryngoscope 2008;118(1):20–3.
11. Frodel JL. Facial suspension with acellular human dermal allograft. Arch Facial Plast Surg 2011;13(1):60–1.
12. Leckenby JI, Harrison DH, Grobbelaar AO. Static support in the facial palsy patient: a case series of 51 patients using tensor fascia lata slings as the sole treatment for correcting the position of the mouth. J Plast Reconstr Aesthet Surg 2014;67(3):350–7.
13. Conley J. Facial rehabilitation: new potentials. Clin Plast Surg 1979;6(3):421–31.
14. Shipchandler TZ, Seth R, Alam DS. Split hypoglossal-facial nerve neurorrhaphy for treatment of the paralyzed face. Am J Otolaryngol 2011;32(6):511–6.
15. Conley J, Baker DC. Hypoglossal-facial nerve anastomosis for reinnervation of the paralyzed face. Plast Reconstr Surg 1979;63(1):63–72.
16. May M, Sobol SM, Mester SJ. Hypoglossal-facial nerve interpositional-jump graft for facial reanimation without tongue atrophy. Otolaryngol Head Neck Surg 1991; 104(6):818–25.
17. Coombs CJ, Ek EW, Wu T, et al. Masseteric-facial nerve coaptation–an alternative technique for facial nerve reinnervation. J Plast Reconstr Aesthet Surg 2009; 62(12):1580–8.
18. Faria JC, Scopel GP, Ferreira MC. Facial reanimation with masseteric nerve: babysitter or permanent procedure? Preliminary results. Ann Plast Surg 2010;64(1): 31–4.
19. Bae YC, Zuker RM, Manktelow RT, et al. A comparison of commissure excursion following gracilis muscle transplantation for facial paralysis using a cross-face nerve graft versus the motor nerve to the masseter nerve. Plast Reconstr Surg 2006;117(7):2407–13.
20. Cheney ML, McKenna MJ, Megerian CA, et al. Early temporalis muscle transposition for the management of facial paralysis. Laryngoscope 1995;105(9 Pt 1): 993–1000.
21. Lee EI, Hurvitz KA, Evans GR, et al. Cross-facial nerve graft: past and present. J Plast Reconstr Aesthet Surg 2008;61(3):250–6.
22. Scaramella LF. Cross-face facial nerve anastomosis: historical notes. Ear Nose Throat J 1996;75(6):343, 347–52, 354.
23. Terzis JK, Tzafetta K. The "babysitter" procedure: minihypoglossal to facial nerve transfer and cross-facial nerve grafting. Plast Reconstr Surg 2009;123(3):865–76.
24. Harii K, Ohmori K, Torii S. Free gracilis muscle transplantation, with microneurovascular anastomoses for the treatment of facial paralysis. A preliminary report. Plast Reconstr Surg 1976;57(2):133–43.
25. Manktelow RT, Tomat LR, Zuker RM, et al. Smile reconstruction in adults with free muscle transfer innervated by the masseter motor nerve: effectiveness and cerebral adaptation. Plast Reconstr Surg 2006;118(4):885–99.
26. Hadlock TA, Malo JS, Cheney ML, et al. Free gracilis transfer for smile in children: the Massachusetts Eye and Ear Infirmary Experience in excursion and quality-of-life changes. Arch Facial Plast Surg 2011;13(3):190–4.
27. Kumar PA, Hassan KM. Cross-face nerve graft with free-muscle transfer for reanimation of the paralyzed face: a comparative study of the single-stage and two-stage procedures. Plast Reconstr Surg 2002;109(2):451–62 [discussion: 463–4].

28. Zuker RM, Goldberg CS, Manktelow RT. Facial animation in children with Mobius syndrome after segmental gracilis muscle transplant. Plast Reconstr Surg 2000; 106(1):1–8 [discussion: 9].
29. Meltzer NE, Byrne PJ. Management of the brow in facial paralysis. Facial Plast Surg 2008;24(2):216–9.
30. Henstrom DK, Lindsay RW, Cheney ML, et al. Surgical treatment of the periocular complex and improvement of quality of life in patients with facial paralysis. Arch Facial Plast Surg 2011;13(2):125–8.
31. Rautio J, Pignatti M. Endoscopic forehead lift for ptosis of the brow caused by facial paralysis. Scand J Plast Reconstr Surg Hand Surg 2001;35(1):51–6.
32. Angelos PC, Stallworth CL, Wang TD. Forehead lifting: state of the art. Facial Plast Surg 2011;27(1):50–7.
33. Yu Y, Sun J, Chen L, et al. Lid loading for treatment of paralytic lagophthalmos. Aesthetic Plast Surg 2011;35(6):1165–71.
34. Razfar A, Afifi AM, Manders EK, et al. Ocular outcomes after gold weight placement and facial nerve resection. Otolaryngol Head Neck Surg 2009;140(1):82–5.
35. Silver AL, Lindsay RW, Cheney ML, et al. Thin-profile platinum eyelid weighting: a superior option in the paralyzed eye. Plast Reconstr Surg 2009;123(6):1697–703.
36. Berghaus A, Neumann K, Schrom T. The platinum chain: a new upper-lid implant for facial palsy. Arch Facial Plast Surg 2003;5(2):166–70.
37. Demirci H, Frueh BR. Palpebral spring in the management of lagophthalmos and exposure keratopathy secondary to facial nerve palsy. Ophthal Plast Reconstr Surg 2009;25(4):270–5.
38. Becker FF. Lateral tarsal strip procedure for the correction of paralytic ectropion. Laryngoscope 1982;92(4):382–4.
39. Golio D, De Martelaere S, Anderson J, et al. Outcomes of periocular reconstruction for facial nerve paralysis in cancer patients. Plast Reconstr Surg 2007;119(4): 1233–7.
40. Krastinova D, Franchi G, Kelly MB, et al. Rehabilitation of the paralysed or lax lower eyelid using a graft of conchal cartilage. Br J Plast Surg 2002;55(1):12–9.
41. Li TG, Shorr N, Goldberg RA. Comparison of the efficacy of hard palate grafts with acellular human dermis grafts in lower eyelid surgery. Plast Reconstr Surg 2005;116(3):873–8 [discussion: 879–80].
42. Marks MW, Argenta LC, Friedman RJ, et al. Conchal cartilage and composite grafts for correction of lower lid retraction. Plast Reconstr Surg 1989;83(4): 629–35.
43. Iyengar SS, Burnstine MA. Treatment of symptomatic facial nerve paralysis with lower eyelid fascia lata suspension. Plast Reconstr Surg 2012;129(3):569e–71e.
44. Olver JM. Raising the suborbicularis oculi fat (SOOF): its role in chronic facial palsy. Br J Ophthalmol 2000;84(12):1401–6.
45. Patel MP, Shapiro MD, Spinelli HM. Combined hard palate spacer graft, midface suspension, and lateral canthoplasty for lower eyelid retraction: a tripartite approach. Plast Reconstr Surg 2005;115(7):2105–14 [discussion: 2115–7].
46. Revenaugh PC, Knott PD, Scharpf J, et al. Simultaneous anterolateral thigh flap and temporalis tendon transfer to optimize facial form and function after radical parotidectomy. Arch Facial Plast Surg 2012;14(2):104–9.

Periocular Reconstruction in Patients with Facial Paralysis

Shannon S. Joseph, MD, MSc[a,1], Andrew W. Joseph, MD, MPH[b,1],
Raymond S. Douglas, MD, PhD[a], Guy G. Massry, MD[c,*]

KEYWORDS

- Facial paralysis • Facial nerve • Paralytic lagophthalmos • Eyelid retraction
- Ectropion • Exposure keratopathy • Synkinesis

KEY POINTS

- Facial nerve injury often results in orbicularis oculi weakness, which impairs eyelid closure and blink, causing potentially serious ocular consequences.
- Patients with inadequate Bell's phenomenon, corneal anesthesia, and decreased tear production are at high risk for exposure keratopathy in the setting of orbicularis oculi weakness and require a thorough ophthalmologic evaluation.
- If the recovery of facial nerve function is likely, then temporary and conservative measures to provide corneal protection and increase ocular surface lubrication are the mainstays of therapy.
- If the recovery of facial nerve function is unlikely or expected to be prolonged, then surgical rehabilitation of the periocular complex should be considered.
- Current surgical reconstructive procedures are most commonly intended to improve coverage of the eye but cannot restore blink.

INTRODUCTION

Facial nerve injury is one of the most serious complications of parotid diseases and parotid surgery. Transient facial paralysis has been reported in as many as 65% of patients after parotidectomy, whereas permanent facial paralysis has been reported in up to 5% of patients.[1–3] The temporal, zygomatic, and buccal branches of the facial

Financial disclosure: None declared.
Conflicts of interest: None declared.
[a] Division of Oculoplastic Surgery, Department of Ophthalmology and Visual Sciences, University of Michigan Medical School, 1000 Wall Street, Ann Arbor, MI 48105, USA; [b] Department of Otolaryngology-Head & Neck Surgery, Johns Hopkins University School of Medicine, 601 North Caroline Street, Baltimore, MD 21287, USA; [c] Ophthalmic Plastic and Reconstructive Surgery, Keck School of Medicine, University of Southern California, 150 North Robertson Boulevard, Suite 314, Beverly Hills, CA 90211, USA
[1] These authors contributed equally to this work.
* Corresponding author.
E-mail address: gmassry@drmassry.com

Otolaryngol Clin N Am 49 (2016) 475–487
http://dx.doi.org/10.1016/j.otc.2015.10.011
0030-6665/16/$ – see front matter © 2016 Elsevier Inc. All rights reserved.

nerve innervate the orbicularis oculi muscle, which is the main protractor of the eyelids. Up to 75% of patients with permanent facial nerve injury following parotidectomy also have orbicularis oculi weakness caused by disruption of its innervation.[1]

Impaired function of the orbicularis oculi manifests as incomplete eyelid closure and reduced blink frequency and amplitude.[4] Blink is essential to effective tear film distribution across the corneal surface. Inadequate blink leads to excessive evaporation of the tear film and desiccation of the cornea. Furthermore, in the setting of orbicularis oculi weakness, the action of the eyelid retractors (levator palpebrae superioris and Müller's muscle for the upper eyelid, and inferior tarsal muscle for the lower eyelid) become more pronounced. This condition manifests as upper and lower eyelid retraction, and widening of the vertical palpebral fissure. Reduced orbicularis oculi tone also means less counteraction against the gravitational pull on the lower eyelid, which may result in paralytic ectropion. Together, these dynamic and static changes of the eyelids lead to increased exposure of the ocular surface. If not managed appropriately, patients may develop corneal epithelial defects, ulcers, perforations, and even endophthalmitis. These ocular complications may cause loss of vision and even loss of the eye. Therefore, it is of paramount importance that patients with facial nerve injury involving the periocular complex undergo a thorough ophthalmologic evaluation and, if indicated, periocular reconstruction.

EVALUATION

A thorough history of the nature and time course of facial nerve injury should be elicited. The likelihood for recovery of facial nerve function should be determined. Patients with a history of facial nerve sacrifice during surgery, facial nerve malignancy, or facial nerve injury longer than 12 months are less likely to recover.[5] The presence of ocular symptoms, including change in vision, eye irritation, pain, foreign body sensation, and tearing, should be documented. A past ophthalmologic medical and surgical history should be obtained. Patients with corneal conditions, including dry eye, have less reserve to withstand increased corneal exposure. Monocular patients with facial paralysis affecting the eye with vision must receive special attention.

Physical examination of the periocular complex should begin with observing the patient at repose with spontaneous blink and then with gentle and forced eyelid closure. The integrity of the main corneal protective mechanisms, including frequency and amplitude of blink, orbicularis oculi strength, Bell's phenomenon, corneal sensation (trigeminal nerve), and tear production, must be assessed (**Table 1**). Bell's phenomenon, not to be confused with Bell's palsy, is the spontaneous upward and outward movement of the eye when an individual attempts to close the eyes. This reflex is present in most patients and is a corneal protective feature for patients with facial paralysis. Visual acuity should be obtained. The ocular surface should be examined with fluorescein dye to identify any corneal epithelial defects or ulcers; conjunctival injection should also be noted because this is often a sign of ocular surface exposure (**Fig. 1**). If one or more of the corneal protective mechanisms are impaired, or if the patient has ocular symptoms, decreased visual acuity, or any signs of ocular surface abnormalities, then an urgent ophthalmology consultation is warranted. An evaluation of the static changes of the periocular complex should also be performed to guide reconstructive management (**Fig. 2, Table 2**).

MANAGEMENT

The goal of management of the periocular complex in patients with facial paralysis is primarily to protect the ocular surface and preserve visual function and secondarily to

Table 1
Examination components to assess the integrity of corneal protective mechanisms in facial paralysis

Examination Component	Details
Blink	Frequency, amplitude, and completeness of involuntary and voluntary blink
Strength of orbicularis oculi	Amount of resistance needed to overcome eyelid closure (the less resistance needed, the weaker the orbicularis oculi)
Bell's phenomenon	Upward rotation of the globe on attempted eyelid closure (minimal or no corneal show on attempted eyelid closure indicates intact Bell's phenomenon)
Corneal sensation	Subjective sensation and reflexive blink in response to touching the cornea with a wisp from a cotton tip applicator
Tear production	Schirmer I test (without anesthesia) measures total tear secretion (basal and reflex): <10 mm is abnormally low

restore facial symmetry. A variety of temporary and long-term measures exist. An individualized approach to management should be implemented based on the duration of facial paralysis, the prognosis of recovery, the extent of dynamic and static dysfunction, the integrity of the corneal protective mechanisms, and the state of the ocular surface.

Temporary Measures

The first line of management for all patients with facial paralysis involving the periocular complex is aggressive ocular surface lubrication. Patients should use preservative-free artificial tears frequently throughout the day, and lubricating ointment before sleep. For patients with mild ocular surface exposure and expected recovery of facial nerve function, such as in the setting of neurapraxia following parotid surgery, lubrication alone in combination with taping of eyes during sleep

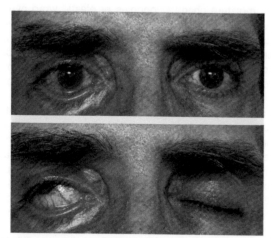

Fig. 1. Patient with right-sided facial paralysis with (*top*) significant conjunctival injection, high tear meniscus, lower eyelid retraction, and paralytic ectropion, with (*bottom*) insufficient Bell's phenomenon.

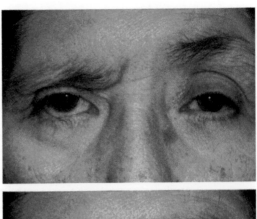

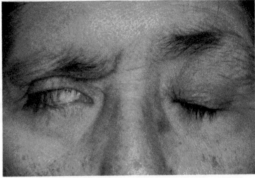

Fig. 2. Examination findings in a patient with right-sided facial paralysis. (*Top*) Note the brow ptosis and lower eyelid retraction, with (*bottom*) significant lagophthalmos, but intact Bell's phenomenon. (*Adapted from* Massry GG. Surgical management of the eye. In: Slattery B, editor. The facial nerve. New York: Thieme Publishers; 2013. p. 165; with permission.)

may be sufficient. If there is moderate to severe ocular surface exposure caused by lagophthalmos, moisture chamber goggles or plastic wrap over the eye should be used during sleep to protect the cornea from desiccation and mechanical trauma. A nighttime humidifier may also be beneficial. Contact lenses, such as the prosthetic replacement of the ocular surface ecosystem (PROSE) device, have been shown to be effective in providing protection and constant hydration of the cornea.[6,7] Patients with low tear production may also benefit from punctal occlusion with plugs or cauterization.

If conservative measures to increase lubrication are insufficient at maintaining the health of the ocular surface, then temporary interventional measures should be implemented. These measures are particularly beneficial for patients in whom the recovery of the facial nerve is expected, or for patients who are poor surgical candidates for other reconstructive measures. Chemodenervation of the levator palpebrae superioris with botulinum toxin-A can induce temporary ptosis for 8 to 12 weeks and effectively reduce upper eyelid retraction and lagophthalmos.[8,9] Care should be taken to avoid inadvertently chemodenervating the superior rectus muscle, which would lead to diplopia and impairment of the protective Bell's phenomenon (**Table 3**).[9] Alternatively, injectable hyaluronic acid filler can be used as temporary upper lid weight, and effectively reduces lagophthalmos and ocular surface exposure (see **Table 3**).[10,11] Similarly, appropriately placed lower eyelid hyaluronic acid filler can three-dimensionally

Table 2
Examination components to assess static periocular changes in facial paralysis

Examination Component	Details
MRD1	Distance between pupillary light reflex to the upper eyelid margin. Upper eyelid normally rests 1 mm below the superior limbus. A high MRD1 reflects upper eyelid retraction, and a low MRD1 reflects blepharoptosis
MRD2	Distance between the pupillary light reflex to the lower eyelid margin. Lower eyelid normally rests at or just above the inferior limbus. A high MRD2 reflects lower eyelid retraction
Lower eyelid laxity	Distraction test: the greater the distance the lower eyelid can be pulled away from the globe, the more laxity is present Snap-back test: if the eyelid cannot snap back to oppose the globe without blink, then laxity is present
Medial and lateral canthal tendon laxity	Medial and lateral distraction test: the greater the displacement of the medial and lateral canthi, the more laxity of the tendons
Lower eyelid malposition	Lower eyelid ectropion or punctal ectropion should be noted
Brow position	Brow ptosis can contribute to decreased superior visual field. Contralateral brow hyperelevation should be noted
Midface ptosis and/or negative vector	Midface ptosis and/or negative vector can exacerbate lower eyelid retraction

Abbreviations: MRD1, margin-reflex distance 1; MRD2, margin-reflex distance 2.

expand, elevate, and support the lower eyelid to reduce lower eyelid malposition and ocular exposure (see **Table 3**).[12]

In some patients with severe ocular surface exposure and impairment of corneal protective mechanisms such as corneal sensation or Bell's phenomenon, a temporary or permanent tarsorrhaphy may be necessary to reduce the exposed ocular surface area, especially if the patient is a poor candidate for more invasive surgical

Table 3
Temporary interventional measures for periorbital reconstruction in facial paralysis

Procedure	Technique
Chemodenervation of the levator palpebrae superioris	Botulinum toxin-A (7.5–15 units) can be injected using a 12.5-mm 30-gauge needle into the levator palpebrae superioris. To avoid the superior rectus muscle, the needle should be placed just behind the superior orbital rim in the midpupillary plane, aiming at the most anterior part of the levator palpebrae superioris muscle[9]
Filler injection to induce upper eyelid ptosis	Hyaluronic acid gel can be injected in the pre–levator aponeurosis plane and/or pretarsal plane[10]
Filler injection to reduce lower eyelid retraction	Hyaluronic acid gel can be injected in a layered approach with multiple fine threadlike injections along the length of the lower eyelid in the area of the orbital septum and orbitomalar ligament[12]
Suture tarsorrhaphy	Horizontal mattress sutures passed through the gray lines of the upper and lower eyelid margins. Adjustable suture tarsorrhaphy with bolsters can also be used if frequent cornea examinations are needed

reconstructive procedures, has inadequate follow-up care, and/or has no anticipated recovery of facial nerve function. The tarsorrhaphy procedure effectively reduces the horizontal palpebral fissure by fusing upper and lower eyelids at the margin over a variable distance, and can be performed medially or laterally (**Fig. 3**). Temporary suture tarsorrhaphy typically lasts only 2 to 3 weeks (see **Table 3**). Permanent tarsorrhaphy involves reapproximating the eyelid margins after deepithelialization, with or without separation of the anterior and posterior lamellae, to allow permanent adhesions to form (**Fig. 4**). These procedures can be reversed, but reversal is usually associated with eyelid margin and eyelash irregularity. Although tarsorrhaphies are simple, fast, and effective, they can be cosmetically objectionable and can cause variable degrees of restriction of the peripheral visual field.

Long-term Measures

Surgical rehabilitation of the periocular complex has been shown to improve the overall quality of life in patients with facial paralysis.[13] All patients with prolonged or unlikely recovery of facial nerve function, especially those with impaired corneal protective mechanisms, should undergo surgical rehabilitation to provide long-term protection of the ocular surface. Most of the current procedures are intended to improve coverage of the ocular surface but cannot restore blink or natural eyelid closure. Further, because persistent effects of gravity lead to continued descent of soft tissue, periorbital surgical reconstruction for patients with facial paralysis is often an ongoing process.

Upper eyelid reconstruction

Upper eyelid loading Upper eyelid loading is one of the most common techniques used to manage upper eyelid retraction and lagophthalmos in patients with facial paralysis. It may be performed at the time of the parotid surgery in cases of planned facial nerve sacrifice. Upper eyelid loading uses the gravitational pull on the upper eyelid and induces mechanical ptosis. This procedure is most effective with the patient in the

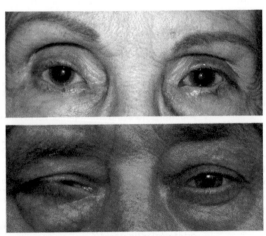

Fig. 3. Permanent lateral tarsorrhaphy. (*Top*) There is 20% lateral tarsorrhaphy on the left side. (*Bottom*) There is 50% lateral tarsorrhaphy on the right side. Note the difference in the horizontal palpebral aperture. ([*Top*] *Adapted from* Massry GG. Surgical management of the eye. In: Slattery B, editor. The facial nerve. New York: Thieme Publishers; 2013. p. 168; with permission.)

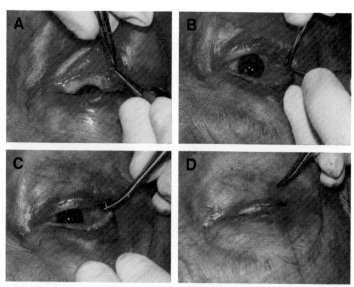

Fig. 4. Permanent tarsorrhaphy procedure. (*A*) The margins of the upper and lower eyelids are deepithelialized to the commissure posterior to the lash line for the desired distance of tarsorrhaphy. (*B*) The anterior and posterior lamellae are split to allow the edges to evert when secured. (*C*) A 5-0 chromic suture is passed between the anterior and posterior lamellae of corresponding parts of the upper and lower eyelid. (*D*) The wound is closed. (*Adapted from* Massry GG. Surgical management of the eye. In: Slattery B, editor. The facial nerve. New York: Thieme Publishers; 2013. p. 168; with permission.)

upright position. Various weights may be tested preoperatively by taping them to the patient's eyelid, selecting the weight inducing the least amount of lagophthalmos and visually significant upper eyelid ptosis. Intraoperatively, the implant is attached to the tarsus at the widest point of the palpebral fissure, usually between the midpupillary line and the medial limbus, and can be sutured either in the pretarsal plane, to the levator aponeurosis, or superior to the tarsus (**Fig. 5**). The senior author (GGM) uses a preaponeurotic fat flap to cover the weight for better cosmesis (Massry GG, unpublished data, 2016). Upper eyelid loading can be performed under local or general anesthesia, and is a reasonable option for patients who are poor surgical candidates.

Gold was the most common material used for eyelid weights, but it was associated with a high incidence of complications, including implant extrusion, migration, wound infection, astigmatism, and poor cosmesis with visibility under the skin.[14] Platinum is now the preferred material because of its higher density, which translates to a slimmer profile and decreased visibility, improved eyelid contour, and overall better cosmesis.[15,16] Compared with gold, platinum is also less inflammatory, which results in lower rates of capsule formation and extrusion.[15,16] The upper eyelid weights can be removed at a later time if facial nerve function recovers.

Upper eyelid müllerectomy Another option to address upper eyelid retraction is müllerectomy (also known as Müller's extirpation). The Müller's muscle is a sympathetically innervated upper eyelid retractor that accounts for 2 to 3 mm of upper eyelid elevation. Müllerectomy involves removal of graded amounts of Müller's muscle, and is performed through a conjunctival incision along the superior tarsal border with the upper eyelid everted. The Müller's muscle is dissected free from the

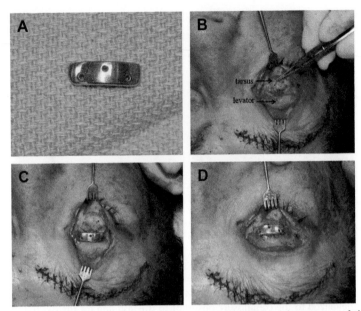

Fig. 5. Upper eyelid weight placement. (*A*) A 1.4-g gold weight. (*B*) Exposure of the tarsus and the levator aponeurosis. (*C*) Gold weight placed above the tarsus and below the recessed levator. (*D*) Gold weight sutured to the tarsus below and the levator above. (*Adapted from* Massry GG. Surgical management of the eye. In: Slattery B, editor. The facial nerve. New York: Thieme Publishers; 2013. p. 171; with permission.)

underlying conjunctiva and the overlying levator aponeurosis. It can then be transected from its insertion on the superior tarsal border and its origin on the inferior surface of the levator. This procedure has been shown to lower the upper eyelid by 1 to 2 mm.[17] The advantage of müllerectomy is that it does not involve implantation of foreign objects into the eyelid, and generally provides good upper eyelid contour. This technique also avoids eyelid crease incisions, which is an important consideration in patients with low eyelid creases, such as the Asian population. However, müllerectomy does not always provide sufficient reduction in upper eyelid retraction.

Upper eyelid blepharotomy Blepharotomy is another technique that has been shown to reduce lagophthalmos and upper eyelid retraction.[18] This procedure can be performed through an eyelid crease skin incision, followed by full-thickness transection of the upper eyelid near the superior border of the tarsus. This approach effectively allows recession of the upper eyelid retractors. Only the skin incision is closed. Alternatively, a transconjunctival incision is made with the upper eyelid everted, and a nearly full-thickness transection is performed, leaving only the skin intact. The length and location of transection depend on the extent and location of upper eyelid retraction. Potential complications of blepharotomy include upper eyelid contour abnormality and ptosis caused by overcorrection.[18] This procedure is less readily reversible compared with upper eyelid loading.

Lower eyelid reconstruction

The development of lower eyelid retraction and malposition in patients with facial paralysis is multifactorial. The lack of orbicularis oculi tone leaves the lower eyelid more susceptible to gravitational pull, which commonly leads to increased horizontal laxity.

Over time, horizontal lengthening of the lower eyelid and canthal tendon occurs. Aging patients with baseline lower eyelid canthal tendon laxity, as well as patients with negative vector globe/eyelid/midface topography (the globe lies anterior to the malar eminence and lower eyelid) are at particularly high risk of developing lower eyelid retraction. Midface ptosis, which is common among patients with facial paralysis, leads to additional tension on the lower eyelid complex, and can exacerbate lower eyelid retraction and paralytic ectropion. The main goal of lower eyelid reconstruction in patients with facial paralysis is to address laxity, create midface support, and correct any eyelid malposition.

Lateral canthal suspension Lateral canthal suspension (LCS) is one of the most commonly performed procedures for lower eyelid reconstruction in patients with facial paralysis. There are many variations of LCS. If horizontal lengthening of the lower eyelid is contributing to lower eyelid laxity, a lateral tarsal strip procedure (canthoplasty) can be performed. This procedure allows for shortening of the lateral lower eyelid over a variable distance depending on the amount of laxity (**Fig. 6**). If laxity is caused by lateral canthal tendon dehiscence but not lower eyelid lengthening, a lateral canthopexy can be performed in which the tendon is reattached to the lateral orbital rim without shortening the lower eyelid. An LCS can also be performed through a minimally invasive lateral upper eyelid crease incision.[19]

Medial canthal tendon plication If there is significant medial canthal laxity that cannot be corrected by lateral tightening alone, medial canthal tendon plication could be performed.[20] The transcaruncular approach can be used by creating a vertical incision through the caruncle, which is then extended inferiorly and superiorly, followed by blunt dissection down to the medial orbital wall, exposing the periosteium.[21] A double-armed suture is then placed through the medial aspect of the tarsus and anchored down to the periosteum superoposteriorly to the posterior lacrimal crest. This suture is then adjusted to the amount of tension necessary to rotate the lower eyelid margin and the punctum superiorly and posteriorly against the globe.

Lower eyelid retraction repair For patients with severe lower eyelid retraction, horizontal tightening alone may be insufficient. In these cases, recession of the lower eyelid retractors along with placement of spacer grafts can be performed to provide vertical height and stability to the lower eyelid. The transconjunctival approach is used to visualize the lower eyelid retractors and release them from the inferior border of the tarsus.[22,23] Spacer grafts can then be secured to the inferior border of the tarsus. Autografts (hard palate mucosa, ear cartilage), allografts (acellular human dermal matrix), and xenografts (acellular porcine dermis) have all been used for this purpose.[24–26] Hard palate mucosa has been shown to provide greater eyelid elevation and lower rate of failure compared with allografts, but it necessitates a second surgical site.[26,27] Patients with lower eyelid retraction as well as midface ptosis and negative vector also benefit from suspension of the suborbicularis oculi fat or the midface to help support the lower eyelid.[28–30]

Brow reconstruction

Facial paralysis can cause ipsilateral brow ptosis over time, especially in aging patients. Brow ptosis can lead to restriction of the superior visual field either directly or indirectly by exacerbating skin hooding from dermatochalasis. Surgical intervention can improve the superior visual field as well as facial asymmetry. External or endoscopic approaches to elevate the brow can be used. Endoscopic brow lift leaves less visible scars but is only effective in providing a small amount of lift. Patients

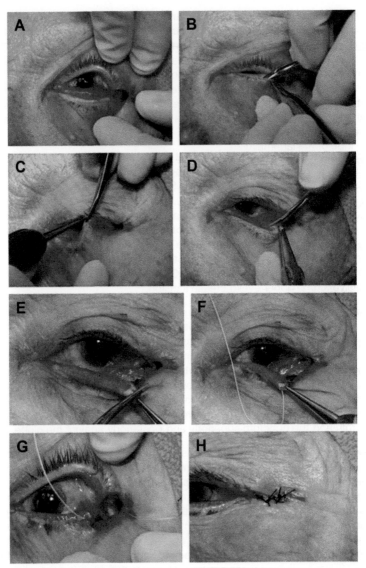

Fig. 6. Lateral tarsal strip procedure. (*A*) A lateral canthotomy skin incision is made. (*B*) The anterior and posterior lamellae are separated. (*C*) The eyelid margin is deepithelialized. (*D*) A subtarsal incision is made. (*E*) The tarsus is shortened. (*F*) A 4-0 Vicryl suture engages the deepithelialized tarsal strip. (*G*) The strip is sutured to the inner orbital rim periosteum at the Whitnall tubercle. (*H*) The skin incision is closed. (*Adapted from* Massry GG. Surgical management of the eye. In: Slattery B, editor. The facial nerve. New York: Thieme Publishers; 2013. p. 169–70; with permission.)

with severe brow ptosis are more likely to benefit from external brow lift, through either the suprabrow or trichophytic incisions, with excision of an ellipse of skin and frontalis muscle.[31] The suprabrow incision is more likely to leave a visible scar than the trichophytic incision, and is less effective at raising the medial brow.

Management of periocular synkinesis

Aberrant facial nerve regeneration after facial paralysis can lead to synkinesis, which produces abnormal facial movements that can occur during facial expressions and at rest. In the periocular region, this commonly manifests as ptosis and reverse ptosis caused by increased orbicularis oculi tone, as well as gustatory tearing (crocodile tears), which is a result of aberrant reinnervation of the lacrimal gland by efferent nerve fibers originating in the superior salivary nucleus. The mainstay of treatment of periocular syn-kinesis is targeted injection of botulinum toxin-A to the orbicularis oculi.[32] Gustatory tearing can be treated with botulinum toxin-A injected transconjunctivally into the palpebral lobe of the lacrimal gland (typical starting dose of 5 units).[33] Neuromuscular retraining plays a significant role as adjunctive therapy to chemodenervation.[32] Patients with severe synkinesis not responsive to the measures discussed earlier may benefit from permanent and highly selective neurectomy of the orbicularis oculi, in which selec-tive branches of the facial nerve are isolated and divided in succession until an adequate reduction in synkinetic movements is achieved without inducing lagophthalmos.[34]

SUMMARY

Facial paralysis is one of the most serious complications of parotid diseases and pa-rotid surgery. When facial paralysis affects the orbicularis oculi, impairment of eyelid closure and blink results in increased exposure of the ocular surface, and serious ocular consequences may ensue. A variety of conservative and interventional man-agement options exist. An individualized and multidisciplinary approach must be used in the management of these patients.

REFERENCES

1. Meier JD, Wenig BL, Manders EC, et al. Continuous intraoperative facial nerve monitoring in predicting postoperative injury during parotidectomy. Laryngo-scope 2006;116:1569–72.
2. Grosheva M, Klussmann JP, Grimminger C, et al. Electromyographic facial nerve monitoring during parotidectomy for benign lesions does not improve the outcome of postoperative facial nerve function: a prospective two-center trial. Laryngoscope 2009;119:2299–305.
3. Sood AJ, Houlton JJ, Nguyen SA, et al. Facial nerve monitoring during parotidec-tomy a systematic review and meta-analysis. Otolaryngol Head Neck Surg 2015; 152:631–7.
4. Sibony PA, Evinger C, Manning KA. Eyelid movements in facial paralysis. Arch Ophthalmol 1991;109:1555–61.
5. Hohman MH, Hadlock TA. Etiology, diagnosis, and management of facial palsy: 2000 patients at a facial nerve center. Laryngoscope 2014;124:E283–93.
6. Gire A, Kwok A, Marx DP. PROSE treatment for lagophthalmos and exposure ker-atopathy. Ophthal Plast Reconstr Surg 2013;29:e38–40.
7. Weyns M, Koppen C, Tassignon MJ. Scleral contact lenses as an alternative to tarsorrhaphy for the long-term management of combined exposure and neurotro-phic keratopathy. Cornea 2013;32:359–61.
8. Yücel OE, Artürk N. Botulinum toxin-A-induced protective ptosis in the treatment of lagophthalmos associated with facial paralysis. Ophthal Plast Reconstr Surg 2012;28:256–60.
9. Naik MN, Gangopadhyay N, Fernandes M, et al. Anterior chemodenervation of levator palpebrae superioris with botulinum toxin type-A (Botox) to induce tempo-rary ptosis for corneal protection. Eye (Lond) 2008;22:1132–6.

10. Mancini R, Taban M, Lowinger A, et al. Use of hyaluronic acid gel in the management of paralytic lagophthalmos: the hyaluronic acid gel 'gold weight'. Ophthal Plast Reconstr Surg 2009;25:23–6.
11. Martín-Oviedo C, García I, Lowy A, et al. Hyaluronic acid gel weight: a nonsurgical option for the management of paralytic lagophthalmos. Laryngoscope 2013;123:E91–6.
12. Goldberg RA, Lee S, Jayasundera T, et al. Treatment of lower eyelid retraction by expansion of the lower eyelid with hyaluronic acid gel. Ophthal Plast Reconstr Surg 2007;23:343–8.
13. Henstrom DK, Lindsay RW, Cheney ML, et al. Surgical treatment of the periocular complex and improvement of quality of life in patients with facial paralysis. Arch Facial Plast Surg 2011;13:125–8.
14. Bergeron C, Moe K. The evaluation and treatment of upper eyelid paralysis. Facial Plast Surg 2008;24:220–30.
15. Silver AL, Lindsay RW, Cheney ML, et al. Thin-profile platinum eyelid weighting: a superior option in the paralyzed eye. Plast Reconstr Surg 2009;123:1697–703.
16. Berghaus A, Neumann K, Schrom T. The platinum chain: a new upper-lid implant for facial palsy. Arch Facial Plast Surg 2003;5:166–70.
17. Hassan AS, Frueh BR, Elner VM. Müllerectomy for upper eyelid retraction and lagophthalmos due to facial nerve palsy. Arch Ophthalmol 2005;123:1221–5.
18. Demirci H, Hassan AS, Reck SD, et al. Graded full-thickness anterior blepharotomy for correction of upper eyelid retraction not associated with thyroid eye disease. Ophthal Plast Reconstr Surg 2007;23:39–45.
19. Taban M, Nakra T, Hwang C, et al. Aesthetic lateral canthoplasty. Ophthal Plast Reconstr Surg 2010;26:190–4.
20. Moe KS, Kao CH. Precaruncular medial canthopexy. Arch Facial Plast Surg 2005;7:244–50.
21. Goldberg RA, Mancini R, Demer JL. The transcaruncular approach: surgical anatomy and technique. Arch Facial Plast Surg 2007;9:443–7.
22. Compton CJ, Clark JD, Nunery WR, et al. Recession and extirpation of the lower eyelid retractors for paralytic lagophthalmos. Ophthal Plast Reconstr Surg 2015;31(4):323–4.
23. Yoo DB, Griffin GR, Azizzadeh B, et al. The minimally invasive, orbicularis-sparing, lower eyelid recession for mild to moderate lower eyelid retraction with reduced orbicularis strength. JAMA Facial Plast Surg 2014;16:140–6.
24. Krastinova D, Franchi G, Kelly MB, et al. Rehabilitation of the paralysed or lax lower eyelid using a graft of conchal cartilage. Br J Plast Surg 2002;55:12–9.
25. McCord C, Nahai FR, Codner MA, et al. Use of porcine acellular dermal matrix (Enduragen) grafts in eyelids: a review of 69 patients and 129 eyelids. Plast Reconstr Surg 2008;122:1206–13.
26. Li TG, Shorr N, Goldberg RA. Comparison of the efficacy of hard palate grafts with acellular human dermis grafts in lower eyelid surgery. Plast Reconstr Surg 2005;116:873–8 [discussion: 879–80].
27. Sullivan SA, Dailey RA. Graft contraction: a comparison of acellular dermis versus hard palate mucosa in lower eyelid surgery. Ophthal Plast Reconstr Surg 2003;19:14–24.
28. Elner VM, Mauffray RO, Fante RG, et al. Comprehensive midfacial elevation for ocular complications of facial nerve palsy. Arch Facial Plast Surg 2003;5:427–33.
29. Graziani C, Panico C, Botti G, et al. Subperiosteal midface lift: its role in static lower eyelid reconstruction after chronic facial nerve palsy. Orbit 2011;30:140–4.

30. Patel MP, Shapiro MD, Spinelli HM. Combined hard palate spacer graft, midface suspension, and lateral canthoplasty for lower eyelid retraction: a tripartite approach. Plast Reconstr Surg 2005;115:2105–14 [discussion: 2115–7].
31. Ueda K, Harii K, Yamada A. Long-term follow-up study of browlift for treatment of facial paralysis. Ann Plast Surg 1994;32:166–70.
32. Husseman J, Mehta RP. Management of synkinesis. Facial Plast Surg 2008;24: 242–9.
33. Falzon K, Galea M, Cunniffe G, et al. Transconjunctival botulinum toxin offers an effective, safe and repeatable method to treat gustatory lacrimation. Br J Ophthalmol 2010;94:379–80.
34. Hohman MH, Lee LN, Hadlock TA. Two-step highly selective neurectomy for refractory periocular synkinesis. Laryngoscope 2013;123:1385–8.

Rare Parotid Gland Diseases

Akshay Sanan, MD, David M. Cognetti, MD*

KEYWORDS

- Rare parotid gland disease • Parotid gland swelling • Sialadenosis • Sialolithiasis
- Sialadenitis • Autoimmune

KEY POINTS

- The majority of nonneoplastic disorders of the parotid gland can be categorized based on clinical history and physical examination.
- Classification of the parotid gland disease process helps to direct treatment and prognosis.
- Diagnosis of autoimmune and granulomatous conditions often requires special laboratory tests and salivary gland biopsy.
- The possibility of underlying neoplastic disorders must be considered while treating nonneoplastic disease processes.
- Newer minimally invasive surgical, medical, and diagnostic options such as sialendoscopy, botulinum toxin injection, and ultrasonography should be considered to complement traditional treatment algorithms.

CLINICAL PRESENTATION

The clinical presentation and history varies for uncommon parotid gland disorders. Swelling is present in nearly all clinical entities and is either nonpainful or painful. Conditions can range from chronic to acute and aggravating factors like eating can direct the differential in a specific way. Other key historical details include constitutional symptoms, unilateral versus bilateral symptoms, history of radioactive iodine treatment, history of measles, mumps, rubella vaccination, and history of autoimmune disease.

SIALADENOSIS

Sialadenosis (sialosis) is a chronic, bilateral, diffuse, noninflammatory, nonneoplastic swelling of the major salivary glands that primarily affects the parotid glands.[1] Sialadenosis can be painless or in some instances tender. Sialadenosis is associated with nutritional and hormonal disturbances, particularly chronic malnutrition, obesity,

Department of Otolaryngology-Head & Neck Surgery, Thomas Jefferson University Hospital, Thomas Jefferson University, 925 Chestnut Street, 6th Floor, Philadelphia, PA 19107, USA
* Corresponding author.
E-mail address: David.Cognetti@jefferson.edu

Otolaryngol Clin N Am 49 (2016) 489–500
http://dx.doi.org/10.1016/j.otc.2015.10.009
0030-6665/16/$ – see front matter © 2016 Elsevier Inc. All rights reserved.

alcoholism, acromegaly, diabetes insipidus, diabetes mellitus, hypothyroidism, liver disease, uremia, and eating disorders.[2] Many medications have been implicated in sialadenosis, most commonly antihypertensives. Some cases of sialadenosis have no underlying cause.

Sialadenosis affects 10% to 50% of patients with bulimia nervosa (**Fig. 1**). Other nutritional deficiencies include beriberi, gastrointestinal disease, malnutrition, Chagas disease, pellagra, and vitamin A deficiency. Diabetes is also an important cause of sialadenosis. In some cases, parotid gland swelling and enlargement precede the diagnosis of diabetes. Some research suggests working up patients for diabetes who present with parotid gland swelling of unknown origin. Sialadenosis is also seen in patients with alcoholism and alcoholic cirrhosis with an estimated incidence of 30% to 86%.

The pathogenesis of sialadenosis is not well-established. It may involve a neuropathic process of the autonomic innervations of the parotid gland in the setting of systemic demyelinating polyneuropathy. Autonomic neuropathies are noted in patients with alcoholism, nonalcoholic liver diseases, and diabetes. Dysfunction of autonomic regulation leads to an imbalance of acinar protein synthesis and protein secretion. Sialadenosis treatment targets the underlying condition with variable resolution of parotid gland symptoms.

Bacterial Sialadenitis

Acute sialadenitis is a bacterial infection of the parotid gland. High bacterial loads in the oral cavity provide opportunity for infection of the glands. Normal salivary flow is protective against retrograde colonization and overgrowth of bacteria in the salivary ducts and parenchyma. Saliva has antimicrobial properties owing to the presence

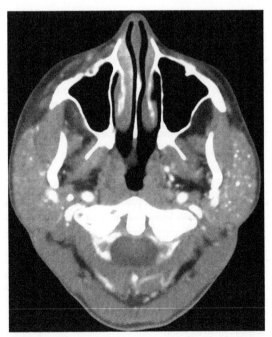

Fig. 1. Axial computed tomography scan showing sialadenosis of bilateral parotid glands in a patient with bulimia nervosa.

of lysosomes, immunoglobulin (Ig)A antibodies, and sialic acid. The current incidence of acute sialadenitis has been reported at 0.02% of hospital admissions, with the parotid gland being most commonly affected.[3]

Salivary stasis, reduced flow, and obstruction can be precipitating events for acute sialadenitis. Acute sialadenitis most frequently occurs in sixth or seventh decades of life. A decrease in saliva production can be caused by multiple medical conditions. Examples include Sjögren syndrome, diuretic therapy for hypertension, osmotic diuresis from diabetes mellitus, and postoperative fluid shift, especially after gastrointestinal procedures.

The classic presentation of acute suppurative parotitis is the sudden onset of diffuse enlargement of the involved gland with associated induration and tenderness (**Fig. 2**). *Staphylococcus aureus* has been attributed as the causative microbe in up to 90% of cases of suppurative sialadenitis. Other aerobic organisms implicated include *Streptococcus pneumoniae*, *Escherichia coli*, and *Haemophilus influenzae*.[4] Initial treatment consists of antibiotics, warm compresses, gland massage, and sialagogues. Empiric treatment with penicillinase-resistant antistaphylococcal antibiotic should be initiated while awaiting cultures. Computed tomography or ultrasound imaging is useful if an abscess or regional spread of infection is suspected. Sialography and sialendoscopy are contraindicated.[5] In the event of abscess formation, incision and drainage is indicated.

Viral Sialadenitis

Mumps
The most common cause of acute viral infection of the parotid gland is mumps. Before the release of the mumps vaccine in 1967, the incidence of mumps in the United States was as high as 300,000 cases per year and it was the most common cause of parotid swelling.[6,7] Subsequent to the development of a vaccine, the demographics of mumps shifted from being a disease of childhood to affecting young adults.

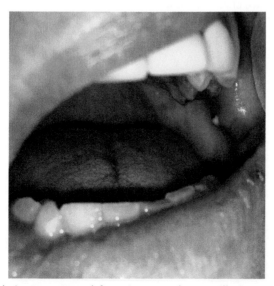

Fig. 2. Purulent drainage expressed from Stensen's duct papilla in a patient with acute bacterial sialadenitis.

Prodromal symptoms include fever, malaise, myalgia, and anorexia. The onset of parotitis usually occurs within 24 hours but may follow up to a week later. Parotitis is generally bilateral, but may be unilateral. The submandibular gland and sublingual gland are involved less frequently.

The diagnosis is made by confirmation of antibodies to the mumps S and V antigens. Amylase can elevate during mumps infection and it is helpful to examine subtypes to distinguish mumps parotitis (amylase-S) and pancreatitis (amylase-P) Diagnosis can also be made by isolating the virus from the cerebrospinal fluid during the first 3 days of clinical symptoms for patients presenting with aseptic meningitis. The mumps virus is also present in the saliva for approximately 1 week starting 2 to 3 days before onset of parotitis. Viral cultures of urine will also be possible for the first 2 weeks of illness. Polymerase chain reaction or viral cultures can also be used to detect the virus.[2] Treatment is symptoms based. Chronic obstructive sialadenitis may develop many years after the acute episode of mumps.

Human immunodeficiency virus

Viral infection with more generalized signs and symptoms as associated with human immunodeficiency virus (HIV) can also cause a focal sialadenitis that may not be appreciated in the acute phase. Diffuse gradual enlargement of the parotid glands may be seen and has been termed HIV-associated salivary gland disease (**Fig. 3**). These findings may be seen at any time in the HIV disease process and may be the presenting symptom. Since the introduction of highly active antiretroviral therapy in the mid 1990s, there has been a decline in the prevalence of oral manifestations of HIV infection. However, the incidence of HIV-associated salivary gland diseases, mostly involving the parotid glands, has remained the same. Parotid gland enlargement reportedly occurs in 1% to 10% of HIV-infected patients. Etiologies of parotid enlargement specific to HIV-seropositive patients include hyperplastic lymphadenopathy, benign lymphoepithelial cysts, and diffuse infiltrative lymphocytosis syndrome. Benign lymphoepithelial cysts occur in 3% to 6% of HIV-positive adults and in 1% to 10% of HIV-positive children, and often presents early in the course of HIV infection with slowly progressive but asymptomatic parotid gland enlargement.[2] A known adverse effect of protease inhibitors is fat accumulation in various parts of the

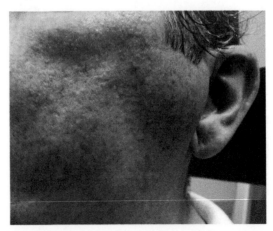

Fig. 3. Diffuse parotid gland enlargement in a patient with human immunodeficiency virus infection.

body. Protease inhibitors have been suggested to cause fatty infiltration of the parotid gland or parotid lipomatosis, resulting in glandular swelling.

Other viral causes

Other viral infections have been implicated in acute viral parotitis including hepatitis C virus, cytomegalovirus, Coxsackie A and B viruses, echoviruses, parainfluenza, adenovirus, and influenza A. Treatment of all viral infections is symptomatic. Added antimicrobial therapy is indicated in the presence of superimposed infections.[8]

Obstructive Sialadenitis

Chronic sialadenitis is characterized by recurrent inflammation and pain in the parotid gland. Factors include the triad of stasis, obstruction, and reduced salivary flow rate. Sialolithiasis, salivary duct stricture, external duct compression, systemic disease, or stasis may be causative. Repeated glandular infection results in permanent damage to the salivary gland characterized by sialectasia, ductal ectasia, and progressive acinar destruction combined with lymphocytic infiltrate. The structural changes with chronic repeated infections result in reduced function. Thus, xerostomia develops in up to 80% of patients.

Patients with chronic sialadenitis present with a history of recurrent painful swelling of the affected parotid gland that is exacerbated with eating. Physical examination confirms asymmetric, firm, and occasionally tender glands. Examination of the oral cavity assesses for xerostomia, quality and consistency of the saliva, patency of the duct opening at the papilla, and bimanual palpation of the glands. Ultrasonography is a valuable adjunct to physical examination and can help to detect salivary stones that are not palpable clinically as well as assess for neoplasms and strictures.

Computed tomography is the preferred diagnostic imaging modality to evaluate for calculi or neoplasms within the gland. Sialography may be useful to detect ductal abnormalities such as ectasia or strictures. A specialized MRI protocol to evaluate the salivary gland ducts, named MR sialography, is a noninvasive technique to evaluate the ductal system.[9] Initial treatment for chronic sialadenitis includes sialogogues, hydration, massage, and antibiotics during an acute exacerbation. When conservative management is insufficient or in cases of sialolithiasis, sialendoscopy can be both diagnostic and therapeutic.[10]

GRANULOMATOUS INFECTIONS OF THE PAROTID GLANDS
Tuberculosis of the Parotid Gland

Tuberculosis is a rare cause of parotid enlargement. It is often mistaken for a parotid tumor. Older children and adults are affected most commonly. Parotid involvement is most common with primary *Mycobacterium tuberculosis* infection, whereas in disseminated pulmonary infections, the submandibular gland is more commonly involved. Most cases of primary tuberculosis of the parotid gland are believed to arise from a focus of infection in the tonsil or teeth.

The presentation is that of an enlarging firm parotid mass that is identical to a neoplasm on imaging.[11] Clinically, it may mimic acute inflammatory sialadenitis and diagnosis requires positive acid-fast salivary stain and purified protein derivative test. Fine needle aspiration can reveal caseous necrosis in some cases. Polymerase chain reaction of the fine needle aspirate is highly sensitive but difficult to obtain.[11] Treatment is the same as for any tuberculosis infection, requiring multidrug therapy. In resistant cases, excision may be necessary and is curative.

Nontuberculous Mycobacterial Infections

Nontuberculous mycobacterial infections are rare in the parotid gland. *M kansasii, M scrofulaceum*, and *M avium* are the most commonly encountered nontuberculous mycobacterial infections and are common in soil, water, and food. These infections are most commonly encountered in children younger than 5 years old. The typical presentation is tender induration in the region of the salivary gland that fails antibiotic therapy. The overlying skin develops thinning and adherence to the infected gland, with a characteristic violaceous hue. Fine needle aspiration biopsy carries a risk of fistula formation. Antibiotic treatment with clarithromycin or other antibiotics can be attempted, but often results in prolonged treatment during which the patient remains symptomatic and fistulization or repeated abscess formation occurs. Thus, recommended treatment is complete gland excision.

Cat-Scratch Disease

Cat-scratch disease is caused by the gram-negative bacillus *Bartonella henselae*. A local infection at the scratch site is followed 1 to 2 weeks later by lymphadenopathy in the draining lymph nodes. Parotid lymph nodes may be involved. Lymph node enlargement progresses over 1 to 2 weeks and can persist for 2 to 3 months. Abscess formation may develop. Reassurance and observation for lymphadenopathy resolution is usually sufficient. If the patient is highly symptomatic, antibiotics like erythromycin, azithromycin, gentamicin, and rifampin are all therapeutic.[12]

Sarcoidosis

Sarcoidosis is a granulomatous disorder with many systemic manifestations encompassing nearly all organ systems. Parotid gland involvement has been reported in 6% to 30% of patients with sarcoidosis.[13] One notable presentation is that of uveoparotid fever, also known as Heerfordt syndrome, which is characterized by uveitis, parotid enlargement, and facial paralysis. This syndrome has been reported to affect 0.3% of patients with sarcoidosis.[14] Parotid swelling can last months to years and eventually resolves spontaneously. Biopsy of the minor salivary glands may establish the diagnosis. Corticosteroids are effective, especially in the acute phase and for the management of facial paralysis.

AUTOIMMUNE
Sjögren Syndrome

Multiple autoimmune diseases may involve the parotid glands. Parotid enlargement is most often seen in Sjögren syndrome, present in up to 55% of Sjögren syndrome patients. Parotid enlargement in Sjögren syndrome can be multicystic and is bilateral 75% of the time. Sjögren syndrome can mimic other causes of recurrent parotitis in that it may present with parotid enlargement that fluctuates in size. Sjögren syndrome is an autoimmune disorder with symptoms including xerostomia, dry eyes, and salivary gland enlargement. Sjögren syndrome affects people of all ages, but is diagnosed typically between the fourth and sixth decades. Primary Sjögren syndrome affects the exocrine glands alone. Secondary Sjögren syndrome is seen in conjunction with another autoimmune condition like lupus or rheumatoid arthritis. Sjögren syndrome patients have been found to have a 44 times greater relative risk of developing lymphoma, which may present early or late in the disease process.[15] Xerostomia is a common presenting complaint. Dry mouth is a debilitating aspect of the disease and heavily impacts quality of life. Physical examination often reveals dry oral mucosa with minimal expression of saliva when the parotid gland is massaged.

The pathophysiology is poorly understood but leads to B-cell–mediated and T-cell–mediated damage of the parotid gland. The histopathologic hallmark of Sjögren syndrome is focal dense lymphocytic infiltration with little or no surrounding edema or fibrosis. CD4$^+$ T cells predominate, with B cells accounting for approximately 20% of cells. The disease begins by immunologic infiltration of surrounding glandular ducts, which expand and replace acinar epithelial cells. Acinar loss leads to decreased glandular function.[16]

Imaging such as computed tomography or MRI of the parotid gland will demonstrate speckled calcifications throughout the affected gland. Long-standing Sjögren syndrome can lead to atrophy of the parotid gland (**Fig. 4**). Treatment for Sjögren syndrome involves symptomatic treatment for xerostomia and prevention of dental damage. The goal is to maximize salivary production of the functioning salivary gland tissue. This can be done with sialogogues and/or muscarinic–cholinergic agonists (pilocarpine, cevimeline).[17] Patients must be encouraged to take frequent sips of water to increase oral secretions. Sialendoscopy with irrigation of the salivary ductal system with or without steroid instillations has been shown to benefit in terms of improvement of salivary gland discomfort, reduced incidence of salivary gland swelling and infection, and improved salivation.

Immunoglobulin G4 Disease

The parotid glands are among the more common sites involved by IgG4-related disease. The majority of entities previously classified as chronic sclerosing sialadenitis, Mikulicz disease, and eosinophilic angiocentric fibrosis are now considered a part of the IgG4-related disease spectrum. An elevated serum IgG4 represents the only valid blood based biomarker. Histology findings include storiform-type fibrosis and

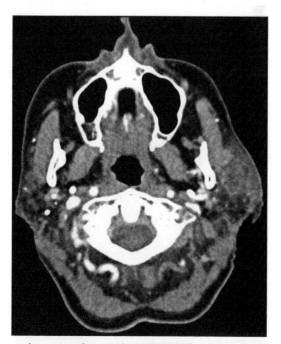

Fig. 4. Axial computed tomography scan in patient with Sjögren syndrome. Note atrophy and vacuole appearance of right parotid gland compared with the left parotid gland.

obliterative phlebitis. Clinically, multicentric lesions that show a rapid response to immunosuppressive therapy characterize the disease (**Fig. 5**).

RADIATION-INDUCED PAROTID GLAND DISEASE
External Beam Radiation

Radiation therapy for head and neck cancer causes radiation-induced xerostomia in 30,000 to 50,000 individuals in the United States annually.[18] Xerostomia occurs when the salivary glands are exposed to radiation doses of greater than 20 Gy.[19] The parotid glands are most susceptible to radiation-induced injury.[20] Salivary gland swelling and pain may develop acutely. The acute inflammatory reaction subsides with standard conservative management (hydration, massage, compresses) when radiation therapy is completed. In the long term, xerostomia exists owing to fibrosis and subsequent atrophy of the gland. Radiation-induced salivary gland tumors are well-documented. Both benign (pleomorphic adenomas, oncocytomas) and malignant neoplasms are increased in incidence.[21]

Radiation-induced parotid gland changes occur in 3 stages. Stage 1 yields mild inflammatory interstitial change with moderate individual gland acinar atrophy. Stage 2 has increased inflammatory infiltrate with fibrosis of the interstitium with epithelial metaplasia in the ductal system. Finally, stage 3 demonstrates cirrhotic parenchymal alteration with clear inflammatory activity with near-complete parenchymal atrophy.

Radioactive Iodine

Sialadenitis is the most common complication of I-131 treatment for well-differentiated thyroid malignancy, with a reported incidence of 10% to 60%.[22] Salivary damage is dose dependent and cumulative with multiple treatments. The sodium–potassium–chloride transporter in salivary tissue concentrates I-131 to levels that are 30 to 40 times greater than plasma levels, which is sufficient to cause glandular damage.[23] The average time to development of late-stage symptoms is 4.8 months. Patients present with xerostomia, frequently with concomitant increase in dental caries, change in taste, infection, stomatitis, and candidiasis.

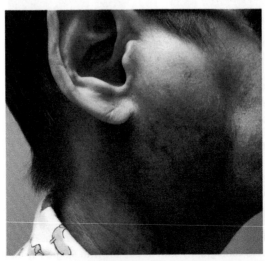

Fig. 5. Parotid gland enlargement in a patient with autoimmune parotid gland disease.

For patients with persistent symptoms, sialendoscopy and irrigation with or without steroid instillations has found to provide symptom relief in majority of patients. Typical examination findings at the time of endoscopy include ductal stenosis, presence of cellular debris and mucous plugs, as well as the absence of vascular marking on the mucosa of the salivary duct with a generalized blanching suggestive of chronic inflammation.

TRAUMA
Penetrating Trauma

Penetrating injuries to the parotid glands may involve the parotid gland or duct. Injuries posterior to the anterior border of the masseter muscle should be thoroughly investigated for ductal injury. Inspection of the wound directly allows for ductal evaluation. If the duct cannot be visualized, a probe may be passed transorally and located in the wound. If the duct has been transected, an end-to-end anastomosis of the duct over a catheter or salivary duct stent should be performed with 6-0 or finer sutures. The catheter or salivary duct is kept in place for 2 weeks and removed subsequently.

Laceration of the parotid parenchyma can usually be managed conservatively. Closing the parenchyma and the parotid capsule with interrupted sutures generally is appropriate. If a salivary cutaneous fistula develops, repeated aspiration and a pressure dressing can generally ensure healing. Resolution may take 1 to 2 weeks to allow for the traumatized ductal system to reopen. Persistence of a fistula strongly suggests duct obstruction rather than parenchymal injury alone.[24] MR sialography or sialendoscopy can be performed in this instance for duct evaluation. If duct obstruction is noted, repair should be performed. If conservative management fails, excision of the parotid gland is curative. Botulinum toxin injection has been shown to be effective in managing refractory salivary gland fistula.[25]

Blunt Trauma

Blunt trauma may also injure the gland with secondary contusion or hematoma. These injuries usually resolve spontaneously, although temporary duct obstruction may occur. A large hematoma should be drained before it becomes organized because subsequent fibrosis and scarring may lead to ductal scarring and obstruction. Rarely, blunt trauma can result in ductal damage that manifests as sialectasia and delayed parotid enlargement (**Fig. 6**).

MISCELLANEOUS DISEASES OF THE PAROTID GLAND
Pneumoparotitis

Pneumoparotitis may occur with any episode of increased intrabuccal pressure. This condition has been reported in glass blowers and after intubation and endoscopy. This condition resolves spontaneously.

Necrotizing Sialometaplasia

Necrotizing sialometaplasia is a disease of unknown origin, although some case reports seem to occur as a reaction to injury. It generally manifests as a mucosal ulceration most commonly found in the hard palate, but it may occur in the parotid gland tissue. Necrotizing sialometaplasia may be mistaken histologically for squamous cell carcinoma or mucoepidermoid carcinoma. The lesion is self-healing and requires no treatment. Clinical correlation with history of duration of illness, risk factors of head and neck cancer, and clinical presentation as well as progression are imperative. If the diagnosis is in doubt, a repeat biopsy should be performed.[26]

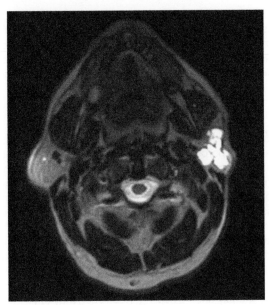

Fig. 6. Axial T2-weighted MRI delineating the marked intraparotid ductal ectasia in a patient with history of blunt trauma to the parotid gland.

Juvenile Recurrent Parotitis

Juvenile recurrent parotitis (JRP) or recurrent parotitis of childhood has similar consequences as sialadenitis in terms of salivary gland damage. JRP is a well-recognized salivary disease in children. The clinical presentation of JRP involves recurrent, nonobstructive, nonsuppurative swelling of either 1 or both of the parotid glands.[27] The condition usually affects children from infancy to age 12 years. Most children will stop having further episodes after puberty, although in some cases this condition continues beyond childhood. Acute flare-ups require intensive treatment with antibiotics and pain control. JRP is idiopathic. Theories of development include a congenital malformation of the Stensen duct, genetic aberrations, viral or bacterial infections, and allergic and autoimmune origins.[28] Diagnosis of JRP is based on clinical presentation and exclusion of other potential etiologies. The treatment for JRP is similar to acute suppurative sialadenitis. Superficial parotidectomy is contraindicated because the disease in most cases is self-remitting. Given its inflammatory nature, surgery carries a greater risk of facial paralysis. Interventional sialendoscopy with duct dilation, irrigation of the gland, instillation of steroid and stent placement have been shown to have therapeutic benefit and long-term symptom relief.[29]

Kimura Disease

Kimura disease is a rare, chronic inflammatory disease that presents with painless soft tissue swelling around the parotid area. Kimura disease is more prevalent in Eastern Asian populations. A unilateral parotid mass is more common; however, bilateral parotid involvement has been reported. Solitary or multiple lesions are found in deep subcutaneous tissue with pruritus in the overlying skin. It is frequently associated with regional lymphadenopathy involving parotid glands and periauricular, axillary and inguinal lymph nodes. Treatment involves observation for asymptomatic lesions or oral corticosteroids. However, parotid gland enlargement recurs after therapy cessation.[2]

Table 1
Diagnosis and management of rare parotid gland diseases

Disease	Features	Management
Sialadenosis	Asymptomatic swelling	Treat underlying cause
Bacterial sialadenitis	Acute inflammation; purulent drainage	Conservative measures, antibiotics
Viral sialadenitis	Acute inflammation; prodromal symptoms	Symptomatic treatment
Obstructive sialadenitis	Painful swelling associated with eating	Removal of stone(s), antibiotics for superinfections
Tuberculosis	Painless, draining mass	Multidrug antibiotic therapy
Cat-scratch disease	Unilateral swelling	Antibiotics
Sarcoidosis	Asymptomatic mass	Conservative measures, immunosuppressive therapy
Sjögren syndrome	Painless swelling of bilateral glands, associated with other autoimmune conditions	Conservative measures, symptomatic treatment, immunosuppressive therapy
Immunoglobulin G4-related disease	Painless swelling	Immunosuppressive therapy
Radiation injury	Painful, recurrent swelling; salivary stasis	Conservative measures, symptomatic treatment
Trauma	Parotid defect secondary to penetrating/blunt trauma	Wound irrigation and duct repair
Juvenile recurrent parotitis	Painless, recurrent swelling	Conservative measures, symptomatic treatment

SUMMARY

A wide range of disease processes can affect the parotid gland and its ductal system. These can be acute or chronic in their presentation. Etiologies can be systemic, glandular, or focal and classification of the disease process is of importance to direct appropriate treatment (**Table 1**).

REFERENCES

1. Scully C, Bagan JV, Eveson JW, et al. Sialosis: 35 cases of persistent parotid swelling from two countries. Br J Oral Maxillofac Surg 2008;46:468–72.
2. Chen S, Paul BC, Myssiorek D. An algorithm approach to diagnosing bilateral parotid enlargement. Otolaryngol Head Neck Surg 2013;148(5):732–9.
3. Perry RS. Recognition and management of acute suppurative parotitis. Clin Pharm 1985;4:566–71.
4. Brook I. Aerobic and anaerobic microbiology of suppurative sialadenitis. J Med Microbiol 2002;51:526–9.
5. Nahlieli O, Nakar LH, Nazarian Y, et al. Sialoendoscopy: a new approach to salivary gland obstructive pathology. J Am Dent Assoc 2006;137:1394–400.
6. What would happen if we stopped vaccinations? 2010. Available at: www.cdc.gov/vaccines/vac-gen/whatifstop.htm#mumps. Accessed July 3, 2015.
7. Utz JP, Houk VN, Alling DW. Clinical and laboratory studies of mumps. N Engl J Med 1964;270:1283–6.

8. Buckley JM, Poche P, McIntosh K. Parotitis and parainfluenza 3 virus. Am J Dis Child 1972;124:789.
9. Su YX, Liao GQ, Kang Z, et al. Application of magnetic resonance virtual endoscopy as a presurgical procedure before sialoendoscopy. Laryngoscope 2006; 116:1899–906.
10. Marchal F, Dulguerov P. Sialolithiasis management: the state of the art. Arch Otolaryngol Head Neck Surg 2003;129:951–6.
11. Kim YH, Jeong WJ, Jung KY, et al. Diagnosis of major salivary gland tuberculosis: experience of eight cases and review of the literature. Acta Otolaryngol 2005;125: 1318–22.
12. Schutze GE. Diagnosis and treatment of Bartonella henselae infections. Pediatr Infect Dis J 2000;19:1185–7.
13. Hamner JE III, Scofield HH. Cervical lymphadenopathy and parotid gland swelling in sarcoidosis: a study of 31 cases. J Am Dent Assoc 1967;74:1224–30.
14. Sugawara Y, Sakayama K, Sada E, et al. Heerfordt syndrome initially presenting with subcutaneous mass lesions: usefulness of gallium-67 scans before and after treatment. Clin Nucl Med 2005;30:732–3.
15. Voulgarelis M, Moutsopoulos HM. Malignant lymphoma in primary Sjögrens syndrome. Isr Med Assoc J 2001;3:761–6.
16. Oxholm P. Primary Sjögren's syndrome—clinical and laboratory markers of disease activity. Semin Arthritis Rheum 1992;22:114–26.
17. Petrone D, Condemi JJ, Fife R, et al. A double-blind, randomized, placebo-controlled study of cevimeline in Sjögren's syndrome patients with xerostomia and keratoconjunctivitis sicca. Arthritis Rheum 2002;46:748–54.
18. Nagler RM, Baum BJ. Prophylactic treatment reduces the severity of xerostomia following radiation therapy for oral cavity cancer. Arch Otolaryngol Head Neck Surg 2003;129:247–50.
19. Saarilahti K, Kouri M, Collan J, et al. Intensity modulated radio-therapy for head and neck cancer: evidence for preserved salivary gland function. Radiother Oncol 2005;74:251–8.
20. Nagler RM. Effects of head and neck radiotherapy on major salivary glands—animal studies and human implications. In Vivo 2003;17:369–75.
21. Rice DH, Batsakis JG, McClatchey KD. Post-irradiation malignant salivary gland tumor. Arch Otolaryngol 1976;102:699–701.
22. Kim JW, Han GS, Lee SH, et al. Sialoendoscopic treatment for radioiodine induced sialadenitis. Laryngoscope 2007;117:133–6.
23. Nakada K, Ishibashi T, Takei T, et al. Does lemon candy decrease salivary gland damage after radioiodine therapy for thyroid cancer? J Nucl Med 2005;46:261–6.
24. Hemenway WG, Bergstrom L. Parotid duct fistula: a review. South Med J 1971;64: 912–8.
25. Breuer T, Ferrazzini A, Grossenbacher R. Botulinum toxin A as a treatment of traumatic salivary gland fistulas. HNO 2006;54:385–90, 392–3.
26. Abrams AM, Melrose RJ, Howell FV. Necrotizing sialometaplasia. A disease simulating malignancy. Cancer 1973;32:130–5.
27. Nahlieli O, Shacham R, Shlesinger M, et al. Juvenile recurrent parotitis: a new method of diagnosis and treatment. Pediatrics 2004;114:9–12.
28. Konno A, Ito E. A study on the pathogenesis of recurrent parotitis in childhood. Ann Otol Rhinol Laryngol Suppl 1979;88:1–20.
29. Schneider H, Koch M, Kunzel J, et al. Juvenile recurrent parotitis: a retrospective comparison of sialendoscopy versus conservative therapy. Laryngoscope 2014; 124:451–5.

Auriculotemporal Syndrome (Frey Syndrome)

Kevin M. Motz, MD, Young J. Kim, MD*

KEYWORDS

- Frey syndrome • Gustatory sweating • Parotidectomy • Botulinum A toxin

KEY POINTS

- Frey syndrome is a common sequela of parotid gland surgery, affecting up to 64% of patients with varying degrees of severity.
- Frey syndrome is secondary to synkinesis of postganglionic parasympathetic nerve fibers within the transected parotid gland reinnervating the overlying sweat glands.
- Many surgical techniques, which are aimed at creating a barrier between the transected parotid gland and the overlying skin, have been used with varying degrees of success to prevent the development of Frey syndrome.
- Subcutaneous injection of botulinum toxin A into affected areas can be used to treat the postoperative symptoms of Frey syndrome.
- Surgical treatment for Frey syndrome refractory to medical management has been described, but clinical data to support its utilization are limited.

INTRODUCTION

Frey syndrome is a postoperative phenomenon following salivary gland surgery and less commonly neck dissection, facelift procedures, and trauma that is characterized by gustatory sweating and flushing. Frey syndrome was first described by Lucie Frey in 1923 and was termed auriculotemporal syndrome. It described sweating and flushing in the preauricular area in response to mastication or a salivary stimulus.[1] Initially thought to be rare, it was later recognized as a common occurrence after salivary gland surgery, occurring in 4% to 62% of postparotidectomy patients 6 to 18 months after surgery.[2–5]

The synkinetic mechanism for Frey syndrome is aberrant reinnervation of postganglionic parasympathetic neurons to nearby denervated sweat glands and cutaneous blood vessels.[6] Consequently, this results in flushing and sweating in the

Otolaryngology–Head and Neck Surgery, Johns Hopkins Hospital, JHOC 6150, 601 North Caroline Street, Baltimore, MD 21231, USA
* Corresponding author.
E-mail address: ykim76@jhmi.edu

Otolaryngol Clin N Am 49 (2016) 501–509
http://dx.doi.org/10.1016/j.otc.2015.10.010
0030-6665/16/$ – see front matter © 2016 Elsevier Inc. All rights reserved.

sympathetically void skin in response to mastication and salivation. The previous sympathetic responses of sweating and flushing are now controlled by postganglionic parasympathetic fibers. Mastication, which releases acetylcholine from the parasympathetic nerve endings,[3,6] now induces sweating and flushing, which was a sympathetic cholinergic response before synkinesis of parasympathetic nerve fibers (**Fig. 1**).

The symptoms of Frey syndrome can include flushing, sweating, burning, neuralgia, and itching. Generally, the symptoms are mild but can result in discomfort as well as social anxiety and avoidance. A survey conducted by Baek and colleagues[7] revealed that Frey syndrome was the most commonly self-perceived consequence of

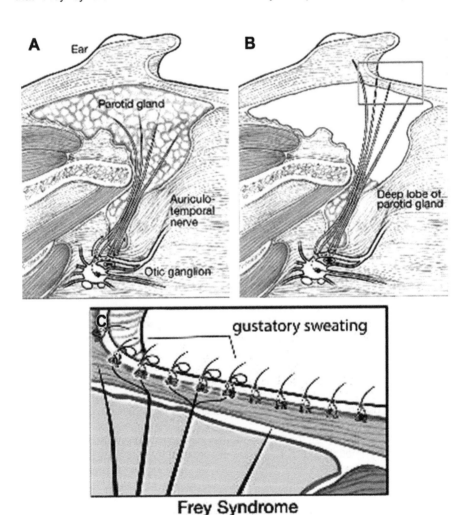

Fig. 1. (*A*) Normal innervation of the parotid gland by the postganglionic parasympathetic nerve fibers from the auriculotemporal nerve. (*B*) Postoperative diagram depicting the regenerated postganglionic parasympathetic nerve fibers extending to the overlying cutaneous tissue. (*C*) Postganglionic parasympathetic nerve fibers innervating the cutaneous sweat gland that results in gustatory sweating. (*From* Hoff S, Mohyuddin N, Yao M. Complications of parotid surgery. Operative Techniques in Otolaryngology–Head and Neck Surgery 2009;20:129; with permission.)

parotidectomy in a group undergoing parotidectomy for benign disease. With significant psychosocial morbidity resulting from Frey syndrome,[8] interventions to prevent the development and to treat this sequela of parotid surgery have been the topic of focus in the literature.

Diagnosis of Frey syndrome is based on clinical history, but confirmatory testing can be done with a Minor starch-iodine test. The starch-iodine test consists of painting the patient's postsurgical affected region with iodine. Once dry, dry starch is then applied to the painted area, and a salivary stimulus is given. The starch turns blue/brown in the presence of iodine and sweat (**Fig. 2**). Patients who underwent parotidectomy had a positive Minor starch-iodine test in 62% of cases, whereas the self-reported incidence of symptoms was only 23% in the same group.[5] These numbers attest both to the high incidence of the synkinesis and to the subclinical nature of Frey syndrome.

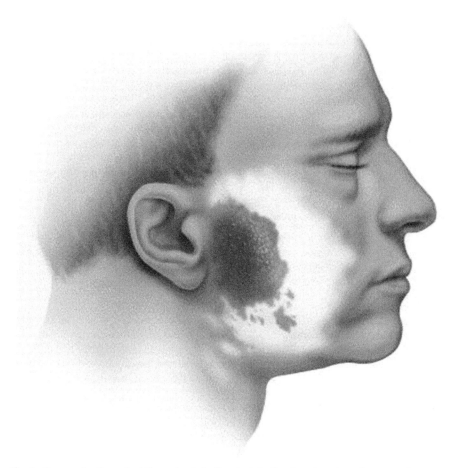

Fig. 2. Demonstration of a Minor starch-iodine test: iodine is painted on the area of interest and allowed to dry. This area is then coated with starch powder. When sweat reacts with iodine, it turns the starch brown. The dark pretragal area demonstrates a positive Minor starch-iodine test, whereas the other lighter areas are considered negative. (*From* Arad A, Blitzer A. Botulinum toxin in the treatment of autonomic nervous system disorders. Operative Techniques in Otolaryngology–Head and Neck Surgery 2004;15:119; with permission.)

SURGICAL METHODS FOR THE PREVENTION OF FREY SYNDROME

Prevention of Frey syndrome has been guided by the alteration of surgical techniques or the addition of procedures focused on preventing synkinesis. The overarching theme for the surgical prevention of Frey syndrome has been the incorporation and maintenance of a barrier between the underlying postganglionic parasympathetic nerve endings within the transected parotid and the overlying cutaneous tissue. Many techniques aimed at accomplishing this have been described and include increased skin flap thickness, local fascia or muscle flaps, and the use of acellular dermal matrix (ADM) or free fat grafts.

Increased Skin Flap Thickness

Within the facial skin, the sweat glands are positioned at the same level or slightly deeper than the base of the hair follicles. Based on this, it has been presumed that increasing the thickness of the elevated skin flap, to keep the sweat glands from being exposed, affords protection from the aberrant parasympathetic nerve regeneration that results in Frey syndrome. Early studies suggested that there was a significant increase in the rate of Frey syndrome when a thin flap was elevated compared with that of a thick flap (12.5 vs 2.6%, $P<.05$).[9] Although this study did lay a foundation for surgical technique, its measurements for flap thickness were crude, and the diagnosis of Frey syndrome lacked objective measurements.[9]

More recent studies, which objectively measured flap thickness and assessed Frey syndrome by clinical symptoms as well as starch-iodine testing, have failed to demonstrate a reduction in the incidence of Frey syndrome with increased flap thickness.[10,11] Although flap thickness did not decrease the incidence of Frey syndrome in these studies, it did show a decrease in the total skin surface area affected and perhaps the overall severity of the disease.[11]

Transposition Muscle or Fascia Flaps

Similar to increasing the thickness of the elevated skin flap to shield the facial sweat glands from aberrant reinnervation, pedicled muscle and fascia flaps have been used to cover the resected parotid gland in an attempt to create a physical barrier between the overlying dermis and the transected nerve fibers within the parotid.

Temporoparietal fascia flap

The temporoparietal fascia flap (TPFF) is a broad, vascularized fascia flap that is based off the superficial temporal artery (**Fig. 3**). It was first described as a composite flap for ear reconstruction in 1976 by Fox and Edgerton[12] and was later adapted to a fascia flap. Given its accessibility, predictable vasculature, and low donor site morbidity, it became a common method for reconstruction of the cheek, ear, nasal cavity, and orbit.

The use of a TPFF was first described in a series of 7 patients undergoing parotidectomy for the prevention of Frey syndrome in 1995 by Sultan and colleagues.[13] The results of this series showed that prophylactic inlay of a TPFF to the parotidectomy defect prevented Frey syndrome as assessed by both clinical history and starch-iodine testing in all 7 patients. In addition, the TPFF allowed for improved cosmetic outcome because it reduced the contour defect.[13] Since its initial description, multiple retrospective studies have confirmed the utility of TPFF for the prevention of Frey syndrome. In these studies, the use of a TPFF decreased the rate of Frey syndrome after parotid surgery, as determined by positive starch-iodine test, to 4% to 17%, and reduced the clinical incidence of gustatory sweating to 4% to 8%.[13,14] This reduced

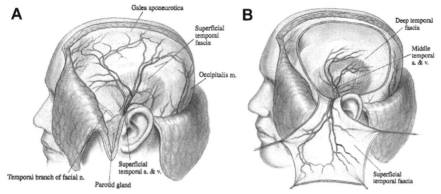

Fig. 3. (*A*) An anatomic drawing of the superficial temporal artery and vein supplying the superficial temporal fascia demonstrating the proximity to the temporal branch of the facial nerve. (*B*) An elevated TPFF. (*From* Larrabee A, Reynolds B, Long C. The temporoparietal fascia flap. Operative Techniques in Otolaryngology–Head and Neck Surgery 1993;4:19; with permission.)

clinical incidence compared with 39% to 57% and 34% to 43%, respectively, for patients who did not undergo TPFF reconstruction.[13,14]

Although this represents an effective technique for the prevention of Frey syndrome, it does require an extended incision, which can generally be hidden in the hairline. In addition, the course of the temporal branch of the facial nerve is at potential risk for injury. Moreover, local flaps increase operative time and can require a second reconstructive team, which may increase overall cost of the procedure.

Sternocleidomastoid muscle flap

The sternocleidomastoid (SCM) muscles flap is a muscular flap with a tripartite blood supply. The occipital artery, which enters the posterior surface of the muscle in the upper third, is the predominant blood supply to the superior SCM flap. This technique has been favored for reconstruction secondary to its proximity and ability to easily rotate into a parotidectomy defect. Although the SCM flap is easy to harvest and can provide adequate cosmetic reconstruction, its ability to prevent Frey syndrome after parotidectomy is unclear. Reports in the literature have supported that the use of an SCM muscle flap decreases the incidence of Frey syndrome. In a retrospective study of 43 patients, Filho and colleagues[15] demonstrated that SCM muscle flap reconstruction following parotidectomy resulted in no cases of Frey syndrome in 24 patients, when assessed clinically and by starch-iodine testing, comparing with 52.6% and 63.2%, respectively, in a control group of patients not undergoing SCM flap reconstruction.[15] In addition, a meta-analysis published in 2009 by Curry and colleagues[16] concluded that SCM flaps decrease the rate of Frey syndrome after parotidectomy. However, other studies have shown that the muscle flaps are ineffective at preventing the sequela of Frey syndrome.[17,18] Unfortunately, given the relatively small number of patients evaluated in the studies and the immense heterogeneity between studies, it is difficult to draw conclusions based on the data available.[18]

Superficial musculoaponeurotic system flap

Another technique, focused on creating a physical barrier between the underlying regenerating auriculotemporal nerve fibers and the overlying dermis, is a superficial musculoaponeurotic system (SMAS) flap. This SMAS flap can be harvested using a standard modified Blair incision or the facelift incision, and the SMAS can be easily separated from the overlying skin and the parotid tissue to be tightly plicated to the ear perichondrium and the SCM muscle, creating a tight surface that prevents the retromandibular collapse for improved contouring. Similar to the other types of local reconstruction, the efficacy data are mixed. Bonanno and colleagues[19] found this technique overwhelmingly effective in preventing the development of Frey syndrome, while other groups failed to demonstrate its ability to do so.[10,20–23] However, although the incidence of postparotidectomy Frey syndrome was not significantly changed in these studies, the severity and overall surface area affected were significantly less.[23] Although this technique does serve to isolate the underlying regenerating nerve fibers, it is more commonly used in clinical practice for cosmetic reasons rather the prevention of Frey syndrome.

Biomaterial and Autologous Implantation

Autologous and biosynthetic material have been used to create the physical barrier between the transected parotid and the overlying cutaneous tissues. Numerous products have been reported, but the most commonly cited are acellular dermal matrix implantation and autologous fat grafting.

Acellular dermal matrix

ADM is a soft tissue matrix graft that is generated by decellularization of tissue that results an intact extracellular matrix. It is commonly used in wound healing and reconstructive surgery because it provides a scaffold for regenerating tissues. Since its development, it has been used in parotidectomy for the prevention of Frey syndrome. As with muscle or fascia flaps, the goal of this graft is to create a biologic barrier between the facial skin flap and the transected parotid gland. In a limited number of studies that have investigated its effectiveness at preventing Frey syndrome, there are limited data that suggest it is effective in reducing both objective and clinical measures of Frey syndrome.[24–26]

Abdominal fat grafting

Abdominal fat implantation to the parotidectomy defect is a commonly used technique for decreasing the postsurgical defect and improving cosmesis. In very limited studies, there have been reports that abdominal fat implantation decreases the occurrence of Frey syndrome. However, this has failed to be substantiated. In addition, abdominal fat harvest requires an additional incision on the abdomen and can frequently be complicated by donor site hematoma and surgical site seroma.

POSTSURGICAL TREATMENT OF FREY SYNDROME
Medical Management

Although intraoperative techniques try to reduce severity and incidence of Frey syndrome, postoperative interventions have been focused on ameliorating symptoms once they develop. Most of the therapies used are given via injection therapy or by topical application. Previous agents have included topical antiperspirants as well as injection with alcohol, scopolamine, glycopyrrolate, or botulinum toxin A (BTA). Currently, BTA is the most widely used agent for intradermal injection. Previous studies have demonstrated that patients undergoing BTA injection demonstrate improvement in symptoms of gustatory sweating and flushing.[27,28] In addition, it has been shown to improve patient quality of life.[28] Unfortunately, with BTA injection, symptomatic recurrence has been demonstrated in up to 27% and 92% of patients at 1 and 3 years, respectively.[29] However, despite a high rate of return symptoms after BTA injection, repeat BTA injection has been shown to be effective.[29] For the studies investigating BTA, the injection dose was between 1.9 and 2.5 U/cm^2 in the involved area.[27–29] Unfortunately, no randomized control studies have been documented, and based on a *Cochrane Review* of the literature, no conclusions can be made on its efficacy.[30]

Surgical Management

Historically, surgical treatment of Frey syndrome has not been used. Reports of surgical transection of the auriculotemporal nerve, tympanic nerve, and greater auricular nerve have been described for the management of Frey syndrome, but they are not commonly practiced. Recently, a cohort of 17 patients with postparotidectomy Frey syndrome who underwent both SCM and temporalis fascia transposition was reported by Dia and colleagues.[31] This report demonstrated that greater than 50% (9/17) of patients who underwent the transposition procedure had complete resolution by starch-iodine testing.[31] In addition, there was a significant reduction in the average surface area of gustatory-sweating–positive skin from 12.80 to 1.32 cm^2 in all patients postoperatively.[31] Although this method is compelling and does appear to be a feasible option for surgical management of Frey syndrome, it does have an increased risk for facial nerve injury. Given the limited number of studies on transposition procedures, no recommendations can be made on its evidence-based efficacy. However, if surgery for Frey syndrome is to be attempted, it should be only be used in cases that are refractory to conservative nonsurgical measures.

SUMMARY

Despite the uncertainty of effectiveness, the above-mentioned intraoperative preventative techniques are low risk and often can also be used to improve cosmetic outcomes. Despite the lack of level 1 evidence-based data, there is likely to be benefit in using an SMAS, SCM, or TPFF reconstruction for both cosmesis and the prevention of Frey syndrome. In addition, ADM represents a suitable alternative to local fascia and muscle flaps for the prevention of Frey syndrome. Of note, local reconstruction with the above techniques is not advised in the presence of malignant disease or gross spillage of benign tumors due to the concern for local recurrence.

In managing symptomatic complaints of Frey syndrome, BTA injection, although not definitive therapy, can significantly decrease the severity and thus morbidity of Frey syndrome. Surgical management of postparotidectomy Frey syndrome should be reserved for severe and refractory cases, as there are limited data to support its use.

REFERENCES

1. Frey L. Le syndrome du nerf auriculo-temporal. Revue Neurologique 1923;2: 92–104.
2. Freedberg A, Shaw R, McManus J. The auriculotemporal syndrome. A clinical and pharmacologic study. J Clin Invest 1948;27(5):669–76.
3. Drummond PD. Mechanisms of gustatory flushing in Frey's syndrome. Clin Auton Res 2002;12:144–6.
4. Rustemeyer J, Eufinger H, Bremerich A. The incidence of Frey's syndrome. J Craniomaxillofac Surg 2008;36:34–7.
5. Neumann A, Rosenberger D, Vorsprach O, et al. The incidence of Frey syndrome following parotidectomy: results of a survey and follow-up. HNO 2011;2:173–8.
6. Gardner WJ, McCubbin JW. Auriculotemporal syndrome: gustatory sweating due to misdirection of regenerated nerve fibers. J Am Med Assoc 1956;160:272–7.

7. Baek C, Chung M, Jeong H, et al. Questionnaire evaluation of sequelae over 5 years after parotidectomy for benign diseases. J Plast Reconstr Aesthet Surg 2009;62(5):633–8.
8. Hartl D, Julieron M, LeRidant A, et al. Botulinum toxin A for quality of life improvement in post-parotidectomy gustatory sweating (Frey's syndrome). J Laryngol Otol 2008;122(10):1100–4.
9. Singleton G, Cassisi N. Frey's syndrome: incidence related to skin flap thickness in parotidectomy. Laryngoscope 1980;90:1636–40.
10. Taylor SM, Yoo J, Matthews TW, et al. Frey's syndrome and parotidectomy flaps: a retrospective cohort study. Otolaryngol Head Neck Surg 2000;122(2):201–3.
11. Durgut O, Basut O, Demir U, et al. Association between skin flap thickness and Frey's syndrome in parotid surgery. Head Neck 2012;35(12):1781–6.
12. Fox J, Edgerton M. The fan flap: an adjunct to ear reconstruction. Plast Reconstr Surg 1976;58:663–7.
13. Sultan M, Wider T, Hugo N. Frey's syndrome: prevention with the temporopartietal fascial flap interposition. Ann Plast Surg 1995;34:292–7.
14. Ahmen O, Kolhe P. Prevention of Frey's syndrome and volume deficit after parotidectomy using the superficial temporal artery fascial flap. Br J Plast Surg 1999;52:256–60.
15. Filho W, Dedivitis R, Rapoport A, et al. Sternocleidomastoid muscle flap preventing Frey syndrome following parotidectomy. World J Surg 2004;28:361–4.
16. Curry J, King N, Reiter D, et al. Meta-analysis of surgical techniques for preventing parotidectomy sequelae. Arch Facial Plast Surg 2009;11(5):327–31.
17. Kornblut A. Sternocleidomastoid muscle transfer in the prevention of Frey's syndrome. Laryngoscope 1991;101:571–2.
18. Sanabria A, Kowalski L, Bradley P, et al. Sternocleidomastoid muscle flap in preventing Frey's syndrome after parotidectomy: a systematic review. Head Neck 2012;34(4):589–98.
19. Bonanno P, Palaia D, Rosenberg M, et al. Prophylaxis against Frey's syndrome in parotid surgery. Ann Plast Surg 2000;44:498–550.
20. Wille-Bischofberger A, Rajan G, Linder T, et al. Impact of the SMAS on Frey's syndrome after parotid surgery: a prospective, long-term study. Plast Reconstr Surg 2007;120:1519–23.
21. Yu L, Hamilton R. Frey's syndrome: prevention with conservative parotidectomy and superficial musculoaponeurotic system preservation. Ann Plast Surg 1992;29:217–22.
22. Allison G, Rappaport I. Prevention of Frey's syndrome with superficial musculoaponeurotic system interposition. Am J Surg 1993;166:407–10.
23. Barbera R, Castillo F, D'oleo C, et al. Superficial musculoaponeurotic system flap in partial parotidectomy and clinical and subclinical Frey's syndrome. Cosmesis and quality of life. Head Neck 2014;36(1):130–6.
24. Govindaraj S, Cohen M, Genden EM, et al. The use of acellular dermis in the prevention of Frey's syndrome. Laryngoscope 2001;111:1993–8.
25. Ye W, Zhu H, Zheng J, et al. Use of allogenic acellular dermal matrix in prevention of Frey's syndrome after parotidectomy. Br J Oral Maxillofac Surg 2008;46:649–52.
26. Wang W, Fan J, Sun C, et al. Systemic evaluation on the use of acellular matrix graft in prevention of Frey syndrome after parotid neoplasm surgery. J Craniofac Surg 2013;24:1526–9.
27. Beerens A, Snow G. Botulinum toxin A in the treatment of patients with Frey syndrome. Br J Surg 2002;89(1):116–9.

28. Tugnoli V, Marchese Ragona R, Eleopra R, et al. The role of gustatory flushing in Frey's syndrome and its treatment with botulinum toxin type A. Clin Auton Res 2002;12(3):174–8.
29. Laccourreye O, Akl E, Gutierrez-Fonseca R, et al. Recurrent gustatory sweating (Frey's syndrome) after intracutaneous injection of botulinum toxin type A: incidence, management, and outcome. Arch Otolaryngol Head Neck Surg 1999; 125(3):283–6.
30. Li C, Wu F, Zhang Q, et al. Interventions for the treatment of Frey's syndrome. Cochrane Database Syst Rev 2015;(3):CD009959.
31. Dia X, Liu H, He J, et al. Treatment of postparotidectomy Frey syndrome with the interposition of temporalis fascia and sternocleidomastoid flaps. Oral Surg Oral Med Oral Pathol Oral Radiol 2015;119(5):514–21.

Index

Note: Page numbers of article titles are in **boldface** type.

A

Acinic cell carcinoma, 355–357
Adenocarcinoma not otherwise specified, 363
Adenoid cystic carcinoma, 301, 352–355
Adenoma(s), basal cell, 303, 304, 337–338
    monomorphic, 336–339
    pleomorphic, 298–299, 303
        benign mixed, 333–336
        recurrent, 398–399
Artery island flap, supraregional, locoregional parotid reconstruction in, 442–443
Auriculotemporal disease. See *Frey syndrome.*

B

Blepharotomy, upper eyelid, 482
Brachial cleft cyst, 294, 295
Brow, reconstruction of, 483–484

C

Carcinoma ex pleomorphic adenoma (malignant mixed tumor), 361–362
Cat-scratch disease, 494

E

Eyelid, lower, reconstruction of, 482–483, 484
    upper, reconstruction of, upper eyelid loading in, 480–481

F

Facial expression, paired muscles of, 280
Facial nerve, and parotid gland, anatomic and functional relationship of, 273–274
    anatomy of, **273–284**
    benign parotid tumors and, 429–431
    branches of, and parotid gland, 426, 427
    extratemporal anatomy of, 282
    injury of, as complication of parotid disease, 475
        evaluation of, 476, 477, 478
        management of, 476–485
    intratemporal and extratemporal course of, 281–282

Otolaryngol Clin N Am 49 (2016) 511–516
http://dx.doi.org/10.1016/S0030-6665(16)00025-6
0030-6665/16/$ – see front matter © 2016 Elsevier Inc. All rights reserved.

oto.theclinics.com

Moving?

Make sure your subscription moves with you!

To notify us of your new address, find your **Clinics Account Number** (located on your mailing label above your name), and contact customer service at:

Email: journalscustomerservice-usa@elsevier.com

800-654-2452 (subscribers in the U.S. & Canada)
314-447-8871 (subscribers outside of the U.S. & Canada)

Fax number: 314-447-8029

Elsevier Health Sciences Division
Subscription Customer Service
3251 Riverport Lane
Maryland Heights, MO 63043

*To ensure uninterrupted delivery of your subscription, please notify us at least 4 weeks in advance of move.

Printed and bound by CPI Group (UK) Ltd, Croydon, CR0 4YY

03/10/2024

01040397-0008